AMERICAN ACADEMY™
OF OPHTHALMOLOGY



# Orbit, Eyelids, and Lacrimal System

*Last major revision 2015–2016*

2017–2018

# BCSC

## Basic and Clinical Science Course™

Protecting Sight. Empowering Lives.™

EB

Published after collaborative review with the European Board of Ophthalmology subcommittee

The American Academy of Ophthalmology is accredited by the Accreditation Council for Continuing Medical Education (ACCME) to provide continuing medical education for physicians.

The American Academy of Ophthalmology designates this enduring material for a maximum of 10 *AMA PRA Category 1 Credits*™. Physicians should claim only the credit commensurate with the extent of their participation in the activity.

CME expiration date: June 1, 2018. *AMA PRA Category 1 Credits*™ may be claimed only once between June 1, 2015, and the expiration date.

BCSC® volumes are designed to increase the physician's ophthalmic knowledge through study and review. Users of this activity are encouraged to read the text and then answer the study questions provided at the back of the book.

To claim *AMA PRA Category 1 Credits*™ upon completion of this activity, learners must demonstrate appropriate knowledge and participation in the activity by taking the posttest for Section 7 and achieving a score of 80% or higher. For further details, please see the instructions for requesting CME credit at the back of the book.

The Academy provides this material for educational purposes only. It is not intended to represent the only or best method or procedure in every case, nor to replace a physician's own judgment or give specific advice for case management. Including all indications, contraindications, side effects, and alternative agents for each drug or treatment is beyond the scope of this material. All information and recommendations should be verified, prior to use, with current information included in the manufacturers' package inserts or other independent sources, and considered in light of the patient's condition and history. Reference to certain drugs, instruments, and other products in this course is made for illustrative purposes only and is not intended to constitute an endorsement of such. Some material may include information on applications that are not considered community standard, that reflect indications not included in approved FDA labeling, or that are approved for use only in restricted research settings. **The FDA has stated that it is the responsibility of the physician to determine the FDA status of each drug or device he or she wishes to use, and to use them with appropriate, informed patient consent in compliance with applicable law.** The Academy specifically disclaims any and all liability for injury or other damages of any kind, from negligence or otherwise, for any and all claims that may arise from the use of any recommendations or other information contained herein.



Cover image: From BCSC Section 5, *Neuro-Ophthalmology.* Fundus photograph showing an arteriovenous malformation (racemose angioma) of the retina in a patient with Wyburn-Mason syndrome. *(Courtesy of Mark J. Greenwald, MD.)*

FSC www.fsc.org MIX Paper from responsible sources FSC® C103061



Printed in the United States of America.

# Basic and Clinical Science Course

Louis B. Cantor, MD, Indianapolis, Indiana, *Senior Secretary for Clinical Education*
Christopher J. Rapuano, MD, Philadelphia, Pennsylvania, *Secretary for Lifelong Learning and Assessment*
George A. Cioffi, MD, New York, New York, *BCSC Course Chair*

## Section 7

### Faculty

Jill Annette Foster, MD, *Chair,* Columbus, Ohio
Keith D. Carter, MD, Iowa City, Iowa
Vikram D. Durairaj, MD, Austin, Texas
Marsha C. Kavanagh, MD, Portsmouth, New Hampshire
Bobby S. Korn, MD, PhD, La Jolla, California
Christine C. Nelson, MD, Ann Arbor, Michigan
Morris E. Hartstein, MD, *Consultant,* Raanana, Israel

The Academy wishes to acknowledge the American Society of Ophthalmic Plastic and Reconstructive Surgery (ASOPRS) for recommending faculty members to the BCSC Section 7 committee.

The Academy also wishes to acknowledge the following committees for review of this edition:

*Committee on Aging:* Paul N. Rosenberg, MD, Webster, New York

*Vision Rehabilitation Committee:* Richard A. Harper, MD, Little Rock, Arkansas

*Practicing Ophthalmologists Advisory Committee for Education:* Robert G. Fante, MD, *Primary Reviewer,* Denver, Colorado; Edward K. Isbey III, MD, *Chair,* Asheville, North Carolina; Alice Bashinsky, MD, Asheville, North Carolina; David J. Browning, MD, PhD, Charlotte, North Carolina; Bradley Fouraker, MD, Tampa, Florida; Dasa Gangadhar, MD, Wichita, Kansas; Steven J. Grosser, MD, Golden Valley, Minnesota; James A. Savage, MD, Memphis, Tennessee

EB

*European Board of Ophthalmology:* Peter Raus, MD, *Chair,* Brussels, Belgium; Artur Klett, MD, FEBO, *Liaison,* Tallinn, Estonia; Maria Borrelli, MD, PhD, Düsseldorf, Germany; Gerd Geerling, MD, PhD, FEBO, Düsseldorf, Germany

## Financial Disclosures

Academy staff members who contributed to the development of this product state that within the past 12 months, they have had no financial interest in or other relationship with any entity discussed in this course that produces, markets, resells, or distributes ophthalmic health care goods or services consumed by or used in patients, or with any competing commercial product or service.

The authors and reviewers state that within the past 12 months, they have had the following financial relationships:*

Dr Browning: Aerpio (S), Alimera Sciences (C), Diabetic Retinopathy Clinical Research (S), Genentech (S), Novartis Pharmaceuticals (S), Pfizer (S), Regeneron Pharmaceuticals (S)

Dr Durairaj: KLS Martin (L), Stryker Corporation/Medical Division (L)

Dr Fante: Ophthalmic Mutual Insurance Company (C, L)

Dr Foster: Allergan (C, L), Merz (C, L)

Dr Fouraker: Addition Technology (C), Alcon Laboratories (C), Keravision (C), Ophthalmic Mutual Insurance Company (C)

Dr Geerling: Allergan (C, L), Bausch + Lomb (C, L), TearLab (C, L, O), TearScience (C, L), Théa Pharma (C, L)

Dr Grosser: Ivantis (O)

Dr Isbey: Alcon Laboratories (S), Allscripts (C), Bausch + Lomb (S), Medflow (C)

Dr Korn: Elsevier (P)

Dr Raus: Allergan (L)

Dr Savage: Allergan (L)

The other authors and reviewers state that within the past 12 months, they have had no financial interest in or other relationship with any entity discussed in this course that produces, markets, resells, or distributes ophthalmic health care goods or services consumed by or used in patients, or with any competing commercial product or service.

*C = consultant fees, paid advisory boards, or fees for attending a meeting; L = lecture fees (honoraria), travel fees, or reimbursements when speaking at the invitation of a commercial sponsor; O = equity ownership/stock options of publicly or privately traded firms (excluding mutual funds) with manufacturers of commercial ophthalmic products or commercial ophthalmic services; P = patents and/or royalties that might be viewed as creating a potential conflict of interest; S = grant support for the past year (all sources) and all sources used for a specific talk or manuscript with no time limitation

## Recent Past Faculty

Warren J. Chang, MD
Roberta E. Gausas, MD
Andrew R. Harrison, MD
John Bryan Holds, MD

In addition, the Academy gratefully acknowledges the contributions of numerous past faculty and advisory committee members who have played an important role in the development of previous editions of the Basic and Clinical Science Course.

## American Academy of Ophthalmology Staff

Dale E. Fajardo, *Vice President, Education*
Beth Wilson, *Director, Continuing Professional Development*
Ann McGuire, *Acquisitions and Development Manager*
Stephanie Tanaka, *Publications Manager*
D. Jean Ray, *Production Manager*
Kimberly Torgerson, *Publications Editor*
Beth Collins, *Medical Editor*
Naomi Ruiz, *Publications Specialist*

American Academy of Ophthalmology
655 Beach Street
Box 7424
San Francisco, CA 94120-7424

# Contents

General Introduction . . . . . . . . . . . . . . . . . . . . . . . xv

**Objectives** . . . . . . . . . . . . . . . . . . . . . . . . . 1

## PART I Orbit . . . . . . . . . . . . . . . . . . . . . . 3

**1 Orbital Anatomy** . . . . . . . . . . . . . . . . . . . . 5

Dimensions . . . . . . . . . . . . . . . . . . . . . . . . 5
Topographic Relationships . . . . . . . . . . . . . . . . . . 5
  Roof of the Orbit . . . . . . . . . . . . . . . . . . . . 6
  Lateral Wall of the Orbit . . . . . . . . . . . . . . . . . 7
  Medial Wall of the Orbit . . . . . . . . . . . . . . . . . 8
  Floor of the Orbit . . . . . . . . . . . . . . . . . . . . 8
Apertures . . . . . . . . . . . . . . . . . . . . . . . . . 9
  Ethmoidal Foramina . . . . . . . . . . . . . . . . . . . . 9
  Superior Orbital Fissure . . . . . . . . . . . . . . . . . 9
  Inferior Orbital Fissure . . . . . . . . . . . . . . . . . 9
  Zygomaticofacial and Zygomaticotemporal Canals . . . . . . . 9
  Nasolacrimal Canal . . . . . . . . . . . . . . . . . . . 10
  Optic Canal . . . . . . . . . . . . . . . . . . . . . . 10
Soft Tissues . . . . . . . . . . . . . . . . . . . . . . . 11
  Periorbita . . . . . . . . . . . . . . . . . . . . . . . 11
  Intraorbital Optic Nerve . . . . . . . . . . . . . . . . 11
  Extraocular Muscles and Orbital Fat . . . . . . . . . . . 11
  Annulus of Zinn . . . . . . . . . . . . . . . . . . . . 12
  Vasculature of the Orbit . . . . . . . . . . . . . . . . 13
  Nerves . . . . . . . . . . . . . . . . . . . . . . . . . 16
  Lacrimal Gland . . . . . . . . . . . . . . . . . . . . . 18
Periorbital Structures . . . . . . . . . . . . . . . . . . 18
  Nose and Paranasal Sinuses . . . . . . . . . . . . . . . 18

**2 Evaluation of Orbital Disorders** . . . . . . . . . . . . 21

History . . . . . . . . . . . . . . . . . . . . . . . . . 21
  Pain . . . . . . . . . . . . . . . . . . . . . . . . . . 21
  Progression . . . . . . . . . . . . . . . . . . . . . . 21
  Periorbital Changes . . . . . . . . . . . . . . . . . . 22
Physical Examination . . . . . . . . . . . . . . . . . . . 23
  Inspection . . . . . . . . . . . . . . . . . . . . . . . 23
  Palpation . . . . . . . . . . . . . . . . . . . . . . . 25
  Auscultation . . . . . . . . . . . . . . . . . . . . . . 26

Primary Studies . . . . . . . . . . . . . . . . . . . . . . 26
Computed Tomography . . . . . . . . . . . . . . . . . . 26
Magnetic Resonance Imaging . . . . . . . . . . . . . . . 28
Comparison of CT and MRI . . . . . . . . . . . . . . . . 29
Ultrasonography . . . . . . . . . . . . . . . . . . . . 31
Secondary Studies . . . . . . . . . . . . . . . . . . . . 32
Venography . . . . . . . . . . . . . . . . . . . . . . 32
Arteriography . . . . . . . . . . . . . . . . . . . . . 32
CT and MR Angiography . . . . . . . . . . . . . . . . . 32
Pathology . . . . . . . . . . . . . . . . . . . . . . . . 32
Laboratory Studies . . . . . . . . . . . . . . . . . . . . 33

**3 Congenital Orbital Anomalies . . . . . . . . . . . . . . . 35**
Anophthalmia . . . . . . . . . . . . . . . . . . . . . . . 35
Microphthalmia . . . . . . . . . . . . . . . . . . . . . . 35
Treatment of Anophthalmia/Microphthalmia . . . . . . . . . . 36
Craniofacial Clefting and Syndromic Congenital Craniofacial Anomalies . . . . . . . . . . . . . . . . . . . 36
Congenital Orbital Tumors . . . . . . . . . . . . . . . . . 39
Hamartomas and Choristomas . . . . . . . . . . . . . . . 39

**4 Orbital Inflammatory and Infectious Disorders . . . . . 43**
Infectious Inflammation . . . . . . . . . . . . . . . . . . 44
Cellulitis . . . . . . . . . . . . . . . . . . . . . . . 44
Necrotizing Fasciitis . . . . . . . . . . . . . . . . . . 48
Orbital Tuberculosis . . . . . . . . . . . . . . . . . . 49
Zygomycosis . . . . . . . . . . . . . . . . . . . . . . 50
Aspergillosis . . . . . . . . . . . . . . . . . . . . . 50
Parasitic Diseases . . . . . . . . . . . . . . . . . . . 51
Noninfectious Inflammation . . . . . . . . . . . . . . . . 51
Thyroid Eye Disease . . . . . . . . . . . . . . . . . . 51
IgG4 Disease . . . . . . . . . . . . . . . . . . . . . 60
Vasculitis . . . . . . . . . . . . . . . . . . . . . . 60
Sarcoidosis . . . . . . . . . . . . . . . . . . . . . . 63
Nonspecific Orbital Inflammation . . . . . . . . . . . . . 63

**5 Orbital Neoplasms and Malformations . . . . . . . . . . . 67**
Vascular Tumors, Malformations, and Fistulas . . . . . . . . 67
Infantile (Capillary) Hemangioma . . . . . . . . . . . . . 67
Cavernous Hemangioma . . . . . . . . . . . . . . . . . . 68
Hemangiopericytoma . . . . . . . . . . . . . . . . . . . 69
Lymphatic Malformation . . . . . . . . . . . . . . . . . 69
Venous Malformation . . . . . . . . . . . . . . . . . . 71
Arteriovenous Malformation . . . . . . . . . . . . . . . 72
Arteriovenous Fistula . . . . . . . . . . . . . . . . . . 72
Orbital Hemorrhage . . . . . . . . . . . . . . . . . . . 74

Neural Tumors . . . . . . . . . . . . . . . . . . . . . . . . 74
Optic Nerve Glioma . . . . . . . . . . . . . . . . . . . . . . 74
Neurofibroma . . . . . . . . . . . . . . . . . . . . . . . 77
Meningioma . . . . . . . . . . . . . . . . . . . . . . . 78
Schwannoma . . . . . . . . . . . . . . . . . . . . . . . 82
Mesenchymal Tumors . . . . . . . . . . . . . . . . . . . . . 82
Rhabdomyosarcoma . . . . . . . . . . . . . . . . . . . . . 82
Miscellaneous Mesenchymal Tumors . . . . . . . . . . . . . . 84
Lymphoproliferative Disorders . . . . . . . . . . . . . . . . 85
Lymphoid Hyperplasia and Lymphoma . . . . . . . . . . . . . 85
Plasma Cell Tumors . . . . . . . . . . . . . . . . . . . . 89
Histiocytic Disorders . . . . . . . . . . . . . . . . . . . 90
Xanthogranuloma . . . . . . . . . . . . . . . . . . . . . 90
Lacrimal Gland Tumors . . . . . . . . . . . . . . . . . . . 91
Epithelial Tumors of the Lacrimal Gland . . . . . . . . . . . 91
Nonepithelial Tumors of the Lacrimal Gland . . . . . . . . . . 94
Secondary Orbital Conditions . . . . . . . . . . . . . . . . . 94
Globe and Eyelid Origin . . . . . . . . . . . . . . . . . . 94
Sinus Disease Affecting the Orbit . . . . . . . . . . . . . . 95
Metastatic Tumors . . . . . . . . . . . . . . . . . . . . . 98
Metastatic Tumors in Children . . . . . . . . . . . . . . . . 98
Metastatic Tumors in Adults . . . . . . . . . . . . . . . . . 99
Management of Orbital Metastases . . . . . . . . . . . . . . 101

**6 Orbital Trauma . . . . . . . . . . . . . . . . . . . . 103**
Midfacial (Le Fort) Fractures . . . . . . . . . . . . . . . . 103
Orbital Fractures . . . . . . . . . . . . . . . . . . . . . . 103
Zygomatic Fractures . . . . . . . . . . . . . . . . . . . . 103
Orbital Apex Fractures . . . . . . . . . . . . . . . . . . . 106
Orbital Roof Fractures . . . . . . . . . . . . . . . . . . . 106
Medial Orbital Fractures . . . . . . . . . . . . . . . . . . 106
Orbital Floor Fractures . . . . . . . . . . . . . . . . . . . 108
Intraorbital Foreign Bodies . . . . . . . . . . . . . . . . . 112
Orbital Hemorrhage . . . . . . . . . . . . . . . . . . . . . 112
Traumatic Vision Loss With Clear Media . . . . . . . . . . . . 112

**7 Orbital Surgery . . . . . . . . . . . . . . . . . . . . 115**
Surgical Spaces . . . . . . . . . . . . . . . . . . . . . . . 115
Orbitotomy . . . . . . . . . . . . . . . . . . . . . . . . . 116
Superior Approach . . . . . . . . . . . . . . . . . . . . . 116
Inferior Approach . . . . . . . . . . . . . . . . . . . . . 118
Medial Approach . . . . . . . . . . . . . . . . . . . . . . 118
Lateral Approach . . . . . . . . . . . . . . . . . . . . . . 120
Orbital Decompression . . . . . . . . . . . . . . . . . . . . 121
Postoperative Care for Orbital Surgery . . . . . . . . . . . . . 124
Special Surgical Techniques in the Orbit . . . . . . . . . . . . 124
Complications of Orbital Surgery . . . . . . . . . . . . . . . 124

**8 The Anophthalmic Socket** . . . . . **127**
Enucleation and Evisceration . . . . . 128
Enucleation . . . . . 128
Evisceration . . . . . 129
Intraoperative Complications of Enucleation and Evisceration . . . . . 130
Orbital Implants . . . . . 131
Prostheses . . . . . 132
Anophthalmic Socket Complications and Treatment . . . . . 132
Deep Superior Sulcus . . . . . 132
Contracture of Fornices . . . . . 133
Exposure and Extrusion of the Implant . . . . . 133
Contracted Sockets . . . . . 134
Anophthalmic Ectropion . . . . . 135
Anophthalmic Ptosis . . . . . 135
Lash Margin Entropion . . . . . 136
Cosmetic Optics . . . . . 136
Exenteration . . . . . 136
Considerations for Exenteration . . . . . 136
Types of Exenteration . . . . . 137

**PART II Periocular Soft Tissues** . . . . . **139**

**9 Facial and Eyelid Anatomy** . . . . . **141**
Face . . . . . 141
Eyelids . . . . . 145
Skin and Subcutaneous Tissue . . . . . 146
Protractors . . . . . 147
Orbital Septum . . . . . 149
Orbital Fat . . . . . 149
Retractors . . . . . 149
Tarsus . . . . . 151
Conjunctiva . . . . . 152
Additional Anatomical Considerations . . . . . 152

**10 Classification and Management of Eyelid Disorders** . . **155**
Congenital Anomalies . . . . . 155
Blepharophimosis–Ptosis–Epicanthus Inversus Syndrome . . . . . 155
Congenital Ptosis of the Upper Eyelid . . . . . 156
Congenital Ectropion . . . . . 156
Euryblepharon . . . . . 156
Ankyloblepharon . . . . . 158
Epicanthus . . . . . 158
Epiblepharon . . . . . 159
Congenital Entropion . . . . . 159
Congenital Distichiasis . . . . . 160
Congenital Coloboma . . . . . 160

Cryptophthalmos . . . . . . . . . . . . . . . . . . . . . . . . . 161
Congenital Eyelid Lesions: Infantile (Capillary) Hemangioma . . . . . 161
Acquired Eyelid Disorders . . . . . . . . . . . . . . . . . . . . . . . 162
Chalazion . . . . . . . . . . . . . . . . . . . . . . . . . . . . . 162
Hordeolum . . . . . . . . . . . . . . . . . . . . . . . . . . . . 163
Eyelid Edema . . . . . . . . . . . . . . . . . . . . . . . . . . . 164
Floppy Eyelid Syndrome . . . . . . . . . . . . . . . . . . . . . . 164
Trichotillomania . . . . . . . . . . . . . . . . . . . . . . . . . 165
Eyelid Neoplasms . . . . . . . . . . . . . . . . . . . . . . . . . . 165
Clinical Evaluation of Eyelid Tumors . . . . . . . . . . . . . . . 165
Benign Eyelid Lesions . . . . . . . . . . . . . . . . . . . . . . . 166
Benign Adnexal Lesions . . . . . . . . . . . . . . . . . . . . . . 169
Benign Melanocytic Lesions . . . . . . . . . . . . . . . . . . . . 172
Premalignant Epidermal Lesions: Actinic Keratosis . . . . . . . . . 175
In Situ Epithelial Malignancies . . . . . . . . . . . . . . . . . . 176
Premalignant Melanocytic Lesions: Lentigo Maligna . . . . . . . . . 177
Malignant Eyelid Tumors . . . . . . . . . . . . . . . . . . . . . 177
Eyelid Trauma . . . . . . . . . . . . . . . . . . . . . . . . . . . . 187
Blunt Trauma . . . . . . . . . . . . . . . . . . . . . . . . . . . 187
Penetrating Trauma . . . . . . . . . . . . . . . . . . . . . . . . 187
Secondary Repair . . . . . . . . . . . . . . . . . . . . . . . . . 189
Dog and Human Bites . . . . . . . . . . . . . . . . . . . . . . . 190
Burns . . . . . . . . . . . . . . . . . . . . . . . . . . . . . . . 190
Eyelid and Canthal Reconstruction . . . . . . . . . . . . . . . . . . 191
Eyelid Defects Not Involving the Eyelid Margin . . . . . . . . . . . 191
Eyelid Defects Involving the Eyelid Margin . . . . . . . . . . . . . 192
Lateral Canthal Defects . . . . . . . . . . . . . . . . . . . . . . 195
Medial Canthal Defects . . . . . . . . . . . . . . . . . . . . . . 195

**11 Periocular Malpositions and Involutional Changes . . . 197**
History and Examination . . . . . . . . . . . . . . . . . . . . . . . 197
Ectropion . . . . . . . . . . . . . . . . . . . . . . . . . . . . . . 197
Involutional Ectropion . . . . . . . . . . . . . . . . . . . . . . . 199
Paralytic Ectropion . . . . . . . . . . . . . . . . . . . . . . . . 201
Cicatricial Ectropion. . . . . . . . . . . . . . . . . . . . . . . . 201
Mechanical Ectropion . . . . . . . . . . . . . . . . . . . . . . . 201
Entropion . . . . . . . . . . . . . . . . . . . . . . . . . . . . . . 202
Congenital Entropion . . . . . . . . . . . . . . . . . . . . . . . 202
Involutional Entropion . . . . . . . . . . . . . . . . . . . . . . . 202
Acute Spastic Entropion . . . . . . . . . . . . . . . . . . . . . . 205
Cicatricial Entropion . . . . . . . . . . . . . . . . . . . . . . . 206
Symblepharon . . . . . . . . . . . . . . . . . . . . . . . . . . . . 208
Trichiasis . . . . . . . . . . . . . . . . . . . . . . . . . . . . . . 208
Management . . . . . . . . . . . . . . . . . . . . . . . . . . . . 208
Blepharoptosis . . . . . . . . . . . . . . . . . . . . . . . . . . . . 209
Evaluation . . . . . . . . . . . . . . . . . . . . . . . . . . . . . 209

Physical Examination . . . . . 209
Ancillary Tests . . . . . 212
Classification . . . . . 213
Treatment of Ptosis . . . . . 218
Eyelid Retraction . . . . . 222
Treatment of Eyelid Retraction . . . . . 223
Facial Paralysis . . . . . 224
Paralytic Ectropion . . . . . 224
Upper Eyelid Paralysis . . . . . 226
Facial Dystonia . . . . . 226
Benign Essential Blepharospasm . . . . . 226
Hemifacial Spasm . . . . . 228
Involutional Periorbital Changes . . . . . 229
Dermatochalasis . . . . . 229
Blepharochalasis . . . . . 230
Blepharoplasty . . . . . 230
Upper Eyelid . . . . . 230
Lower Eyelid . . . . . 230
Preoperative Evaluation for Blepharoplasty . . . . . 231
Techniques . . . . . 232
Complications . . . . . 233
Brow Ptosis . . . . . 234
Treatment of Functional Brow Ptosis . . . . . 234
Facial Rejuvenation . . . . . 235
Pathogenesis of the Aging Face . . . . . 236
Physical Examination of the Aging Face . . . . . 236
Nonsurgical Facial Rejuvenation . . . . . 237
Laser Skin Resurfacing . . . . . 237
Cosmetic Uses of Botulinum Toxin . . . . . 238
Soft Tissue Dermal Fillers . . . . . 239
Facial Rejuvenation Surgery . . . . . 241
Forehead Rejuvenation . . . . . 241
Midface Rejuvenation . . . . . 241
Lower Face and Neck Rejuvenation . . . . . 245
Conclusion . . . . . 247

**PART III Lacrimal System . . . . . 249**

**12 Anatomy, Development, and Physiology of the Lacrimal Secretory and Drainage Systems . . . . . 251**
Normal Anatomy . . . . . 251
Secretory System . . . . . 251
Drainage System . . . . . 252
Development . . . . . 255
Secretory System . . . . . 255
Drainage System . . . . . 255
Physiology . . . . . 255

**13 Abnormalities of the Lacrimal Secretory and Drainage Systems . . . 257**
Developmental Abnormalities . . . 257
Lacrimal Secretory System . . . 257
Lacrimal Drainage System . . . 257
Congenital Lacrimal Drainage Obstruction . . . 259
Evaluation . . . 259
Punctal and Canalicular Agenesis and Dysgenesis . . . 259
Congenital Nasolacrimal Duct Obstruction . . . 260
Dacryocystocele . . . 265
Acquired Lacrimal Drainage Obstruction . . . 267
Evaluation . . . 267
Punctal Disorders . . . 272
Canalicular Obstruction . . . 273
Acquired Nasolacrimal Duct Obstruction . . . 276
Therapeutic Closure of the Lacrimal Drainage System . . . 281
Trauma . . . 282
Canaliculus . . . 282
Lacrimal Sac and Nasolacrimal Duct . . . 284
Infection . . . 284
Dacryoadenitis . . . 284
Canaliculitis . . . 284
Dacryocystitis . . . 285
Neoplasm . . . 286
Lacrimal Gland . . . 286
Lacrimal Drainage System . . . 287

Basic Texts . . . 289
Related Academy Materials . . . 291
Requesting Continuing Medical Education Credit . . . 293
Study Questions . . . 295
Answer Sheet for Section 7 Study Questions . . . 301
Answers . . . 303
Index . . . 307

# General Introduction

The Basic and Clinical Science Course (BCSC) is designed to meet the needs of residents and practitioners for a comprehensive yet concise curriculum of the field of ophthalmology. The BCSC has developed from its original brief outline format, which relied heavily on outside readings, to a more convenient and educationally useful self-contained text. The Academy updates and revises the course annually, with the goals of integrating the basic science and clinical practice of ophthalmology and of keeping ophthalmologists current with new developments in the various subspecialties.

The BCSC incorporates the effort and expertise of more than 90 ophthalmologists, organized into 13 Section faculties, working with Academy editorial staff. In addition, the course continues to benefit from many lasting contributions made by the faculties of previous editions. Members of the Academy Practicing Ophthalmologists Advisory Committee for Education, Committee on Aging, and Vision Rehabilitation Committee review every volume before major revisions. Members of the European Board of Ophthalmology, organized into Section faculties, also review each volume before major revisions, focusing primarily on differences between American and European ophthalmology practice.

## Organization of the Course

The Basic and Clinical Science Course comprises 13 volumes, incorporating fundamental ophthalmic knowledge, subspecialty areas, and special topics:

1 Update on General Medicine
2 Fundamentals and Principles of Ophthalmology
3 Clinical Optics
4 Ophthalmic Pathology and Intraocular Tumors
5 Neuro-Ophthalmology
6 Pediatric Ophthalmology and Strabismus
7 Orbit, Eyelids, and Lacrimal System
8 External Disease and Cornea
9 Intraocular Inflammation and Uveitis
10 Glaucoma
11 Lens and Cataract
12 Retina and Vitreous
13 Refractive Surgery

In addition, a comprehensive Master Index allows the reader to easily locate subjects throughout the entire series.

## References

Readers who wish to explore specific topics in greater detail may consult the references cited within each chapter and listed in the Basic Texts section at the back of the book.

These references are intended to be selective rather than exhaustive, chosen by the BCSC faculty as being important, current, and readily available to residents and practitioners.

## Videos

This edition of Section 7, *Orbit, Eyelids, and Lacrimal System,* includes videos related to topics covered in the book. The videos were selected by members of the BCSC faculty and are available to readers of the print and electronic versions of Section 7 (www.aao.org/bcscvideo_section07). Mobile-device users can scan the QR code below (a QR-code reader must already be installed on the device) to access the video content.

## Study Questions and CME Credit

Each volume of the BCSC is designed as an independent study activity for ophthalmology residents and practitioners. The learning objectives for this volume are given on page 1. The text, illustrations, and references provide the information necessary to achieve the objectives; the study questions allow readers to test their understanding of the material and their mastery of the objectives. Physicians who wish to claim CME credit for this educational activity may do so by following the instructions given at the end of the book.

## Conclusion

The Basic and Clinical Science Course has expanded greatly over the years, with the addition of much new text, numerous illustrations, and video content. Recent editions have sought to place greater emphasis on clinical applicability while maintaining a solid foundation in basic science. As with any educational program, it reflects the experience of its authors. As its faculties change and medicine progresses, new viewpoints emerge on controversial subjects and techniques. Not all alternate approaches can be included in this series; as with any educational endeavor, the learner should seek additional sources, including Academy Preferred Practice Pattern Guidelines.

The BCSC faculty and staff continually strive to improve the educational usefulness of the course; you, the reader, can contribute to this ongoing process. If you have any suggestions or questions about the series, please do not hesitate to contact the faculty or the editors.

The authors, editors, and reviewers hope that your study of the BCSC will be of lasting value and that each Section will serve as a practical resource for quality patient care.

# Objectives

Upon completion of BCSC Section 7, *Orbit, Eyelids, and Lacrimal System,* the reader should be able to

- describe the normal anatomy and function of orbital and periocular tissues
- identify general and specific pathophysiologic processes (including congenital, infectious, inflammatory, traumatic, neoplastic, and involutional) that affect the structure and function of these tissues
- select appropriate examination techniques and protocols for diagnosing disorders of the orbit, eyelids, and lacrimal system
- select from among the various imaging and ancillary studies available those that are most useful for the particular patient
- describe appropriate differential diagnoses for disorders of the orbital and periocular tissues
- state the indications for enucleation, evisceration, and exenteration
- describe functional and cosmetic indications in the surgical management of eyelid and periorbital conditions
- state the principles of medical and surgical management of conditions affecting the orbit, eyelids, and lacrimal system
- identify the major postoperative complications of orbital, eyelid, and lacrimal system surgery

# PART I

# Orbit

CHAPTER 1

# Orbital Anatomy

BCSC Section 2, *Fundamentals and Principles of Ophthalmology,* also discusses ocular anatomy and includes many illustrations.

## Dimensions

The orbits are the bony cavities that contain the globes, extraocular muscles, nerves, fat, and blood vessels. Each bony orbit is pear shaped, tapering posteriorly to the apex and the optic canal. The medial orbital walls are approximately parallel and are separated by 25 mm in the average adult. The widest dimension of the orbit is approximately 1 cm behind the anterior orbital rim. Average measurements of the adult orbit are shown in Table 1-1. The intraorbital segment of the optic nerve is slightly S-curved and moves with the eye. The normal redundancy of the optic nerve allows the eye to rotate and move forward without damaging the nerve.

## Topographic Relationships

The orbital septum arises from the orbital rims anteriorly. The paranasal sinuses are either rudimentary or very small at birth, and they increase in size through adolescence. They lie adjacent to the floor, medial wall, and anterior portion of the orbital roof. The orbital walls are composed of 7 bones: ethmoid, frontal, lacrimal, maxilla (maxillary), palatine, sphenoid, and zygomatic. The composition of each of the 4 walls and their location in relation

**Table 1-1 Average Dimensions of the Adult Orbit**

| | |
|---|---|
| Volume | 30 $cm^3$ |
| Entrance height | 35 mm |
| Entrance width | 40–45 mm |
| Medial wall length | 40–45 mm |
| Distance from posterior globe to optic foramen | 18 mm |
| Length of orbital segment of optic nerve | 25–30 mm |

to adjacent extraorbital structures are shown in Figures 1-1, 1-2, and 1-3 and summarized in the following sections.

## Roof of the Orbit

- composed of the orbital plate of the frontal bone and the lesser wing of the sphenoid bone
- important landmarks: the *lacrimal gland fossa,* which contains the orbital lobe of the lacrimal gland; the *fossa for the trochlea of the superior oblique tendon,* located 5 mm behind the superior nasal orbital rim; and the *supraorbital notch,* or *foramen,* which transmits the supraorbital vessels and the supraorbital branch of the frontal nerve
- located adjacent to the anterior cranial fossa and frontal sinus

A

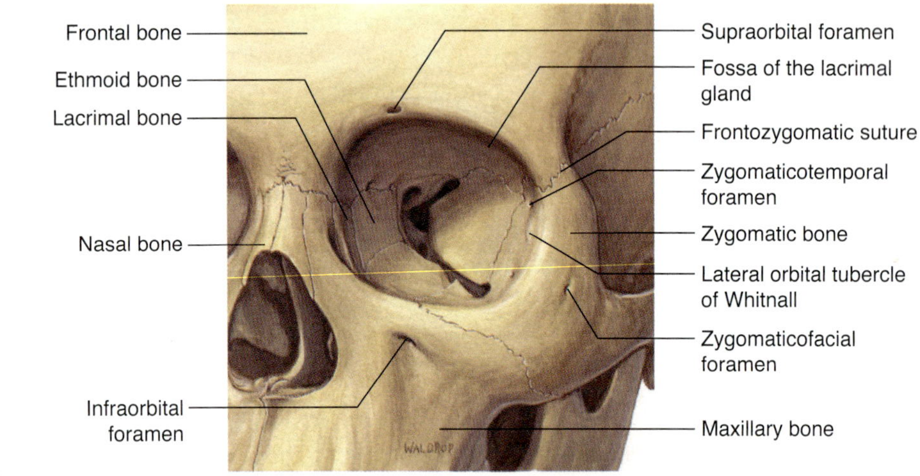


B

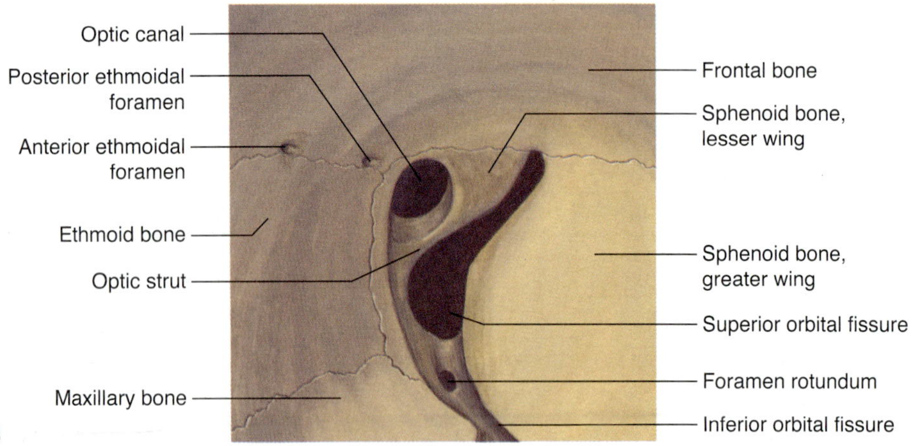


**Figure 1-1** **A,** Orbital bones, frontal view. **B,** Orbital bones, apex. *(Reproduced with permission from Dutton JJ.* Atlas of Clinical and Surgical Orbital Anatomy. *Philadelphia: Saunders; 1994:8.)*

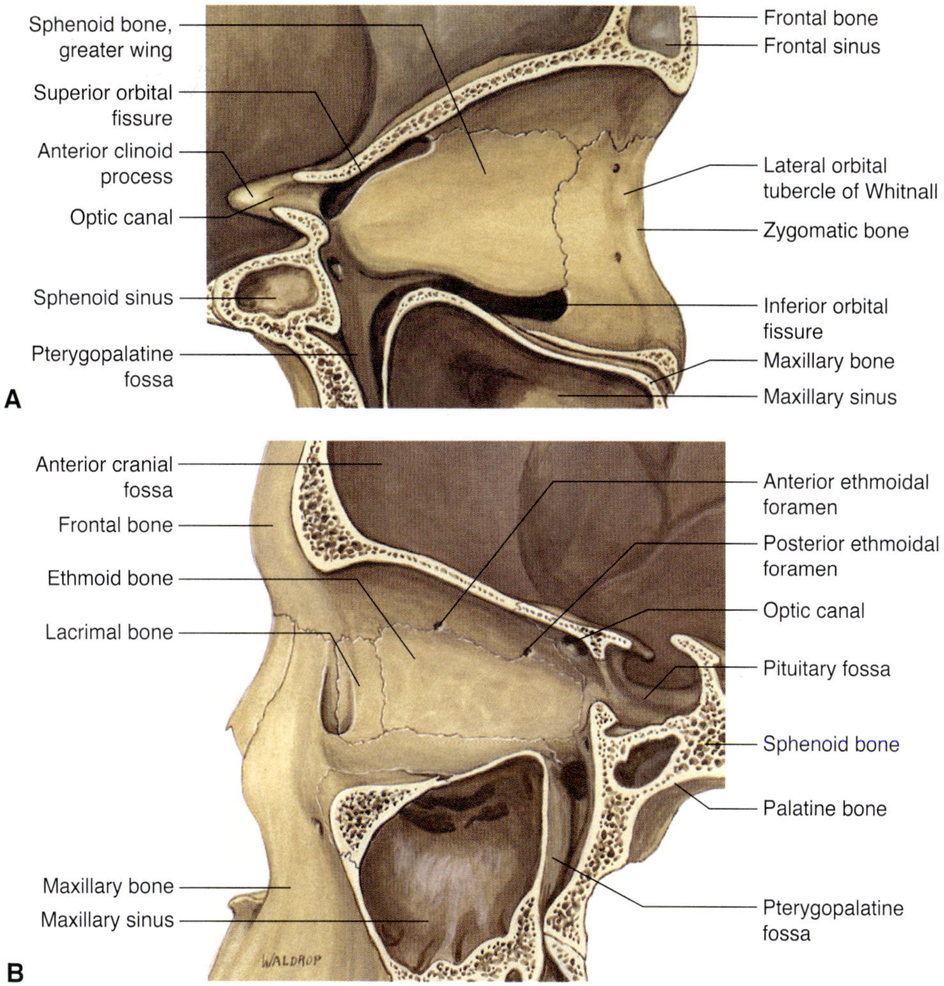


**Figure 1-2** **A,** Orbital bones, lateral wall, internal view. **B,** Orbital bones, medial wall, internal view. *(Reproduced with permission from Dutton JJ.* Atlas of Clinical and Surgical Orbital Anatomy. *Philadelphia: Saunders; 1994:9–10.)*

## Lateral Wall of the Orbit

- composed of the zygomatic bone and the greater wing of the sphenoid bone; separated from the lesser wing (portion of the orbital roof) by the superior orbital fissure
- important landmarks: the *lateral orbital tubercle of Whitnall,* with multiple attachments, including the lateral canthal tendon, the lateral horn of the levator aponeurosis, the check ligament of the lateral rectus, the Lockwood ligament (the suspensory ligament of the globe), and the Whitnall ligament; and the *frontozygomatic suture,* located 1 cm above the tubercle
- located adjacent to the middle cranial fossa and the temporal fossa

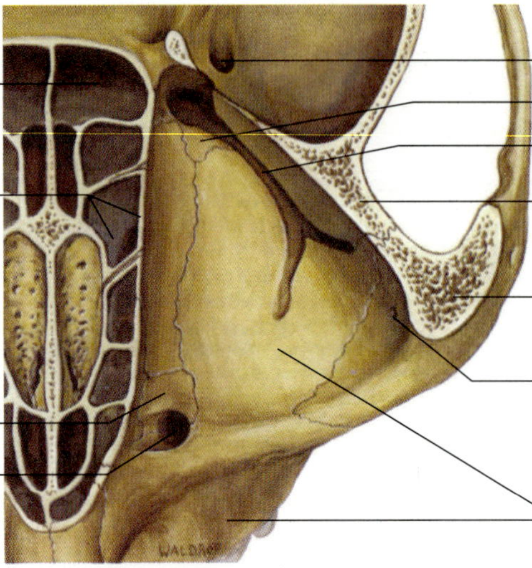


**Figure 1-3** Orbital bones, orbital floor, internal view. *(Modified with permission from Dutton JJ.* Atlas of Clinical and Surgical Orbital Anatomy. *Philadelphia: Saunders; 1994:11.)*

- commonly extends anteriorly to the equator of the globe, helping to protect the posterior half of the eye while still allowing wide peripheral vision
- is the thickest and strongest of the orbital walls

## Medial Wall of the Orbit

- composed of the orbital plate of the ethmoid bone, the lacrimal bone, the frontal process of the maxillary bone, and the lesser wing of the sphenoid bone
- important landmark: the *frontoethmoidal suture,* marking the approximate level of the cribriform plate, the roof of the ethmoids, the floor of the anterior cranial fossa, and the entry of the anterior and posterior ethmoidal arteries into the orbit
- located adjacent to the ethmoid and sphenoid sinuses and nasal cavity
- medial wall of the optic canal is formed by the lesser wing of the sphenoid, and this is also the lateral wall of the sphenoid sinus
- only the lacrimal bone exists wholly within the orbital confines

The thinnest walls of the orbit are the *lamina papyracea,* between the orbit and the ethmoid sinuses along the medial wall, and the *maxillary bone,* particularly in its posteromedial portion. These are the bones most frequently fractured as a result of indirect, or blowout, fractures (see Chapter 6). Infections of the ethmoid sinuses may extend through the lamina papyracea to cause orbital cellulitis and proptosis.

## Floor of the Orbit

- composed of the maxillary bone, palatine bone, and the orbital plate of the zygomatic bone

- forms the roof of the maxillary sinus; does not extend to the orbital apex but instead ends at the pterygopalatine fossa; hence, it is the shortest of the orbital walls
- important landmarks: the *infraorbital groove* and *infraorbital canal,* which transmit the infraorbital artery and the maxillary division of the trigeminal nerve

Dutton JJ. *Atlas of Clinical and Surgical Orbital Anatomy.* 2nd ed. Philadelphia: Saunders; 2011.

## Apertures

The orbital walls are perforated by several important apertures (see Figs 1-1 through 1-3).

### Ethmoidal Foramina

The anterior and posterior ethmoidal arteries pass through the corresponding ethmoidal foramina in the medial orbital wall along the frontoethmoidal suture. These foramina provide a potential route of entry into the orbit for infections and neoplasms from the sinuses and also serve as a surgical landmark for the superior extent of medial wall surgery. Limiting manipulation of the medial orbital wall below the level of the foramina helps prevent inadvertent entry into the cranial vault. Disruption of the medial wall above the level of the foramina may disrupt a plane superior to the cribriform plate.

### Superior Orbital Fissure

The superior orbital fissure separates the greater and lesser wings of the sphenoid bone and transmits cranial nerves III, IV, and VI; the first (ophthalmic) division of cranial nerve (CN) V; and sympathetic nerve fibers. Most of the venous drainage from the orbit passes through this fissure by way of the superior ophthalmic vein to the cavernous sinus (Fig 1-4; see also Fig 1-1).

### Inferior Orbital Fissure

The inferior orbital fissure is bounded by the sphenoid, maxillary, and palatine bones and lies between the lateral orbital wall and the orbital floor. It transmits the second (maxillary) division of CN V, including the zygomatic nerve, and branches of the inferior ophthalmic vein leading to the pterygoid plexus. The maxillary nerve ($V_2$) exits the skull through the foramen rotundum and travels through the pterygopalatine fossa to enter the orbit at the infraorbital groove. After giving off the zygomatic branch, the nerve becomes the infraorbital nerve and travels anteriorly in the floor of the orbit through the infraorbital canal, emerging on the face of the maxilla 1 cm below the inferior orbital rim. The infraorbital nerve carries sensation from the lower eyelid, cheek, upper lip, upper teeth, and gingiva.

### Zygomaticofacial and Zygomaticotemporal Canals

The zygomaticofacial canal and zygomaticotemporal canal transmit vessels and branches of the zygomatic nerve through the lateral orbital wall to the cheek and the temporal fossa, respectively.

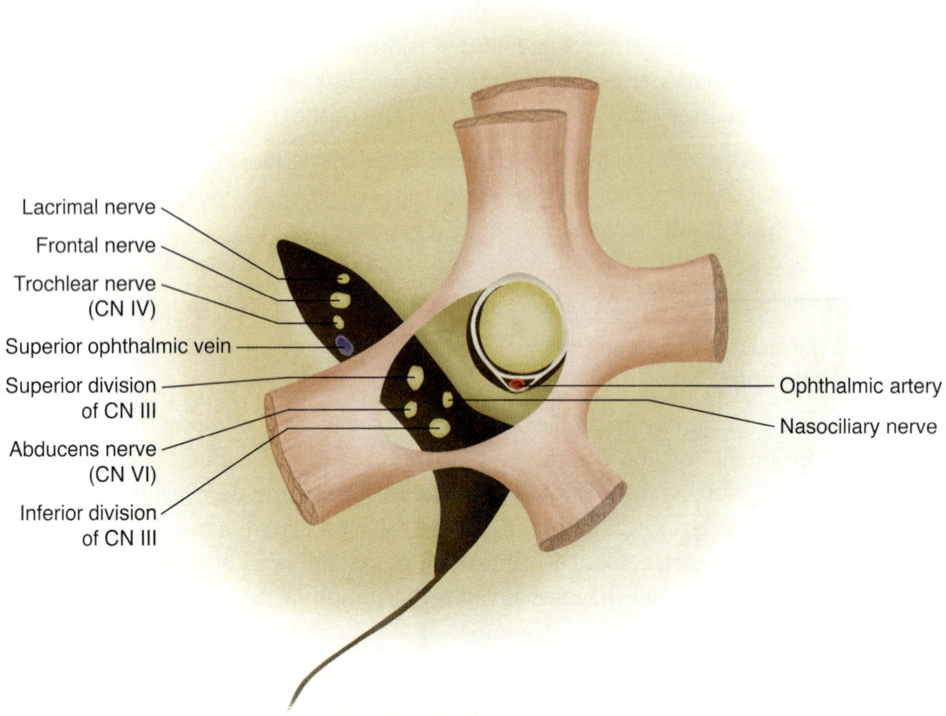


**Figure 1-4** View of orbital apex, right orbit. The ophthalmic artery enters the orbit through the optic canal, whereas the superior and inferior divisions of cranial nerve (CN) III, CN VI, and the nasociliary nerve enter the muscle cone through the oculomotor foramen. Cranial nerve IV, the frontal and lacrimal nerves, and the ophthalmic vein enter through the superior orbital fissure and thus lie within the periorbita but outside the muscle cone. Note that the presence of many nerves and arteries along the lateral side of the optic nerve mandates a superonasal surgical approach to the optic nerve in the orbital apex. *(Illustration by Cyndie C. H. Wooley.)*

## Nasolacrimal Canal

The nasolacrimal canal extends from the lacrimal sac fossa to the inferior meatus beneath the inferior turbinate in the nose. This canal transmits the nasolacrimal duct, which is continuous from the lacrimal sac to the nasal mucosa (see Part III, Lacrimal System).

## Optic Canal

The optic canal is 8–10 mm long and is located within the lesser wing of the sphenoid bone. This canal is separated from the superior orbital fissure by the bony optic strut. The optic nerve, ophthalmic artery, and sympathetic nerves pass through this canal. The orbital end of the canal is the optic foramen, which normally measures less than 6.5 mm in diameter in adults. Optic canal enlargement accompanies the expansion of the nerve, as seen with optic nerve gliomas. Narrowing of the canal occurs in disorders such as fibrous dysplasia. Blunt trauma may cause an optic canal fracture or shearing of the nerve at the foramen, resulting in optic nerve damage.

## Soft Tissues

### Periorbita

The periorbita is the periosteal covering of the orbital bones. At the orbital apex, it fuses with the dura mater covering the optic nerve. Anteriorly, the periorbita is continuous with the orbital septum and the periosteum of the facial bones. The line of fusion of these layers at the orbital rim is called the *arcus marginalis*. The periorbita adheres loosely to the bone except at the orbital margin, sutures, fissures, foramina, tubercles, and canals. In an exenteration, the periorbita can be easily separated except where these firm attachments are present. Subperiosteal fluid, such as pus or blood, is usually loculated within these boundaries. The periorbita is richly innervated by sensory nerves.

### Intraorbital Optic Nerve

The intraorbital portion of the optic nerve is approximately 30 mm long. The nerve is somewhat longer than the orbit, allowing eye movement without traction on the nerve. The optic nerve is 4 mm in diameter and surrounded by the pia mater, arachnoid, and dura mater, which are continuous with the same layers covering the brain. The dura mater covering the posterior portion of the intraorbital optic nerve fuses with the annulus of Zinn at the orbital apex and is continuous with the periosteum of the optic canal.

### Extraocular Muscles and Orbital Fat

The extraocular muscles are responsible for the movement of the eye and for synchronous movements of the eyelids. All of the extraocular muscles, except the inferior oblique muscle, originate at the orbital apex and travel anteriorly to insert onto the eye or eyelid. The 4 rectus muscles (superior, medial, lateral, and inferior recti) originate in the annulus of Zinn. The levator palpebrae superioris muscle arises above the annulus on the lesser wing of the sphenoid bone. The superior oblique muscle originates slightly medial to the levator muscle origin, and travels anteriorly through the trochlea on the superomedial orbital rim, where it turns posterolaterally toward the eye. The inferior oblique muscle originates in the anterior orbital floor lateral to the lacrimal sac and travels posterolaterally within the lower eyelid retractors to insert inferolateral to the macula.

In the anterior portion of the orbit, the rectus muscles are connected by a membrane known as the *intermuscular septum*. When viewed in the coronal plane, this membrane forms a ring that divides the orbital fat into the *intraconal fat (central surgical space)* and the *extraconal fat (peripheral surgical space)*. These anatomical designations on a magnetic resonance (MR) or computed tomography (CT) scan are helpful for describing the location of a mass. A knowledge of these spaces helps direct the surgical dissection to the mass.

The orbit is further divided by many fine fibrous septa that unite and support the globe, optic nerve, and extraocular muscles (Fig 1-5). Accidental or surgical orbital trauma can disrupt this supporting system and contribute to globe displacement

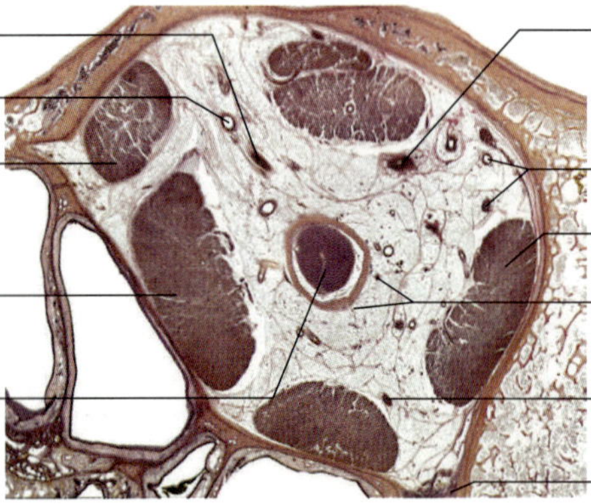


**Figure 1-5** Cross section of the orbit at mid-orbit and at the widest extent of the extraocular muscles. Note the pink-stained fibrous tissue septae in the intraconal space. *(Modified with permission from Dutton JJ.* Atlas of Clinical and Surgical Orbital Anatomy. *Philadelphia: Saunders; 1994:151.)*

and restriction. In some cases of diplopia after fracture, restriction of eye movement is caused by the entrapment of the orbital connective tissue rather than by the muscles themselves.

The motor innervation of the extraocular muscles arises from cranial nerves III, IV, and VI. The superior rectus and levator muscles are supplied by the superior division of CN III (oculomotor nerve). The inferior rectus, medial rectus, and inferior oblique muscles are supplied by the inferior division of CN III. The lateral rectus is supplied by CN VI (abducens nerve). The cranial nerves to the rectus muscles enter the orbit posteriorly through the superior orbital fissure and travel through the intraconal fat to enter the muscles' intraconal surface at the junction of the posterior third and anterior two-thirds. Cranial nerve IV (trochlear nerve) crosses over the levator muscle and innervates the superior oblique on the superior surface at its posterior third. The nerve to the inferior oblique muscle travels anteriorly on the lateral aspect of the inferior rectus to enter the muscle on its posterior surface.

## Annulus of Zinn

The annulus of Zinn is the fibrous ring formed by the common origin of the 4 rectus muscles (Fig 1-6). The ring encircles the optic foramen and the central portion of the superior orbital fissure. The superior origin of the lateral rectus muscle separates the superior orbital fissure into 2 compartments. The portion of the orbital apex enclosed by the annulus is called the *oculomotor foramen.* This opening transmits CN III (upper and lower divisions), CN VI, and the nasociliary branch of the ophthalmic division of CN V (trigeminal). The superior and lateral aspect of the superior orbital fissure external to the muscle cone transmits CN IV as well as the frontal and lacrimal branches of the ophthalmic division of CN V. Cranial nerve IV is the only nerve that innervates an extraocular muscle and does not pass directly into the muscle cone when entering the orbit. Cranial nerves III and VI pass directly into the muscle cone through the oculomotor foramen. The

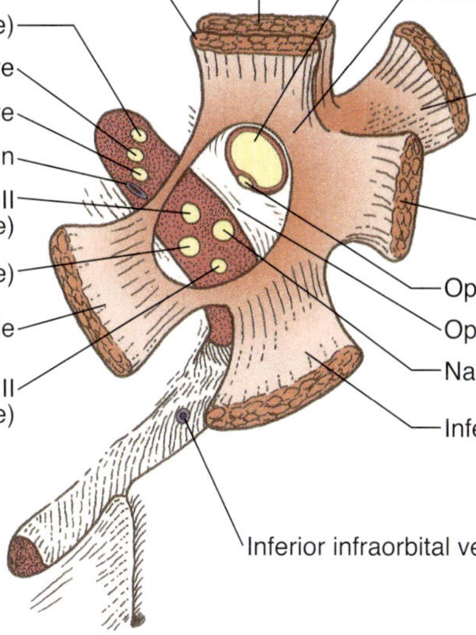


**Figure 1-6** Anterior view of the right orbital apex showing the distribution of nerves as they enter through the superior orbital fissure and optic canal. This view also shows the annulus of Zinn, the fibrous ring formed by the common origin of the 4 rectus muscles. *(Reproduced with permission from Nerad JA.* Techniques in Ophthalmic Plastic Surgery. *Philadelphia: Saunders; 2010.)*

superior ophthalmic vein passes through the superior and lateral portion of the superior orbital fissure outside the oculomotor foramen.

## Vasculature of the Orbit

The blood supply to the orbit arises primarily from the ophthalmic artery (Figs 1-7, 1-8), which is a branch of the internal carotid artery. Smaller contributions come from the external carotid artery by way of the internal maxillary and facial arteries. The ophthalmic artery travels underneath the intracranial optic nerve through the dura mater along the optic canal to enter the orbit. The major branches of the ophthalmic artery are the

- branches to the extraocular muscles
- central retinal artery (to the optic nerve and retina)
- posterior ciliary arteries (long to the anterior segment and short to the choroid)

Terminal branches of the ophthalmic artery travel anteriorly and form rich anastomoses with branches of the external carotid in the face and periorbital region (Fig 1-9).

The superior ophthalmic vein provides the main venous drainage of the orbit (see Figs 1-7, 1-8). This vein originates in the superonasal quadrant of the orbit and extends posteriorly through the superior orbital fissure into the cavernous sinus. Frequently, the superior ophthalmic vein appears on axial orbital CT scans as the only structure coursing

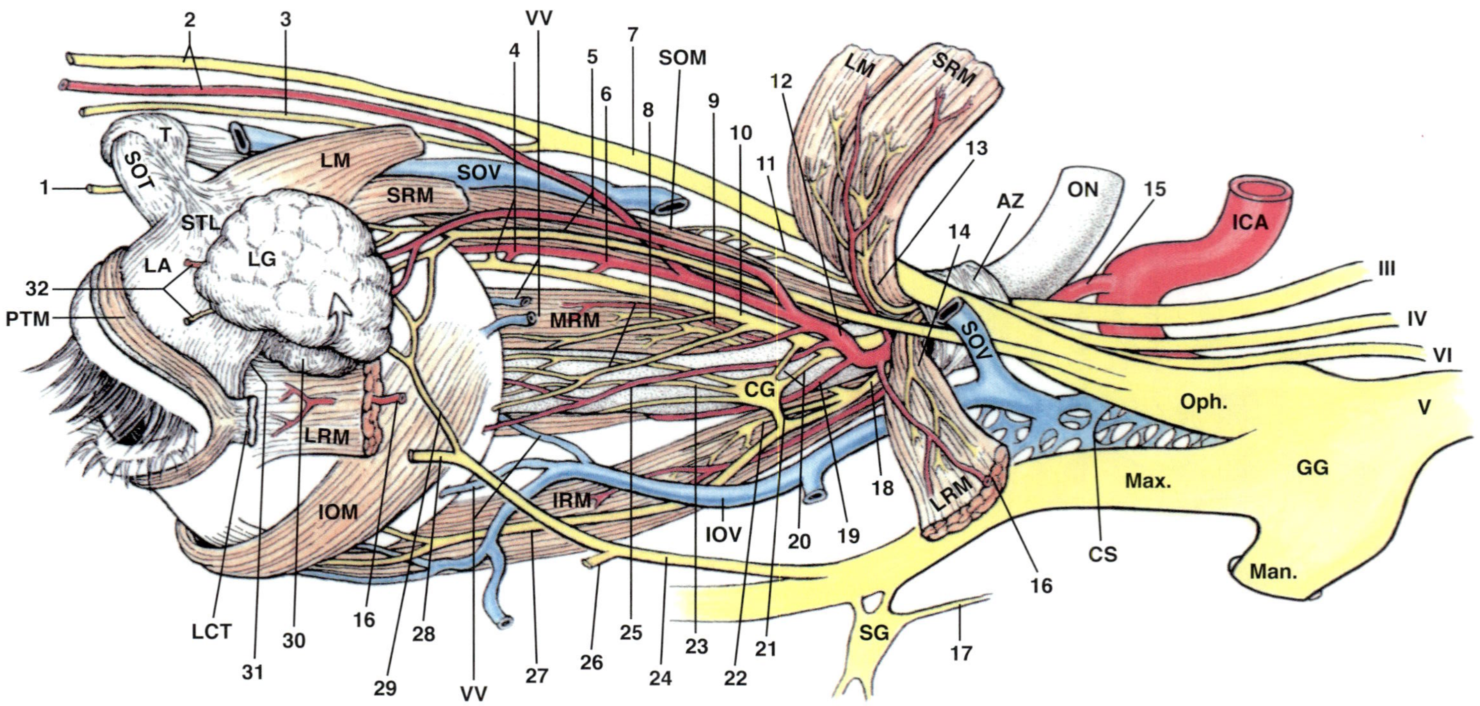


**Figure 1-7** Side view of left orbit. *AZ,* annulus of Zinn; *CG,* ciliary ganglion; *CS,* cavernous sinus; *GG,* Gasserian ganglion; *ICA,* internal carotid artery; *IOM,* inferior oblique muscle; *IOV,* inferior ophthalmic vein; *IRM,* inferior rectus muscle; *LA,* levator aponeurosis; *LCT,* lateral canthal tendon; *LG,* lacrimal gland; *LM,* levator muscle; *LRM,* lateral rectus muscle; *Man.,* mandibular nerve; *Max.,* maxillary nerve; *MRM,* medial rectus muscle; *ON,* optic nerve; *Oph.,* ophthalmic nerve; *PTM,* pretarsal muscle; *SG,* sphenopalatine ganglion; *SOM,* superior oblique muscle; *SOT,* superior oblique tendon; *SOV,* superior ophthalmic vein; *SRM,* superior rectus muscle; *STL,* superior transverse ligament; *T,* trochlea; *VV,* vortex veins; *1,* infratrochlear nerve; *2,* supraorbital nerve and artery; *3,* supratrochlear nerve; *4,* anterior ethmoid nerve and artery; *5,* lacrimal nerve and artery; *6,* posterior ethmoid artery; *7,* frontal nerve; *8,* long ciliary nerves; *9,* branch of CN III to medial rectus muscle; *10,* nasociliary nerve; *11,* CN IV; *12,* ophthalmic (orbital) artery; *13,* superior ramus of CN III; *14,* CN VI; *15,* ophthalmic artery, origin; *16,* anterior ciliary artery; *17,* vidian nerve; *18,* inferior ramus of CN III; *19,* central retinal artery; *20,* sensory branches from ciliary ganglion to nasociliary nerve; *21,* motor (parasympathetic) nerve to ciliary ganglion from nerve to inferior oblique muscle; *22,* branch of CN III to inferior rectus muscle; *23,* short ciliary nerves; *24,* zygomatic nerve; *25,* posterior ciliary arteries; *26,* zygomaticofacial nerve; *27,* nerve to inferior oblique muscle; *28,* zygomaticotemporal nerve; *29,* lacrimal secretory nerve; *30,* lacrimal gland–palpebral lobe; *31,* lateral horn of levator aponeurosis; *32,* lacrimal artery and nerve terminal branches. *(Reproduced from Stewart WB, ed.* Ophthalmic Plastic and Reconstructive Surgery. *4th ed. San Francisco: American Academy of Ophthalmology Manuals Program; 1984.)*

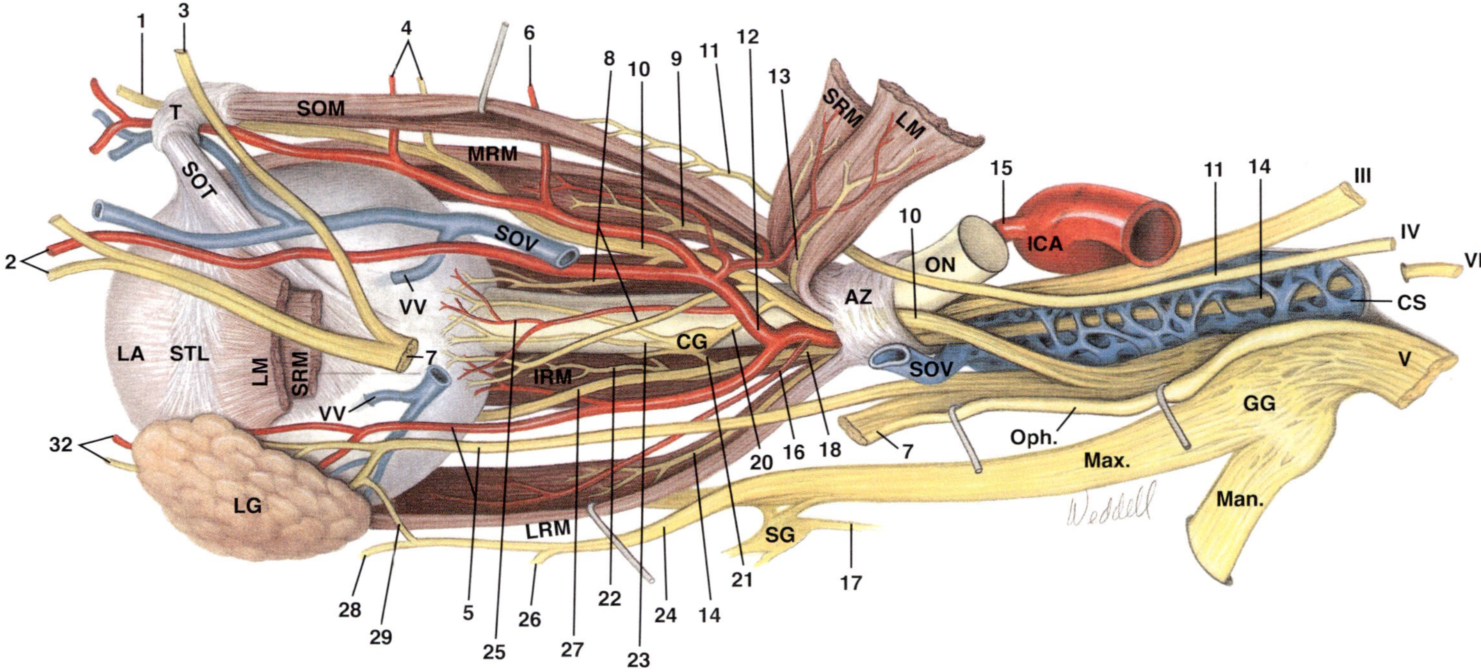


**Figure 1-8** Top view of left orbit. *AZ,* annulus of Zinn; *CG,* ciliary ganglion; *CS,* cavernous sinus; *GG,* Gasserian ganglion; *ICA,* internal carotid artery; *IRM,* inferior rectus muscle; *LA,* levator aponeurosis; *LG,* lacrimal gland; *LM,* levator muscle; *LRM,* lateral rectus muscle; *Man.,* mandibular nerve; *Max.,* maxillary nerve; *MRM,* medial rectus muscle; *ON,* optic nerve; *Oph.,* ophthalmic nerve; *SG,* sphenopalatine ganglion; *SOM,* superior oblique muscle; *SOT,* superior oblique tendon; *SOV,* superior ophthalmic vein; *SRM,* superior rectus muscle; *STL,* superior transverse ligament; *T,* trochlea; *VV,* vortex veins; *1,* infratrochlear nerve; *2,* supraorbital nerve and artery; *3,* supratrochlear nerve; *4,* anterior ethmoid nerve and artery; *5,* lacrimal nerve and artery; *6,* posterior ethmoid artery; *7,* frontal nerve; *8,* long ciliary nerves; *9,* branch of CN III to medial rectus muscle; *10,* nasociliary nerve; *11,* CN IV; *12,* ophthalmic (orbital) artery; *13,* superior ramus of CN III; *14,* CN VI; *15,* ophthalmic artery, origin; *16,* anterior ciliary artery; *17,* vidian nerve; *18,* inferior ramus of CN III; *20,* sensory branches from ciliary ganglion to nasociliary nerve; *21,* motor (parasympathetic) nerve to ciliary ganglion from nerve to inferior oblique muscle; *22,* branch of CN III to inferior rectus muscle; *23,* short ciliary nerves; *24,* zygomatic nerve; *25,* posterior ciliary arteries; *26,* zygomaticofacial nerve; *27,* nerve to inferior oblique muscle; *28,* zygomaticotemporal nerve; *29,* lacrimal secretory nerve; *32,* lacrimal artery and nerve terminal branches. *(Reproduced from Stewart WB, ed.* Ophthalmic Plastic and Reconstructive Surgery. *4th ed. San Francisco: American Academy of Ophthalmology Manuals Program; 1984.)*

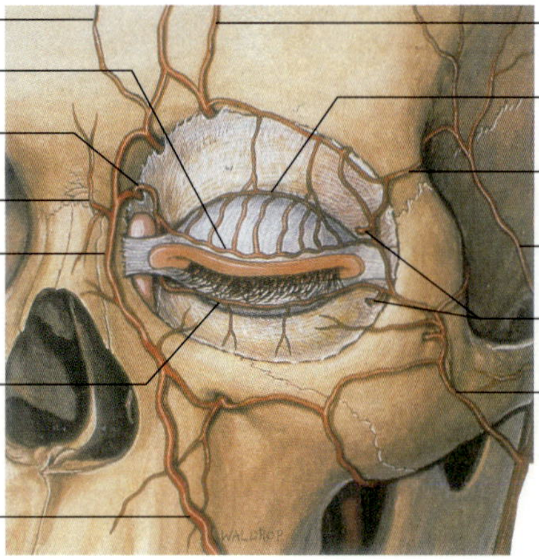


**Figure 1-9** Periorbital and eyelid arteries, frontal view. *(Reproduced with permission from Dutton JJ.* Atlas of Clinical and Surgical Orbital Anatomy. *Philadelphia: Saunders; 1994.)*

diagonally through the superior orbit. Many anastomoses occur anteriorly with the veins of the face as well as posteriorly with the pterygoid plexus.

## Nerves

Sensory innervation to the periorbital area is provided by the ophthalmic and maxillary divisions of CN V (Fig 1-10). After branching off at the trigeminal ganglion, the ophthalmic division of CN V travels in the lateral wall of the cavernous sinus, where it divides into 3 main branches: frontal, lacrimal, and nasociliary. The frontal and lacrimal nerves enter the orbit through the superior orbital fissure above the annulus of Zinn (see Fig 1-6) and travel anteriorly in the extraconal fat to innervate the medial canthus (supratrochlear branch), upper eyelid (lacrimal and supratrochlear branches), and forehead (supraorbital branch). The nasociliary branch enters the orbit through the superior orbital fissure within the annulus of Zinn, entering the intraconal space and traveling anteriorly to innervate the eye via the ciliary branches. The short ciliary nerves penetrate the sclera after passing through the ciliary ganglion without synapse. The long ciliary nerves pass by the ciliary ganglion and enter the sclera, where they extend anteriorly to supply the iris, cornea, and ciliary muscle.

The muscles of facial expression, including the orbicularis oculi, procerus, corrugator superciliaris, and frontalis muscles, receive their motor supply by way of branches of CN VII (the facial nerve) that enter on the undersurface of each muscle.

The parasympathetic innervation, which controls accommodation, pupillary constriction, and lacrimal gland stimulation, follows a complicated course. Parasympathetic innervation enters the eye as the short posterior ciliary nerves after synapsing within the ciliary ganglion. Parasympathetic innervation to the lacrimal gland originates in the lacrimal nucleus of the pons and eventually joins the lacrimal nerve to enter the lacrimal gland.

Sympathetic activity originates in the hypothalamus, with sympathetic fibers descending through the brainstem to the spinal cord, where they continue. Fibers destined for the orbit synapse in the ciliospinal center of Budge-Waller and then travel with branches of

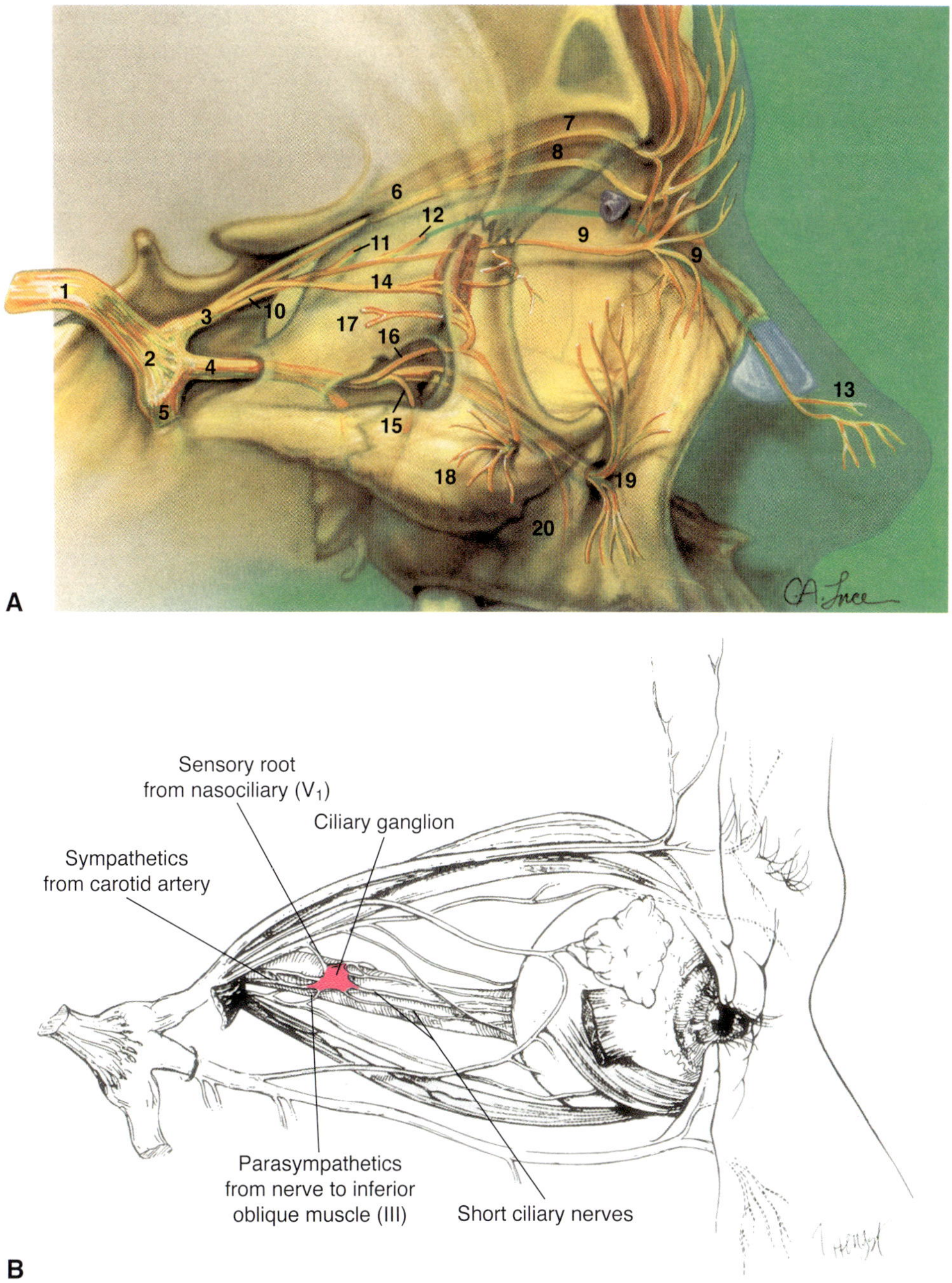


**Figure 1-10** **A,** Sensory nerves. *1,* CN V (trigeminal); *2,* trigeminal ganglion; *3,* ophthalmic division of CN V ($V_1$); *4,* maxillary division of CN V ($V_2$); *5,* mandibular division of CN V ($V_3$); *6,* frontal nerve; *7,* supraorbital nerve; *8,* supratrochlear nerve (trochlea noted by *purple*); *9,* infratrochlear nerve; *10,* nasociliary nerve; *11,* posterior ethmoidal nerve; *12,* anterior ethmoidal nerve; *13,* external or dorsal nasal nerve; *14,* lacrimal nerve; *15,* posterior superior alveolar nerve; *16,* zygomatic nerve; *17,* zygomaticotemporal nerve; *18,* zygomaticofacial nerve; *19,* infraorbital nerve; *20,* anterior superior alveolar nerve. **B,** Contributions to the ciliary ganglion. *(Part A reproduced with permission from Zide BM, Jelks GW, eds.* Surgical Anatomy of the Orbit. *New York: Raven; 1985:12. Part B reproduced with permission from Doxanas MT, Anderson RL.* Clinical Orbital Anatomy. *Baltimore: Williams & Wilkins; 1984.)*

the carotid artery to enter the orbit. The sympathetic nerves carry innervation for pupillary dilation, vasoconstriction, smooth muscle function of the eyelids and orbit, and hidrosis. The nerve fibers follow the arterial supply to the pupil, eyelids, and orbit and travel anteriorly in association with the long ciliary nerves. Interruption of this innervation results in the familiar signs of Horner syndrome: ptosis of the upper eyelid, elevation of the lower eyelid, miosis, anhidrosis, and vasodilation. See Chapter 1 in BCSC Section 5, *Neuro-Ophthalmology,* for detailed discussion of neuro-ophthalmic anatomy.

### Lacrimal Gland

The lacrimal gland is composed of a larger orbital lobe and a smaller palpebral lobe. The gland is located within a fossa of the frontal bone in the superotemporal orbit. Ducts from both lobes pass through the palpebral lobe and empty into the upper conjunctival fornix. Frequently, a portion of the palpebral lobe is visible on slit-lamp examination with the upper eyelid everted. Biopsy is generally not performed on the palpebral lobe or temporal conjunctival fornix because it can interfere with lacrimal drainage. The orbital lobe of the lacrimal gland may prolapse inferiorly out of the fossa and present as a mass in the lateral upper eyelid.

## Periorbital Structures

### Nose and Paranasal Sinuses

The bones forming the medial, inferior, and superior orbital walls are close to the nasal cavity and are pneumatized by the paranasal sinuses, which arise from and drain into the nasal cavity. The sinuses decrease the weight of the skull and function as resonators for the voice. The sinuses also support the nasal passages in trapping irritants and in warming and humidifying the air. Pathophysiologic processes in these spaces that secondarily affect the orbit include sinonasal carcinomas, inverted papillomas, zygomycoses, granulomatosis with polyangiitis (Wegener granulomatosis), and mucoceles as well as sinusitis, which may cause orbital cellulitis or abscess.

The nasal cavity is divided into 2 nasal fossae by the nasal septum. The lateral wall of the nose has 3 bony projections: the superior, middle, and inferior conchae (turbinates). The turbinates are covered by nasal mucosa, and they overhang the corresponding meatuses. Just cephalad to the superior concha is the sphenoethmoidal recess, into which the sphenoid sinus drains. The frontal sinus, the maxillary sinus, and the anterior and middle ethmoid air cells drain into the middle meatus. The nasolacrimal duct opens into the inferior meatus. The nasal cavity is lined by a pseudostratified, ciliated columnar epithelium with copious goblet cells. The mucous membrane overlying the lateral alar cartilage is hair bearing and therefore less suitable for use as a composite graft in eyelid reconstruction than the mucoperichondrium over the nasal septum.

The frontal sinuses develop from evaginations of the frontal recess and cannot be seen radiographically until the sixth year of life. Pneumatization of the frontal bone continues through childhood and is complete by early adulthood (Fig 1-11). The sinuses can develop

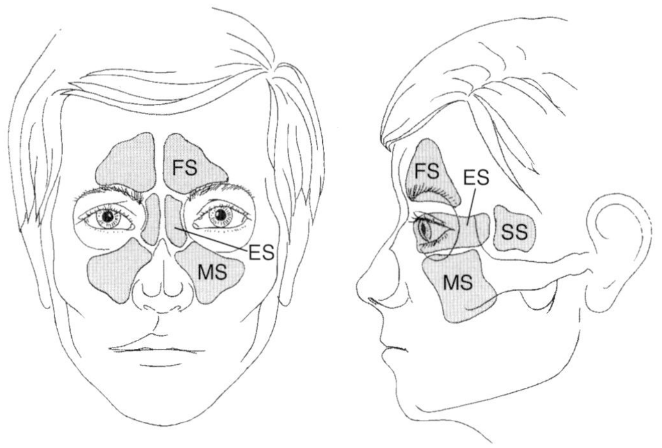


**Figure 1-11** Relationship of the orbits to the paranasal sinuses: FS, frontal sinus; ES, ethmoid sinus; MS, maxillary sinus; SS, sphenoid sinus.

asymmetrically and vary greatly in size and shape. Each frontal sinus drains through separate frontonasal ducts and empties into the anterior portion of the middle meatus.

The ethmoid air cells are thin-walled cavities that lie between the medial orbital wall and the lateral wall of the nose. They are present at birth and expand as the child grows. Ethmoid air cells can extend into the frontal, lacrimal, and maxillary bones and may extend into the orbital roof *(supraorbital ethmoids).* The numerous small, thin-walled air cells of the ethmoid sinus are divided into anterior, middle, and posterior. The anterior and middle air cells drain into the middle meatus; the posterior air cells, into the superior meatus. Sinusitis in the ethmoids is a common cause of orbital cellulitis and medial orbital subperiosteal effusions or abscesses when the inflammation or infection spreads through the thin bone or the vascular foramina of the medial orbital wall.

The sphenoid sinus evaginates from the posterior nasal roof to pneumatize the sphenoid bone. It is rudimentary at birth and reaches full size after puberty. The sinus drains into the sphenoethmoidal recess of each nasal fossa. The optic canal is located immediately superolateral to the sinus wall. Vision loss and visual field abnormalities can be direct sequelae of pathologic processes involving the sphenoid sinus.

The maxillary sinuses are the largest of the paranasal sinuses. The roof of each maxillary sinus forms the floor of each orbit. The maxillary sinuses extend posteriorly in the maxillary bone to the inferior orbital fissure. The infraorbital nerve and artery travel along the roof of the sinus from posterior to anterior. The bony nasolacrimal canal lies within the medial wall. The sinus drains into the middle meatus of the nose by way of the maxillary ostium. Orbital blowout fractures commonly disrupt the floor of the orbit medial to the infraorbital canal, where the bone is thinnest. The infraorbital nerve is often compromised, causing hypoesthesia of the cheek, upper lip, and maxillary teeth.

Jordan DR, Anderson RA. *Surgical Anatomy of the Ocular Adnexa: A Clinical Approach.* Ophthalmology Monograph 9. San Francisco: American Academy of Ophthalmology; 1996.

CHAPTER 2

# Evaluation of Orbital Disorders

The evaluation of an orbital disorder should distinguish orbital from periorbital and intraocular lesions. The orbit has a somewhat limited repertoire of ways it can respond to pathologic conditions. Orbital disease can be categorized into 5 basic clinical patterns: (1) inflammatory (acute, subacute, and chronic), (2) mass effect (causing globe displacement with axial or nonaxial proptosis), (3) structural (congenital or acquired change in the bony orbital structure), (4) vascular (venous or arterial lesions with characteristic dynamic changes), and (5) functional (sensory and/or motor dysfunction of neurovascular structures). This classification provides a framework for development of a differential diagnosis. The evaluation begins with a detailed history.

## History

The history establishes a probable diagnosis and guides the initial workup and therapy. Such a history should include

- onset, course, and duration of symptoms (eg, pain, altered sensation, diplopia, changes in vision) and signs (eg, erythema, palpable mass, globe displacement)
- prior disease (such as thyroid eye disease or sinus disease) and therapy
- injury (especially head or facial trauma)
- systemic disease (especially cancer)
- family history
- old photographs for establishing a timeline of the process

### Pain

Pain may be a symptom of inflammatory or infectious lesions, orbital hemorrhage, malignant lacrimal gland tumors, invasion from adjacent nasopharyngeal carcinoma, or metastatic lesions.

### Progression

The rate of progression can be a helpful diagnostic indicator. Disorders with onset occurring over days to weeks are usually caused by nonspecific orbital inflammation (NSOI), scleritis, myositis, dacryoadenitis, orbital cellulitis, hemorrhage, thrombophlebitis, fulminant neoplasia (rhabdomyosarcoma, neuroblastoma), or metastatic tumors. Conditions with onset occurring over months to years are usually caused by dermoid cyst, benign mixed tumor, neurogenic tumor, cavernous hemangioma, lymphoma, fibrous histiocytoma, fibrous dysplasia, or osteoma.

## Periorbital Changes

Periorbital changes may provide clues indicative of the underlying disorders. For example, ecchymosis of the eyelid skin may be a sign of metastatic neuroblastoma (Fig 2-1), leukemia, or amyloidosis. Another example is optociliary shunt vessels on the disc that are suggestive of a meningioma. These vessels represent a communication between veins and should be called *retinociliary venous collaterals* (Fig 2-2). Table 2-1 lists various periorbital signs and their common causes.

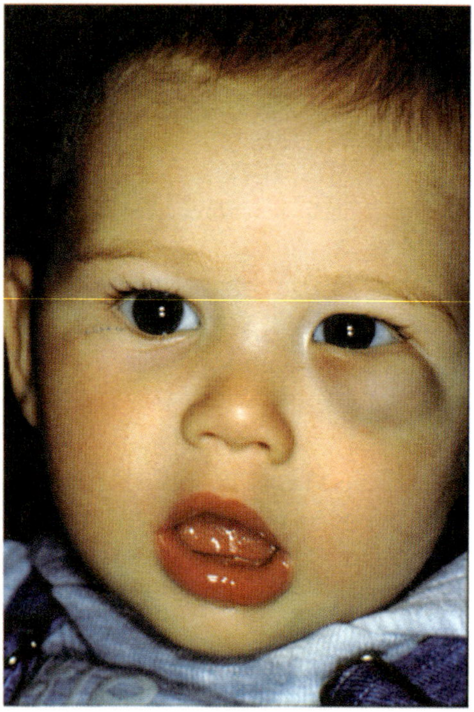

**Figure 2-1** Left lower eyelid ecchymosis in child with metastatic neuroblastoma. *(Courtesy of Keith D. Carter, MD.)*

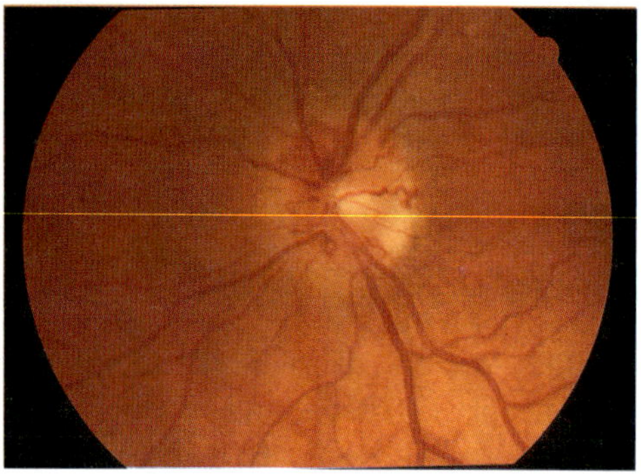

**Figure 2-2** Optociliary shunt vessels (retinociliary venous collaterals) secondary to an optic nerve meningioma. *(Courtesy of Sohan Hayreh, MD.)*

**Table 2-1 Periorbital Changes Associated With Orbital Disease**

| Sign | Etiology |
|---|---|
| A salmon-colored mass in the cul-de-sac | Lymphoma (see Fig 5-14) |
| Eyelid retraction and lid lag | Thyroid eye disease (see Fig 4-5) |
| Vascular congestion over the insertions of the rectus muscles (particularly the lateral rectus) | Thyroid eye disease (see Fig 4-6A) |
| Corkscrew conjunctival vessels | Arteriovenous fistula (see Fig 4-6B) |
| Vascular anomaly of eyelid skin | Lymphatic malformation, varix, or hemangioma (see Fig 5-1) |
| S-shaped eyelid | Plexiform neurofibroma (see Fig 5-8) or lacrimal gland mass |
| Eczematous lesions of the eyelids | Mycosis fungoides (T-cell lymphoma) |
| Ecchymosis of eyelid skin | Metastatic neuroblastoma, leukemia, or amyloidosis (see Fig 2-1) |
| Prominent temple | Sphenoid wing meningioma (see Fig 5-9A), metastatic neuroblastoma |
| Edematous swelling of lower eyelid | Meningioma, inflammatory tumor, metastases |
| Optociliary shunt vessels (retinociliary venous collaterals) on disc | Meningioma (see Fig 2-2) |
| Frozen globe | Metastases or zygomycosis |
| Black-crusted lesions in nasopharynx | Phycomycosis |
| Facial asymmetry | Fibrous dysplasia (see Fig 5-12A) or neurofibromatosis |

# Physical Examination

Special attention should be given to visual acuity, pupillary responses, ocular motility, globe position, and ophthalmoscopy. Diagnostic and imaging studies are often required in addition to the basic workup.

## Inspection

Globe displacement is the most common clinical manifestation of an orbital abnormality. It usually results from a tumor, a vascular abnormality, an inflammatory process, or a traumatic event.

Several terms are used to describe the position of the eye and orbit. *Proptosis* or *exophthalmos* denotes a forward displacement or protrusion of the eye. *Exorbitism* refers to an angle between the lateral orbital walls that is greater than 90°, which may also be associated with shallow orbital depth. This condition contrasts with *hypertelorism,* or *telorbitism,* which refers to a wider-than-normal separation between the medial orbital walls. Generally, exorbitism and hypertelorism are congenital or traumatic abnormalities. *Telecanthus* denotes an abnormal increased distance between the medial canthi. The eye may also be displaced vertically (hyperglobus or hypoglobus) or horizontally by an orbital mass. Retrodisplacement of the eye into the orbit, called *enophthalmos,* may occur as a result of volume expansion of the orbit (fracture), in association with orbital varix or secondary to sclerosing orbital tumors (eg, metastatic breast carcinoma).

Proptosis often indicates the location of a mass because the globe is usually displaced away from the site of the mass. Axial displacement is usually indicative of an intraconal mass behind the globe; such lesions include cavernous hemangioma, glioma, meningioma, metastases, and arteriovenous malformations. Nonaxial displacement is caused by lesions with a prominent component outside the muscle cone. Superior displacement is produced by maxillary sinus tumors invading the orbital floor and pushing the globe upward. Inferomedial displacement can result from orbital dermoid cysts and lacrimal gland tumors. Inferolateral displacement can result from frontoethmoidal mucoceles, abscesses, osteomas, and ethmoid sinus carcinomas. Bilateral proptosis in adults is caused most often by thyroid eye disease (TED); however, other disorders, such as lymphoma, vasculitis, NSOI, metastatic tumors, carotid-cavernous fistulas, cavernous sinus thrombosis, and leukemic infiltrates, can also produce bilateral proptosis. Unilateral proptosis in adults is also most frequently caused by TED. In children with bilateral proptosis, the clinician should consider TED, NSOI, metastatic neuroblastoma, or leukemic infiltrates.

Exophthalmometry is a measurement of the anterior-posterior position of the globe, generally from the lateral orbital rim to the anterior corneal surface (Hertel exophthalmometry, Fig 2-3A). The Naugle exophthalmometer uses the frontal and maxillary bones as its reference structure (Fig 2-3B). This exophthalmometer is useful in fracture patients when the lateral canthus has been displaced. On average, the globes are more prominent in men than in women and more prominent in black patients than in white patients. An asymmetry of greater than 2 mm between an individual patient's eyes suggests proptosis or enophthalmos. Proptosis may best be appreciated clinically when the examiner looks up from below with the patient's head tilted back (the so-called worm's-eye view; Fig 2-4).

Pseudoproptosis is either the simulation of abnormal prominence of the eye or a true asymmetry that is not the result of increased orbital contents. Diagnosis should be postponed until a mass lesion has been ruled out. Causes of pseudoproptosis are

- enlarged globe (eg, myopia)
- contralateral enophthalmos (silent sinus syndrome)

A 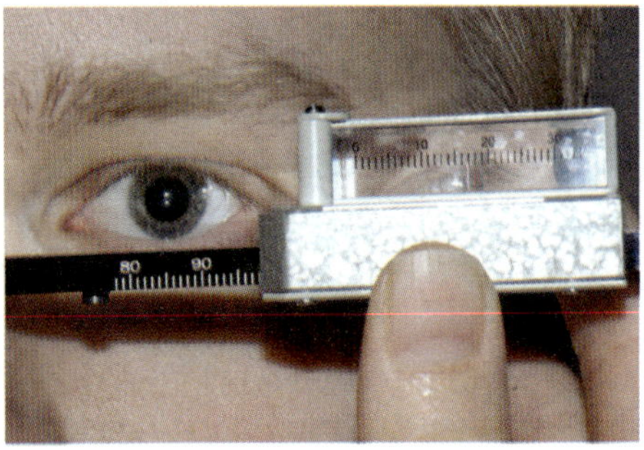
B 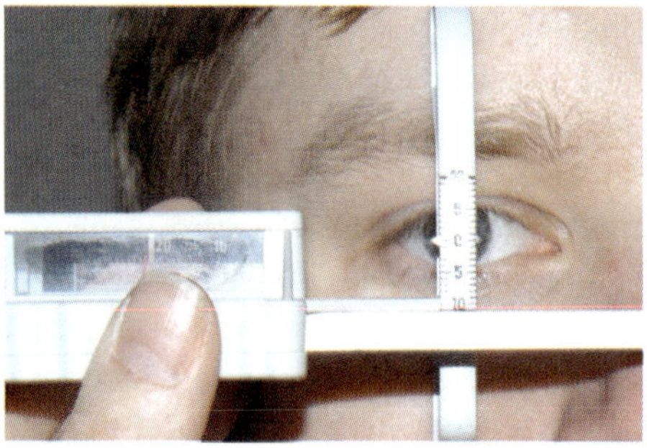

**Figure 2-3** The Hertel exophthalmometer **(A)** uses the lateral canthus as its reference point. The Naugle exophthalmometer **(B)** uses the frontal and maxillary bones as its reference point. It can measure both proptosis and hyperglobus or hypoglobus. *(Courtesy of University of Iowa.)*

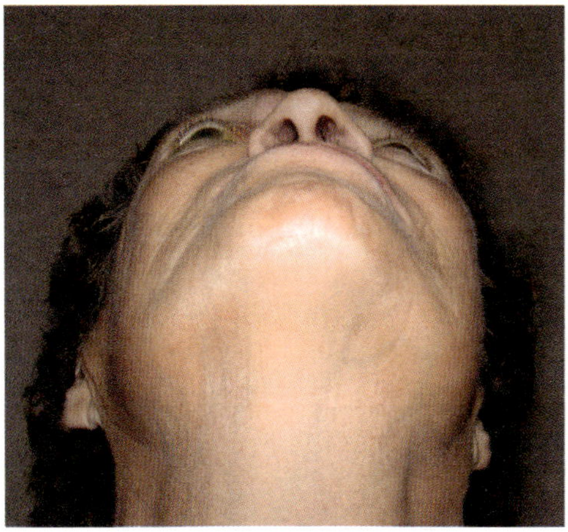

**Figure 2-4** "Worm's-eye view" position. Note proptosis of the right eye. *(Courtesy of Keith D. Carter, MD.)*

- asymmetric orbital size
- asymmetric palpebral fissures (usually caused by ipsilateral eyelid retraction, facial nerve paralysis, or contralateral ptosis)

Ocular movements may be restricted in a specific direction of gaze by neoplasm or inflammation. In TED, the inferior rectus is the muscle most commonly affected; this mechanically limits globe elevation and may cause hypotropia in primary gaze and restriction of upgaze. A large or rapidly enlarging orbital mass can also impede ocular movements, even in the absence of direct muscle invasion.

Eyelid abnormalities are common in TED. The von Graefe sign is a delay in the upper eyelid's descent ("lid lag") during downgaze and is highly suggestive of a diagnosis of TED. In fact, such lid lag and the retraction of the upper and lower eyelids are the most common physical signs of TED (see Chapter 4).

Garrity JA, Henderson JW. *Henderson's Orbital Tumors.* 4th ed. Philadelphia: Lippincott Williams & Wilkins; 2007.

Rootman J, ed. *Diseases of the Orbit: A Multidisciplinary Approach.* 2nd ed. Philadelphia: Lippincott Williams & Wilkins; 2003.

## Palpation

Palpation around the globe may disclose the presence of a mass in the anterior orbit, especially if the lacrimal gland is enlarged. Increased resistance to retrodisplacement of the globe is a nonspecific abnormality that may result either from a retrobulbar tumor or from diffuse inflammation such as that seen in TED. The physician should also palpate regional lymph nodes.

The differential diagnosis for a palpable mass in the superonasal quadrant may include mucocele, mucopyocele, encephalocele, neurofibroma, dermoid cyst, rhabdomyosarcoma, or lymphoma. A palpable mass in the superotemporal quadrant may be a prolapsed lacrimal gland, a dermoid cyst, a lacrimal gland tumor, lymphoma, or NSOI. A lesion behind the equator of the globe is usually not palpable.

Pulsations of the eye are caused by transmission of the vascular pulse through the orbit. This may result from either abnormal vascular flow or transmission of normal intracranial pulsations through a bony defect in the orbital walls. Abnormal vascular flow may be caused by arteriovenous communications, such as carotid-cavernous fistulas. Defects in the bony orbital walls may result from sinus mucoceles, surgical removal of bone, trauma, or developmental abnormalities, including encephalocele, meningocele, or sphenoid wing dysplasia (associated with neurofibromatosis).

### Auscultation

Auscultation with a stethoscope over the globe or on the mastoid bone may detect bruits in cases of carotid-cavernous fistula. The patient may also subjectively describe an audible bruit. Patients with such arteriovenous communications often have tortuous dilated epibulbar vessels (see Chapter 4, Fig 4-6B).

## Primary Studies

Computed tomography (CT) and magnetic resonance imaging (MRI) are the primary studies for evaluation of orbital disorders. Ultrasonography (echography) may be helpful for some disorders.

### Computed Tomography

Computed tomography is essential in the management of orbital disorders. The tissues in a tomographic plane are assigned a density value proportional to their coefficient of absorption of x-rays. Either 2- or 3-dimensional images are digitally constructed from these density measurements. CT is the most valuable technique for delineating the shape, location, extent, and character of lesions in the orbit (Fig 2-5). CT helps refine the differential diagnosis, and when orbitotomy is indicated, CT helps guide the selection of the surgical approach by showing the relationship of the lesion to the surgical space or spaces of the orbit. The resolution and soft-tissue contrast of CT are adequate to visualize nearly

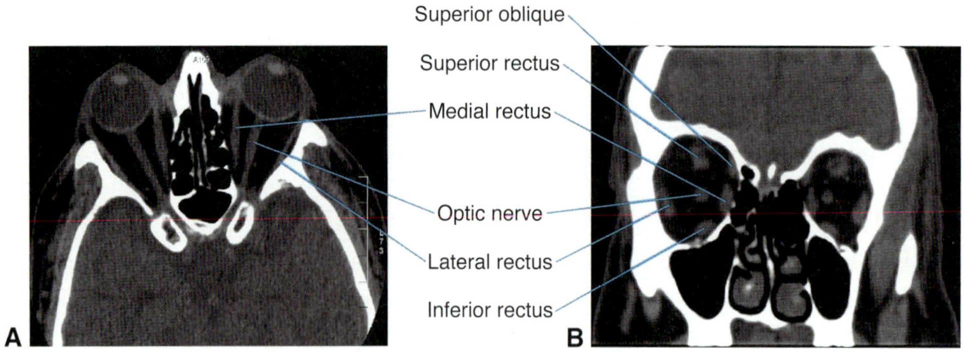


**Figure 2-5** CT views of the orbit demonstrating normal anatomy. **A,** Axial. **B,** Coronal. *(Courtesy of Thomas Y. Hwang, MD, PhD, and Timothy J. McCulley, MD.)*

all orbital pathologic processes, and the bony resolution is superior to that provided by all other modalities, making CT the imaging technique of choice for orbital trauma and bony tumors. Orbital CT scans are usually obtained in 3-mm sections (as opposed to the thicker 5-mm sections typically utilized in head CT scans). For greater detail, fine cuts at 1.5-mm intervals may be requested.

The visualization of tumors that are highly vascularized (eg, meningioma) or that have altered vascular permeability is improved by the use of intravenous contrast-enhancing agents. Contrast is also helpful to identify an orbital abscess. If desired, contrast must be specifically ordered as part of the study. CT has resolution and tissue-contrast capabilities that allow imaging of not only bones but also soft tissue and foreign bodies.

Orbital images can be obtained in the axial plane, parallel to the course of the optic nerve; in the coronal plane, showing the eye, optic nerve, and extraocular muscles in cross section; or in the sagittal plane, parallel to the nasal septum. Current CT scanners use software to reconstruct (reformat) any section in any direction (axial, coronal, or sagittal). Modern spiral (helical) CT scanners have multiple detector ports, and the scanner and the collecting tube move in a spiral fashion around the patient, generating a continuous data set. This results in rapid acquisition of a larger volume of data that, in combination with modern software, allows highly detailed reconstructions in all imaging planes. Direct coronal scans are ideal for evaluation of the optic nerve and extraocular muscles and the bony roof and floor of the orbit. Three-dimensional CT allows reformatting of CT information into 3-dimensional projections of the bony orbital walls (Fig 2-6). Because this type of imaging requires thin sections and additional computer time, 3-dimensional CT is typically reserved to assist in preparation for craniofacial surgery or repairs of complex orbital fractures.

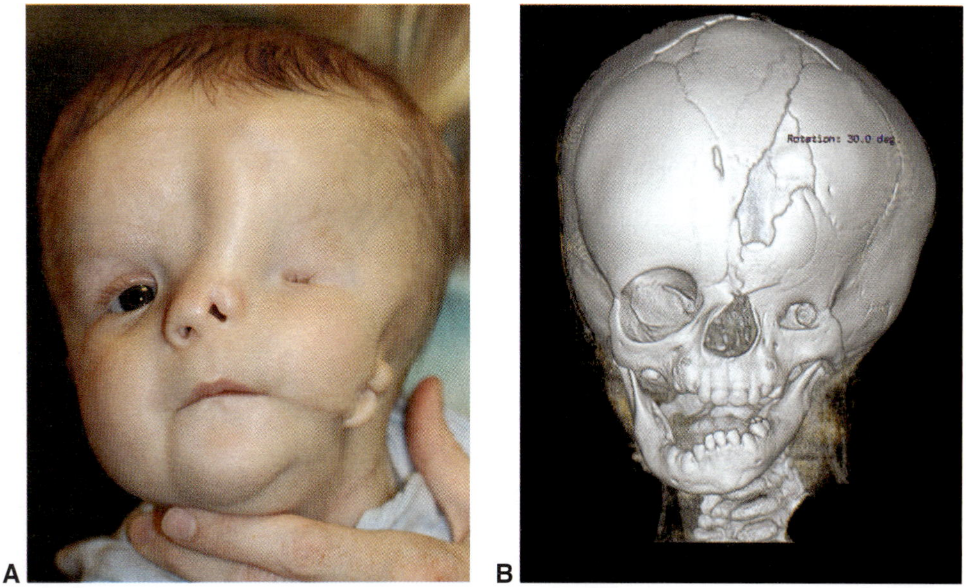


**Figure 2-6** **A,** Patient with hemifacial microsomia. **B,** Three-dimensional CT reconstruction of same patient. *(Courtesy of Jill Foster, MD.)*

## Magnetic Resonance Imaging

MRI is a noninvasive imaging technique that does not employ ionizing radiation and has no known adverse biological effects (Fig 2-7). MRI is based on the interaction of 3 physical components: atomic nuclei possessing an electrical charge, radiofrequency (RF) waves, and a powerful magnetic field.

When a tissue containing hydrogen atoms is placed in the magnetic field, individual nuclei align themselves in the direction of the magnetic field. These aligned nuclei can be excited by an RF pulse emitted from a coil lying within the magnetic field. Excited nuclei align themselves against the static magnetic field; as the RF pulse is terminated, the nuclei flip back to their original magnetized position. The time it takes for this realignment to occur (the relaxation time) can be measured.

Each orbital tissue has specific magnetic resonance (MR) parameters that provide the information used to generate an image. These parameters include tissue proton density and relaxation times. Proton density is determined by the number of protons per unit volume of tissue. Fat has greater proton density per unit volume than bone and, therefore, greater signal intensity. *T1,* or longitudinal relaxation time, is the time required for the net bulk magnetization to realign itself along the original axis. *T2,* or transverse relaxation time, is the mean relaxation time based on the interaction of hydrogen nuclei within a given tissue, an indirect measure of the effect the nuclei have on each other. Each tissue has different proton density and T1 and T2 characteristics, providing the image contrast necessary to differentiate tissues. Healthy tissues can have imaging characteristics different from those of diseased tissue, a good example being the bright signal associated with tissue edema seen on T2-weighted scans.

MRI is usually performed with images created from both T1 and T2 parameters. T1-weighted images generally offer the best anatomical detail of the orbit. T2-weighted images have the advantage of showing methemoglobin brighter than melanin, whereas these substances have the same signal intensity on T1-weighted images. The difference

A 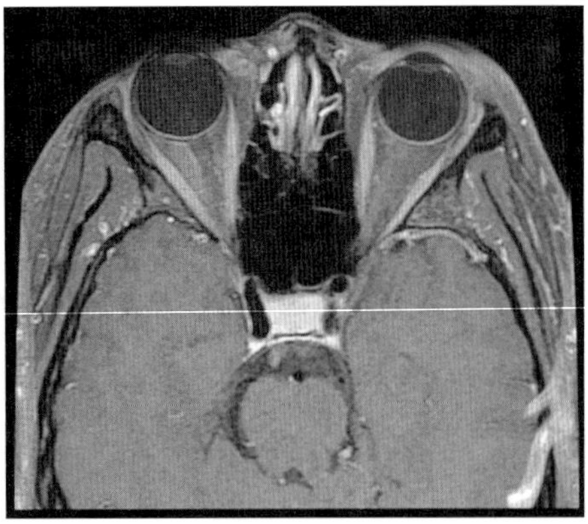 B 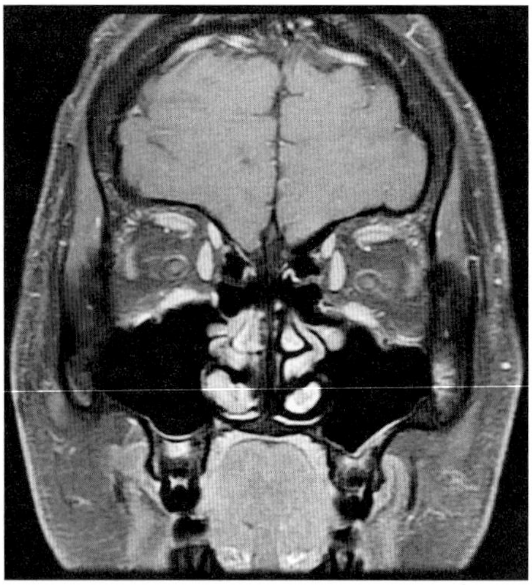

**Figure 2-7** T1-weighted magnetic resonance (MR) images of the orbit, with fat suppression. **A,** Axial. **B,** Coronal. *(Courtesy of Thomas Y. Hwang, MD, PhD, and Timothy J. McCulley, MD.)*

in brightness seen on T2 images can be helpful in differentiating melanotic lesions from hemorrhagic processes. Gadolinium, a paramagnetic contrast agent given intravenously, allows enhancement of vascularized lesions so that they exhibit the same density as fat. It also demonstrates enhancement of lesions with abnormal vascular permeability. Special MR sequences have been developed to suppress the normal bright signal of fat on T1 images (fat suppression; see Fig 2-7) and the bright signal of cerebrospinal fluid on T2 images (fluid-attenuated inversion recovery, or FLAIR). Gradient echo sequences may reveal hemorrhage in vascular malformations that might be missed on T1- and T2-weighted images.

## Comparison of CT and MRI

Although both CT and MRI are important modalities for the detection and characterization of orbital and ocular diseases, CT is currently the primary and single most-useful orbital imaging technique. Compared with MRI, it is faster, less expensive, and less sensitive to movement artifact. In general, CT provides better spatial resolution, allowing precise localization of a lesion. MRI generally provides better tissue contrast than CT; however, in most orbital conditions, the orbital fat provides sufficient natural tissue contrast to allow ready visualization of orbital tumors on CT. Each of the techniques has advantages in specific situations, some of which are discussed in the following text and in Table 2-2.

**Table 2-2 Comparison of CT and MRI in Orbital Disease**

| CT | MRI |
|---|---|
| Good technique for most orbital conditions, especially trauma and thyroid eye disease | Better technique for orbitocranial junction or intracranial imaging |
| Good view of bone and calcium | No view of bone or calcification |
| Limited definition of the orbital apex | Good view of orbital apex soft tissues unimpeded by bone |
| Better spatial resolution | More soft tissue detail |
| Reformatting or rescanning required to image in multiple planes | Simultaneous imaging of multiple planes |
| Improved imaging with contrast in many cases | Improved imaging with contrast in many cases |
| Less motion artifact because of shorter scanning time | More motion artifact because of longer scanning time |
| Less claustrophobic environment in scanner | Tighter confines in scanner; "open scanners" now available but have lower resolution |
| Good technique for patients with metallic foreign bodies | More contraindications (eg, patients with ferromagnetic metallic foreign bodies, aneurysm clips, pacemakers) |
| Contraindicated in pregnancy; use should be limited with children | Can safely be used with pregnant women and children |
| Less expensive technique | More expensive technique |
| Contrast contraindicated in patients with allergy to iodine or with renal dysfunction | Use of gadolinium carries risk of nephrogenic systemic fibrosis in patients with severe renal failure (stage 4 or 5; GFR <30 mL/min/1.73 $m^2$) |

CT = computed tomography; GFR = glomerular filtration rate; MRI = magnetic resonance imaging.

MRI offers advantages over CT in some situations. It allows the direct display of anatomical information in multiple planes (sagittal, axial, coronal, and any oblique plane). MRI provides better soft-tissue definition than does CT, a capability that is especially helpful in the evaluation of demyelination and in vascular and hemorrhagic lesions (Fig 2-8). As with CT, contrast agents are available to improve MRI detail.

Compared with CT, MRI also provides better tissue contrast of structures in the orbital apex, intracanalicular portion of the optic nerve, structures in periorbital spaces, and orbitocranial tumors, as there is no artifact from the skull base bones. Bone and calcification produce low signal on MRI. Bony structures may be evaluated by visualization of the signal void left by the bone. However, this is not possible when the bone is adjacent to structures that also create a signal void, such as air, rapidly flowing blood, calcification, and dura mater. Thus, CT is superior to MRI for the evaluation of fractures, bone destruction, and tissue calcification.

MRI is contraindicated in patients who have ferromagnetic metallic foreign bodies in the orbit or periorbital soft tissue, ferromagnetic vascular clips from previous surgery, magnetic intravascular filters, or electronic devices in the body such as cardiac pacemakers. If necessary, the presence of such foreign material can be ruled out with plain films or CT. Certain types of eye makeup can produce artifacts and should be removed prior to MRI. Dental amalgam is not a ferromagnetic substance and is not a

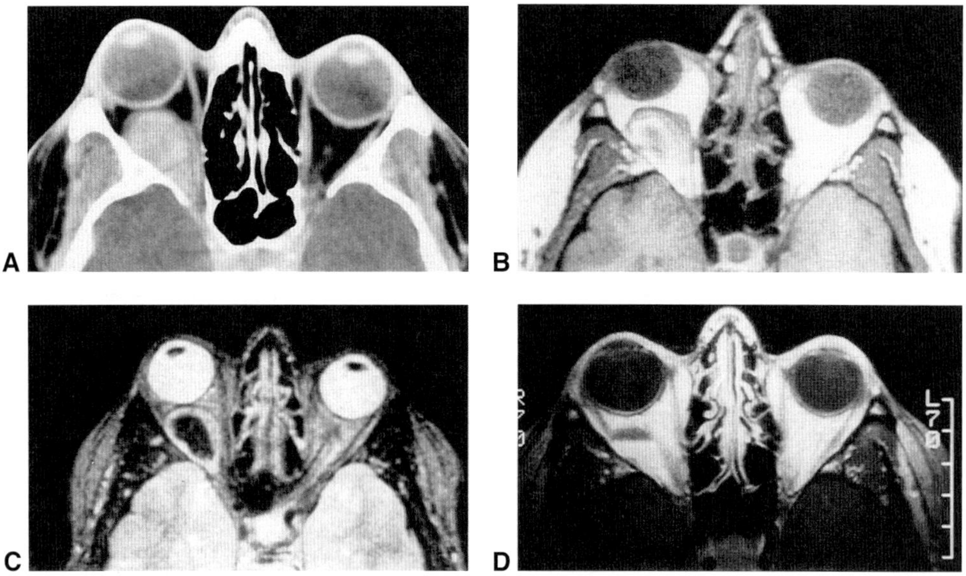

**Figure 2-8** **A,** CT scan of a patient with acute right exophthalmos resulting from a spontaneous orbital hemorrhage. The hematoma exhibits discrete margins, homogeneous consistency, and a radiodensity similar to that of blood vessels and muscle. **B,** T1 MR scan obtained 4 days after the hemorrhage demonstrates the transient bull's-eye pattern characteristic of a hematoma beginning to undergo physical changes and biochemical hemoglobin degradation. **C,** T2 MR scan obtained the same day as the T1 study shows a characteristic ring pattern. **D,** T1 MR scan performed 3 months later shows that the hematoma has decreased in size. There is layering of the degraded blood components.

contraindication to MRI, but this material does produce artifacts and degrades the images on both MRI and CT.

Although CT and MRI yield different images, it is not unusual for both techniques to be required in the evaluation of an orbital disorder. The choice between these modalities should be based on the specific patient's condition. In most cases, CT is the more effective and economical choice (see Table 2-2). MRI is the better primary technique for imaging the orbitocranial junction and brain, but CT scanning may enhance the assessment by providing better bone images. When the orbitocranial junction or brain is involved, CT scanning and MRI may be complementary and, in some cases, both are required to evaluate complex lesions.

Ben Simon GJ, Annunziata CC, Fink J, Villablanca P, McCann JD, Goldberg RA. Rethinking orbital imaging: establishing guidelines for interpreting orbital imaging studies and evaluating their predictive value in patients with orbital tumors. *Ophthalmology.* 2005; 112(12):2196–2207.

Dutton JJ. *Radiology of the Orbit and Visual Pathways.* Philadelphia: Saunders Elsevier; 2010.

Miglioretti DL, Johnson E, Williams A, et al. The use of computed tomography in pediatrics and the associated radiation exposure and estimated cancer risk. *JAMA Pediatr.* 2013; 167(8):700–707.

## Ultrasonography

Orbital ultrasonography may be used to examine patients with orbital disorders. The size, shape, and position of normal and abnormal orbital tissues can be determined by means of contemporary ultrasound techniques. Two-dimensional images of these tissues can be obtained with B-scan ultrasonography. Standardized A-scan ultrasonography provides one-dimensional images of the orbital soft tissues characterized by a series of spikes of varying height and width that demonstrate the particular echogenic characteristics of each tissue. Areas of edema can sometimes be used to discern the degree of disease activity. Ultrasonography has high resolution in the area of the sclera and optic nerve insertion and is useful for evaluating scleritis and other anterior inflammation that produces fluid in the sub-Tenon space. Localization of foreign bodies is possible with ultrasonography. *Doppler ultrasonography* can provide specific information regarding blood flow and can demonstrate arterialization, retrograde flow in the orbital veins in cases of dural cavernous fistula or arteriovenous malformation, or vascular abnormalities associated with increased blood flow. Vascular tumors can be identified by active pulsation or, in the case of venous lesions, by compressibility and change in size with the Valsalva maneuver.

However, ultrasonographic analysis of orbital tissues and diseases requires specialized equipment and experienced personnel, and office-based equipment is generally not suitable for this purpose. Ultrasonography is of limited value in assessing lesions of the posterior orbit (because of sound attenuation) or the sinuses or intracranial space (because sound does not pass well through air or bone).

Aburn NS, Sergott RC. Orbital colour Doppler imaging. *Eye (Lond).* 1993;7(Pt 5):639–647.

Williamson TH, Harris A. Color Doppler ultrasound imaging of the eye and orbit. *Surv Ophthalmol.* 1996;40(4):255–267.

## Secondary Studies

Secondary studies that are performed for specific indications include venography and arteriography. These studies are rarely used but may be helpful in specific cases.

### Venography

Before the era of CT and MRI, orbital venography was used in the diagnosis and management of orbital varices and in the study of the cavernous sinus. Contrast material is injected into the frontal or the angular vein to reveal a venous abnormality. Subtraction and magnification techniques have been used to increase the resolution of venography. Because moving blood generates a signal void during MR imaging, larger venous abnormalities and structures can be visualized well on MR venography. Some orbitocranial vascular malformations or fistulas are best accessed via the superior ophthalmic vein.

### Arteriography

Arteriography is the gold standard for diagnosis of an arterial lesion such as an aneurysm or arteriovenous malformation. Retrograde catheterization of the cerebral vessels is accomplished through the femoral artery. However, since there is a small risk of serious neurologic and vascular complications (1%–2%), because the technique requires installation of the catheter and injection of radiopaque dye into the arterial system, the test is reserved for patients with a high probability of having a lesion.

Visualization can be maximized by the use of selective injection of the internal and external carotid arteries, magnification to allow viewing of the smaller caliber vessels, and subtraction techniques to radiographically eliminate bone. An additional benefit of arteriography is the ability to simultaneously treat and image a lesion.

### CT and MR Angiography

The development of better hardware and software has made possible precise CT and MR imaging of arteriovenous malformations, aneurysms, and arteriovenous fistulas without the expense, discomfort, and risks associated with intravascular catheterization and injection of contrast material. However, MR angiography is less sensitive than direct angiography for identifying carotid-cavernous sinus fistulas. When determining which test to use, the ophthalmologist may consult with a radiologist to discuss the suspected lesion and to ensure selection of the imaging modality best suited for the patient.

## Pathology

The diagnosis of an orbital lesion usually requires analysis of tissue obtained through an orbitotomy. Appropriate handling of the tissue specimen is necessary to ensure an accurate diagnosis. Most tissue samples are placed in formalin for permanent section analysis. If a lymphoproliferative lesion is suspected, some fresh tissue should be sent for analysis of flow cytometry. Frozen section evaluation may be performed at the time of surgery, but it is generally not used for definitive diagnosis of an orbital tumor. However, when the area of proposed biopsy is not obvious, frozen sections are helpful to confirm that appropriate tissue has been obtained for permanent section analysis. Frozen section analysis is also used intraoperatively to determine tumor margins and ensure complete tumor removal. Tissue removed for frozen section analysis should be placed in a dampened saline gauze and promptly sent to the frozen section laboratory.

Because of the vast array of possible unusual tumor types in the orbit, preoperative consultation with a pathologist familiar with orbital disease may be helpful to maximize the information gained from any orbital biopsy. In many cases, fresh tissue should be obtained and frozen for cell-surface marker studies. Cell-marker studies are required in the analysis of all orbital lymphoid lesions. These studies may permit differentiation of reactive lymphoid hyperplasia from lymphoma. Such studies may also indicate the presence of estrogen receptors in cases of metastatic prostate or breast carcinoma and thus provide useful information about sensitivity to hormonal therapy. Marker studies are also useful in the diagnosis of poorly differentiated tumors when light microscopy alone cannot yield a definitive diagnosis. Although cell-marker studies have largely replaced electron microscopy in the diagnosis of undifferentiated tumors, it may nevertheless be worthwhile in these cases to preserve fresh tissue in glutaraldehyde for possible electron microscopy. In noncohesive tumors (hematologic or lymphoid), a touch prep may permit a diagnosis.

All biopsy specimens must be treated delicately so that crush and cautery artifacts, which can confuse interpretation, are minimized. Permanent section tissue biopsy specimens should be placed in fixatives promptly. If fine-needle aspiration biopsy is planned, a cytologist or trained technician must be available to handle the aspirate. In special cases, the biopsy can be performed under either ultrasonographic or CT control. Although a fine-bore needle occasionally yields a sufficient cell block, the specimen is usually limited to cytologic study. This technique may not permit as firm a diagnosis as is possible with larger biopsy specimens, in which light and electron microscopy can be used to evaluate the histologic pattern.

See BCSC Section 4, *Ophthalmic Pathology and Intraocular Tumors,* for a more extensive discussion of pathology.

## Laboratory Studies

Screening for abnormal thyroid function commonly includes $T_4$ and thyroid-stimulating hormone (TSH) tests. Results of these serum tests are abnormal in 90% of patients with TED. However, if thyroid disease is strongly suspected and these results are normal, additional endocrine studies such as thyroid-stimulating immunoglobulins or TSH-receptor antibodies can be considered as tests with greater sensitivity for detecting thyroid disease.

Granulomatosis with polyangiitis (Wegener granulomatosis; see Chapter 4) should be considered in patients with sclerokeratitis or coexisting sinus disease and orbital mass lesions. A useful test for this uncommon disease is the antineutrophil cytoplasmic antibody (ANCA) serum assay, which shows a cytoplasmic staining pattern (c-ANCA) in granulomatosis with polyangiitis. The test results may be negative initially in localized disease. Biopsy of affected tissues classically shows vasculitis, granulomatous inflammation, and tissue necrosis, although necrotizing vasculitis is not always present in orbital biopsies.

Testing for serum angiotensin-converting enzyme (ACE) and lysozyme may be helpful in the diagnosis of sarcoidosis. This multisystem granulomatous inflammatory condition may present with lacrimal gland enlargement, conjunctival granulomas, extraocular muscle or optic nerve infiltration, or solitary orbital granulomas. Diagnosis is confirmed through biopsy of one or more affected organs.

CHAPTER 3

# Congenital Orbital Anomalies

Developmental defects of the orbit manifest clinically at any time from conception until late in life. Most significant congenital anomalies of the eye and orbit are apparent on ultrasonography before birth. As a rule, the more profound the abnormality, the earlier in development it occurred. Identifying the embryologic origin of the congenital malformation helps us understand and classify the physical changes in the patient. If an anomaly is caused by a slowing or cessation of a normal stage of development, the resulting deformity can be considered a pure arrest. An example is microphthalmia. However, a superimposed aberrant growth usually follows the original arrest, and the resulting deformity does not represent any previous normal stage of development. An example of this latter condition is formation of an orbital cyst following incomplete closure of the fetal fissure.

In the examination of the child with an ocular or craniofacial malformation, the clinician should focus on carefully defining the severity of the defect and identifying associated changes. Some syndromes may have specific associated ocular changes or secondary ocular complications such as exposure keratitis or strabismus related to orbital maldevelopment. See BCSC Section 2, *Fundamentals and Principles of Ophthalmology,* Part II (Embryology); and Section 6, *Pediatric Ophthalmology and Strabismus,* for detailed discussion, including illustrations, of many of the topics covered in this chapter.

## Anophthalmia

True anophthalmia is defined as a total absence of tissues of the eye. Three types of anophthalmia have been described. *Primary anophthalmia* is rare and usually bilateral. It occurs when the primary optic vesicle fails to grow out from the cerebral vesicle at the 2-mm stage of embryonic development. *Secondary anophthalmia* is rare and lethal and results from a gross abnormality in the anterior neural tube. *Consecutive anophthalmia* presumably results from a secondary degeneration of the optic vesicle.

Because orbital development is partially dependent on the size and growth of the globe, the bones of the orbit, the eyelids, and also the adnexal structures fail to develop and remain hypoplastic in anophthalmia. Intervention requires measures that address all of these issues, not just the missing eye.

## Microphthalmia

Microphthalmia is much more common than anophthalmia and is defined by the presence of a small eye with axial length that is at least 2 standard deviations below the mean axial length for age. Microphthalmic eyes vary in size depending on the severity of the defect. Most infants with a unilateral small orbit and no visible eye actually have a microphthalmic globe. The defect may be isolated, or it may occur with a constellation of abnormalities as part of a well-defined syndrome. Because multiple genetic mutations have been reported in anophthalmia/microphthalmia, microphthalmia is considered a developmental phenotype that results from several different genetic rearrangements.

## Treatment of Anophthalmia/Microphthalmia

All children with microphthalmia have hypoplastic orbits. Most microphthalmic eyes have no potential for vision, and therefore treatment focuses on achieving a cosmetically acceptable appearance that is reasonably symmetrical. Treatment begins shortly after birth and consists of socket expansion with progressively larger conformers, which are used until the patient can be fitted with a prosthesis. Enucleation is usually not necessary for the fitting of a conformer or an ocular prosthesis and is ordinarily avoided because it may worsen the bony hypoplasia. Orbital volume may be augmented with autogenous materials such as dermis-fat grafts or with synthetic implants. When placed at an early age, dermis-fat grafts may grow with the child, resulting in progressive socket expansion. In cases of severe bony asymmetry, intraorbital tissue expanders may be progressively inflated to enlarge the hypoplastic orbit.

For severe microphthalmia or anophthalmia or for older children with previously untreated microphthalmia, craniofacial techniques have been used to reposition and resize the orbit. Such repairs are complex, as noted in the following discussion of craniofacial clefting.

*Microphthalmia with orbital cyst* results from failure of the choroidal fissure to close in the embryo. This condition is usually unilateral but may be bilateral. The presence of an orbital cyst may be beneficial for stimulating normal growth of the involved orbital bone and eyelids. In some cases, the orbital cyst may be removed to allow for fitting of an ocular prosthesis.

Hayashi N, Repka MX, Ueno H, Iliff NT, Green WR. Congenital cystic eye: report of two cases and review of the literature. *Surv Ophthalmol.* 1999;44(2):173–179.

McLean CJ, Ragge NK, Jones RB, Collin JR. The management of orbital cysts associated with congenital microphthalmos and anophthalmos. *Br J Ophthalmol.* 2003;87(7):860–863.

Semerci CN, Kalay E, Yıldırım C, et al. Novel splice-site and missense mutations in the *ALDH1A3* gene underlying autosomal recessive anophthalmia/microphthalmia. *Br J Ophthalmol.* 2014;98(6):832–840.

## Craniofacial Clefting and Syndromic Congenital Craniofacial Anomalies

Craniofacial clefts occur as a result of a developmental arrest or mechanical disruption of development. Etiologic theories include a failure of neural crest cell migration and a failure of fusion or movement of facial processes. Facial clefts in the skeletal structures are distributed around the orbit and maxilla; clefts in the soft tissues are most apparent around the eyelids and lips. Examples of clefting syndromes affecting the orbit and eyelids are the oculoauriculovertebral spectrum, which includes hemifacial microsomia, oculoauriculovertebral dysplasia (Goldenhar syndrome), and mandibulofacial dysostosis (Treacher Collins–Franceschetti syndrome, Fig 3-1); and some forms of midline clefts with hypertelorism.

The bones of the skull or orbit may also have congenital clefts through which the intracranial contents can herniate. These protruding contents can be the meninges *(meningocele),* brain tissue *(encephalocele),* or both meninges and brain tissue *(meningoencephalocele).* When these herniations involve the orbit, they most commonly present anteriorly with a protrusion subcutaneously near the medial canthus or over the bridge of the nose. Straining or crying may increase the size of the mass, and the globe may be displaced temporally and downward (inferolaterally). Such herniations less commonly move into the posterior orbit; these lesions may cause anterior displacement and pulsation of the globe. Treatment is surgical and should be carried out in collaboration with a neurosurgeon. Meningoceles and encephaloceles adjacent to the orbit are frequently associated with anomalies of the optic disc, such as morning glory disc.

Craniosynostosis can occur as an isolated abnormality or in conjunction with other anomalies as part of a genetic syndrome. *Syndromic craniosynostosis* is the premature closure of 1 or more sutures in the bones of the skull and results in various skeletal deformities, including orbital defects. Ophthalmic problems include strabismus, astigmatism, ptosis, exophthalmos, nasolacrimal duct obstruction, and amblyopia. Secondary intracranial hypertension can be a complication. Hypertelorism and proptosis are frequently observed in craniosynostosis syndromes such as Crouzon syndrome (craniofacial dysostosis; Fig 3-2) and Apert syndrome (acrocephalosyndactyly; Fig 3-3). Syndromic craniosynostosis is a

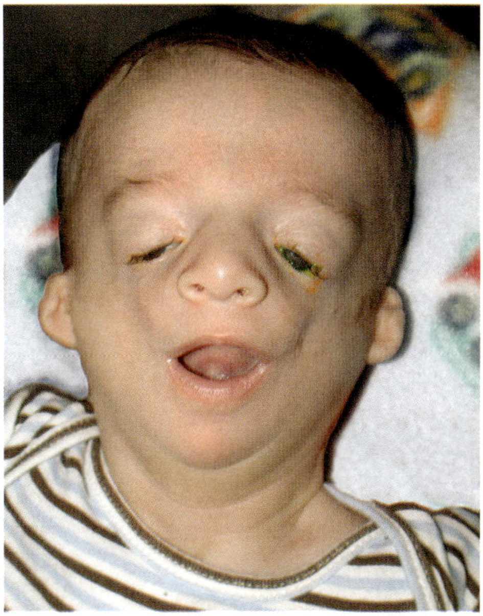

**Figure 3-1** Treacher Collins–Franceschetti syndrome (mandibulofacial dysostosis). *(Courtesy of Jill Foster, MD.)*

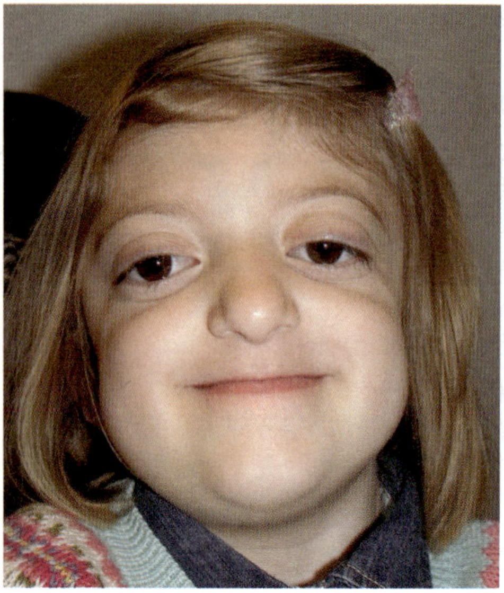

**Figure 3-2** Crouzon syndrome (craniofacial dysostosis). *(Courtesy of Jill Foster, MD.)*

genetically heterogeneous disorder, with mutations identified in several genes, predominantly the fibroblast growth factor receptor genes.

The severe orbital and facial defects associated with craniofacial disorders can sometimes be improved with surgery. Bony and soft tissue reconstruction is generally necessary. Such operations are often staged and usually require a team approach with multiple subspecialists.

Jadico SK, Huebner A, McDonald-McGinn DM, Zackai EH, Young TL. Ocular phenotype correlations in patients with TWIST versus FGFR3 genetic mutations. *J AAPOS.* 2006; 10(5):435–444.

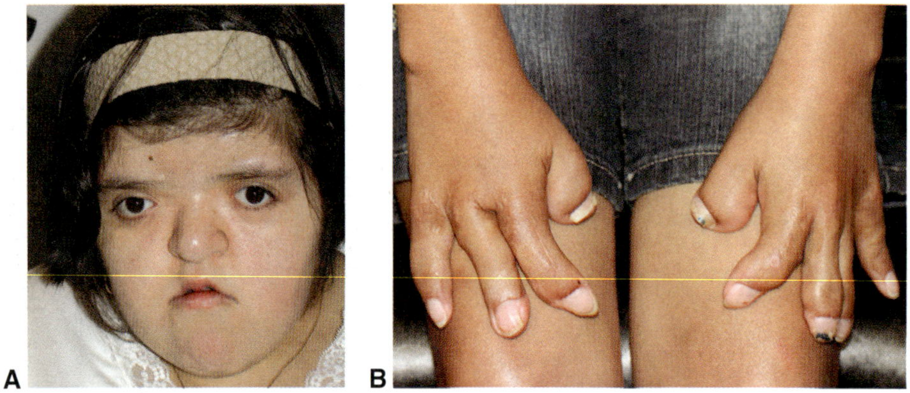

**Figure 3-3** **A,** Apert syndrome. **B,** Syndactyly in Apert syndrome. *(Courtesy of Jill Foster, MD.)*

## Congenital Orbital Tumors

### Hamartomas and Choristomas

*Hamartomas* are anomalous growths of tissue consisting only of mature cells normally found at the involved site. Classic examples are infantile (capillary) hemangiomas and the characteristic lesions of neurofibromatosis. *Choristomas* are tissue anomalies characterized by types of cells not normally found at the involved site. Classic examples are dermoid cysts, epidermoid cysts, dermolipomas, and teratomas. These congenital and juvenile tumors are discussed further in BCSC Section 6, *Pediatric Ophthalmology and Strabismus.*

#### *Dermoid cyst*

Dermoid and epidermoid cysts are among the most common orbital tumors of childhood. These cysts are present congenitally and enlarge progressively. The more superficial cysts usually become symptomatic in childhood, but deeper orbital dermoids may not become clinically evident until adulthood. *Dermoid cysts* are lined by keratinizing epithelium and contain dermal appendages, such as hair follicles and sebaceous glands. They contain an admixture of oil and keratin. In contrast, *epidermoid cysts* are lined by epidermis only and are usually filled with keratin; they do not contain dermal appendages.

Orbital dermoid cysts occur most commonly in the area of the lateral brow adjacent to the frontozygomatic suture (Fig 3-4A); less often they may be found in the medial upper eyelid adjacent to the frontoethmoidal suture. Dermoid cysts commonly present as palpable smooth, painless, oval masses that enlarge slowly. They may be freely mobile or they may be fixed to periosteum at the underlying suture. If the dermoid occurs in the temporal fossa, computed tomography (CT) is often indicated to rule out dumbbell expansion

A

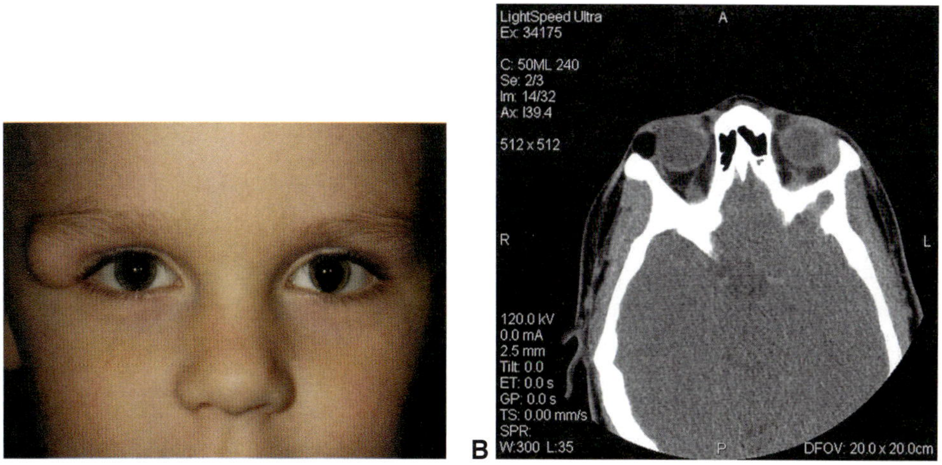


**Figure 3-4** **A,** Young child with a dermoid tumor (epithelial choristoma), characteristically located at the frontozygomatic suture line. **B,** Computed tomography scan of a lateral dermoid in the axial plane. Note the well-defined borders and hypointense central area characteristic of a dermoid. *(Part A courtesy of Keith D. Carter, MD; part B courtesy of Jill Foster, MD.)*

through the suture into the underlying orbit. A dumbbell dermoid cyst such as this can cause pulsating proptosis with mastication, a highly specific feature of this condition. CT is also useful to evaluate medial lesions and to distinguish dermoids from congenital encephaloceles, dacryoceles, and vascular lesions that might also occur in this location. With CT, an orbital dermoid cyst is typically well defined, and it has an enhancing wall and a nonenhancing lumen (Fig 3-4B). A partially calcified margin or rim is visible in most cases. With magnetic resonance imaging, the lesion is best appreciated on fat-suppression sequences and appears as a well-defined round to ovoid structure of variable size. Most dermoids are relatively hypointense with respect to orbital fat on T1-weighted images and relatively hyperintense on T2-weighted images. Enhancement is minimal due to the lack of blood vessels in the cyst.

Dermoid cysts that do not present until adulthood often are not palpable because they are situated posteriorly in the orbit, usually in the superior and temporal portions adjacent to the bony sutures. The globe and adnexa may be displaced, causing progressive proptosis, and erosion or remodeling of bone can occur. Long-standing dermoids may erode the orbital bones. In some cases, the clinical presentation of orbital dermoids may be orbital inflammation, which is incited by leakage of oil and keratin from the cyst. Expansion of the dermoid cyst and inflammatory response to leakage may result in an orbitocutaneous fistula, which may also occur following incomplete surgical removal.

**Management** Dermoid cysts are usually removed surgically. Because dermoids that present in childhood are often superficial, they can be excised through an incision placed in the upper eyelid crease or directly over the lesion. If possible, the cyst wall should be maintained during surgery. Rupture of the cyst can lead to an acute inflammatory process if part of the cyst wall or any of the contents remain within the eyelid or orbit. If the cyst wall is ruptured, the surgeon should remove the cyst contents. Complete surgical removal may be difficult if the cyst has leaked preoperatively and adhesions have developed.

Ahuja R, Azar NF. Orbital dermoids in children. *Semin Ophthalmol.* 2006;21(3):207–211.

Shields JA, Kaden IH, Eagle RC Jr, Shields CL. Orbital dermoid cysts: clinicopathologic correlations, classification, and management. *Ophthal Plast Reconstr Surg.* 1997;13(4): 265–276.

Shields JA, Shields CL. Orbital cysts of childhood—classification, clinical features, and management. *Surv Ophthalmol.* 2004;49(3):281–299.

### *Dermolipoma*

Dermolipomas are solid tumors usually located in and beneath the conjunctiva over the globe's lateral surface (Fig 3-5). These benign lesions may have deep extensions that can extend to the levator aponeurosis and extraocular muscles. Superficially, dermolipomas may have fine hairs that can be irritating to patients. These tumors typically require no treatment unless the lesion is large and/or cosmetically objectionable. In these cases, only the anterior, visible portion should be excised; when possible, the overlying conjunctiva should be preserved. Care must be taken to avoid damage to the lacrimal gland ducts, extraocular muscles, and the levator aponeurosis. Lesions that may simulate dermolipomas include prolapsed orbital fat, prolapsed palpebral lobe of the lacrimal gland, and lymphomas (such processes are generally found only in adults).

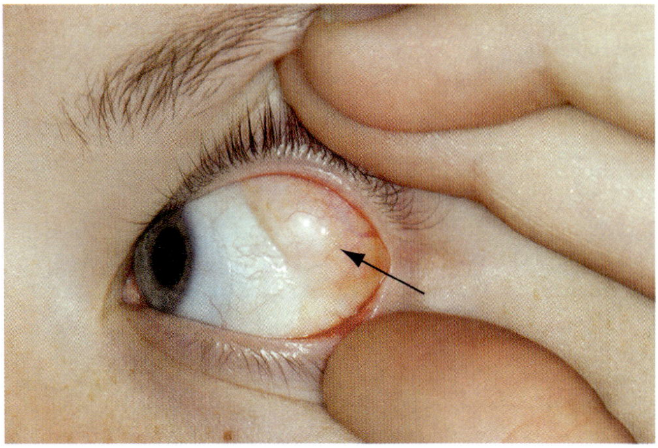

**Figure 3-5** Dermolipoma of left lateral orbit. There are fine hairs on the surface of the tumor *(arrow)*. *(Courtesy of Keith D. Carter, MD.)*

Fry CL, Leone CR Jr. Safe management of dermolipomas. *Arch Ophthalmol.* 1994;112(8): 1114–1116.

### *Teratoma*

Teratomas are rare tumors that arise from all 3 germinal layers (ectoderm, mesoderm, and endoderm) and are usually cystic. Histologically, teratoma is characterized by a complex arrangement of various tissues, including clear cysts lined by either epidermis or gastrointestinal or respiratory epithelium. Islands of hyaline cartilage, cerebral tissue, epidermal cysts, and choroid plexus are frequently found. A child with an orbital teratoma characteristically presents with severe unilateral proptosis at birth. As a consequence, the globe and optic nerve may be maldeveloped. The proptosis may increase over the first few days or weeks, and compression of the globe can result in corneal exposure and vision loss. When the lesion is smaller, the globe is often normal. Although teratomas in other parts of the body have been known to undergo malignant transformation, teratomas confined to the orbit are generally benign; for those that are malignant, exenteration may be necessary. However, some cystic teratomas can be removed and ocular function preserved.

CHAPTER 4

# Orbital Inflammatory and Infectious Disorders

Orbital inflammatory disease comprises a broad range of disorders that can be divided conceptually into specific and nonspecific inflammations; in other words, those that have an identifiable cause and those that do not. For example, an infection or autoimmune disease can be considered a specific cause of orbital inflammation. In contrast, *nonspecific orbital inflammation* is defined as a benign inflammatory process of the orbit without a known local or systemic cause. It is therefore a diagnosis of exclusion after all specific causes of inflammation have been eliminated. Table 4-1 shows a limited differential diagnosis of orbital inflammatory disease. This chapter presents an overview of the major

**Table 4-1 Differential Diagnosis of Major Orbital Inflammations**

**Infectious (identify as preseptal or orbital cellulitis)**
- Bacterial (identify the source)
  - Direct inoculation (trauma, surgery)
  - Spread from adjacent tissue (sinusitis, dacryocystitis, dacryoadenitis)
  - Spread from distant focus (bacteremia, pneumonia)
  - Opportunistic infection (necrotizing fasciitis, tuberculosis)
- Fungal
  - Zygomycosis
  - Aspergillosis
- Parasitic
  - Echinococcosis
  - Cysticercosis

**Autoimmune**
- Thyroid eye disease (TED)
- Immunoglobulin G4 (IgG4) disease

**Vasculitic**
- Giant cell arteritis
- Granulomatosis with polyangiitis
- Polyarteritis nodosa
- Vasculitis associated with connective tissue disorders

**Granulomatous**
- Sarcoidosis

**Nonspecific orbital inflammation (NSOI) (diagnosis of exclusion)**

causes of specific and nonspecific orbital inflammation, with the goal of providing a working knowledge of the most common of these disorders.

Gordon LK. Orbital inflammatory disease: a diagnostic and therapeutic challenge. *Eye (Lond).* 2006;20(10):1196–1206.

## Infectious Inflammation

### Cellulitis

The most common cause of cellulitis is bacterial infection. However, in each clinical setting, the physician must first define the etiology of the cellulitis; failure to do so may result in delay in the identification and effective treatment of noninfectious (eg, autoimmune, malignant, foreign-body) etiologies.

Bacterial infections of the orbit or periorbital soft tissues originate from 3 primary sources:

- direct spread from adjacent sinusitis, dacryocystitis, or dacryoadenitis
- direct inoculation following trauma or skin infection
- hematologic spread from a distant focus (eg, otitis media, pneumonia)

Although periorbital infections are typically classified as being either preseptal cellulitis (involvement anterior to the orbital septum) or orbital cellulitis (involvement posterior to the septum), they often represent a continuum, with common underlying causes requiring similar treatment regimens. It must be emphasized that infectious cellulitis—whether preseptal or orbital—is most commonly caused by underlying sinusitis, particularly if no obvious source of inoculation is noted.

#### *Preseptal cellulitis*

Preseptal cellulitis occurs anterior to the orbital septum. Eyelid edema, erythema, and inflammation may be severe, but the globe is uninvolved. Therefore, pupillary reaction, vision, and ocular motility are not disturbed; pain on eye movement and chemosis are absent.

Although preseptal cellulitis in adults is usually due to penetrating cutaneous trauma or dacryocystitis, in children, a common cause is underlying sinusitis leading to preseptal inflammation. Historically, preseptal cellulitis in infants and children younger than 5 years was often associated with bacteremia, septicemia, and meningitis caused by *Haemophilus influenzae.* The *H influenzae* type b vaccine has significantly diminished this etiology. Now, most pediatric cases are the result of infection with gram-positive cocci.

**Treatment** When infection is thought to be the cause of the process, antibiotics should be initiated as promptly as possible. The workup should proceed quickly, particularly in children, and include computed tomography (CT) of the orbit and sinuses if the eyelid swelling is profound enough to preclude examination of the globe and thereby exclude orbital cellulitis. It may be helpful to consult the primary care physician or a specialist in infectious diseases when developing the treatment plan and choosing antibiotics.

In children, oral antibiotics (eg, cephalexin for an anterior etiology, amoxicillin clavulanate for an infection originating in the sinuses), frequent warm compresses, and nasal decongestants (eg, oxymetazoline nasal spray), in cases of associated sinusitis, are typically effective therapy; this approach is chosen if the examination of the child is reliable and follow-up examinations can be ensured. If community-acquired methicillin-resistant *Staphylococcus aureus* (CA-MRSA) is a possible etiologic agent, trimethoprim-sulfamethoxazole (TMP-SMX) may be considered. Hospitalization and intravenous (IV) antibiotics (eg, ceftriaxone, vancomycin) are indicated in some infants or if the cellulitis progresses despite outpatient therapy, as preseptal infection can progress to orbital cellulitis.

In teenagers and adults, preseptal cellulitis usually arises from a superficial source and responds quickly to appropriate oral antibiotics (eg, ampicillin-sulbactam, TMP-SMX, doxycycline, clindamycin) and warm compresses. Initial antibiotic selection is based on the history, clinical findings, and initial laboratory studies. Prompt sensitivity studies are indicated so that the antibiotic selection can be revised, if necessary. *Staphylococcus aureus* is the most common pathogen in patients with preseptal cellulitis resulting from trauma. The infection usually responds rapidly to a penicillinase-resistant penicillin, such as methicillin or ampicillin-sulbactam. However, *methicillin-resistant S aureus (MRSA),* previously recognized as a cause of severe nosocomial infections, is now increasingly encountered in the community setting as well. CA-MRSA infections tend to present as a fluctuant abscess with surrounding cellulitis. The pain associated with the lesion is often out of proportion to its appearance. CA-MRSA is often susceptible to a range of antibiotics (including TMP-SMX, rifampin, or clindamycin), whereas hospital-associated MRSA is sensitive only to vancomycin and linezolid. However, both types of MRSA may result in acute morbidity and long-term disability. MRSA has also been associated with necrotizing fasciitis, orbital cellulitis, endogenous endophthalmitis, panophthalmitis, and cavernous sinus thrombosis. Because of the potentially aggressive nature of this pathogen, successful management demands a high degree of clinical suspicion and prompt medical and surgical intervention. In addition, consultation with specialists in infectious diseases may be warranted.

In older adults, infections behave differently. These patients may not manifest the typical signs of inflammation, increased erythema and calor, as seen in younger patients. Furthermore, severe infections may not be associated with febrile reactions. Response to antibiotics may also be delayed, and surgical intervention to excise devitalized tissue may be necessary to clear an infection.

Imaging studies should be performed to rule out underlying sinusitis if no direct inoculation site is identified. If the patient does not respond to oral antibiotics within 48 hours or if orbital involvement becomes evident, prompt hospital admission, CT, and IV antibiotics are usually indicated.

Surgical drainage may be necessary if preseptal cellulitis progresses to a localized abscess. Incision and drainage can usually be performed directly over the abscess, but care should be taken to avoid damaging the levator aponeurosis in the upper eyelid. To avoid contaminating the orbital soft tissues, the surgeon should not open the orbital septum.

Pelton RW, Klapper SR. Preseptal and orbital cellulitis. *Focal Points: Clinical Modules for Ophthalmologists.* San Francisco: American Academy of Ophthalmology; 2008, module 11.

Rutar T, Chambers HF, Crawford JB, et al. Ophthalmic manifestations of infections caused by the USA300 clone of community-associated methicillin-resistant *Staphylococcus aureus. Ophthalmology.* 2006;113(8):1455–1462.

### *Orbital cellulitis*

Orbital cellulitis involves structures posterior to the orbital septum, and in the majority of cases, it occurs as a secondary extension of acute or chronic bacterial sinusitis (Table 4-2). Clinical findings include fever, leukocytosis (75% of cases), erythema, proptosis, chemosis, ptosis, and restriction of and pain with ocular movement (Fig 4-1). Decreased vision, impaired color vision, restricted visual fields, and pupillary abnormalities suggest optic neuropathy that demands immediate investigation and aggressive management. Delay in treatment may result in blindness, cavernous sinus thrombosis, cranial neuropathy, brain abscess, or death.

In the presence of postseptal findings, imaging of the orbit and paranasal sinuses is essential. Identification of sinusitis is an indication for otolaryngologic consultation.

**Table 4-2 Causes of Orbital Cellulitis**

| |
|---|
| **Extension from periorbital structures** |
| Paranasal sinuses (sinusitis) |
| Face and eyelids, infection of |
| Lacrimal sac (dacryocystitis) |
| Teeth (dental infection) |
| **Exogenous causes** |
| Trauma (rule out foreign bodies) |
| Surgery (after any orbital or periorbital surgery) |
| **Endogenous causes** |
| Bacteremia with septic embolization |
| **Intraorbital causes** |
| Endophthalmitis |
| Dacryoadenitis |

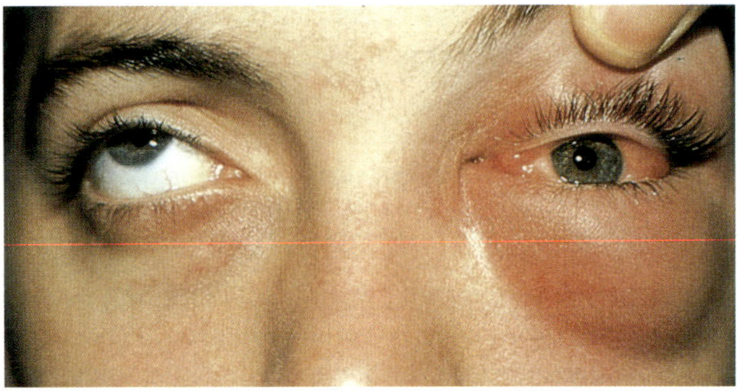

**Figure 4-1** Left-sided orbital cellulitis with marked erythema, proptosis, and ptosis. Chemosis is also present, along with associated impairment of vertical ductions. *(Courtesy of Jeffrey A. Nerad, MD.)*

Antibiotic therapy should provide broad-spectrum coverage because infections in adults usually involve multiple organisms that may include gram-positive cocci, such as *H influenzae* and *Moraxella catarrhalis,* and anaerobes. Although nasal decongestants may help to promote spontaneous drainage of the infected sinus, early surgical intervention to drain the involved sinus is usually indicated, especially if orbital findings progress during IV antibiotic therapy. In contrast, orbital cellulitis in children is more often caused by a single gram-positive organism and is less likely to require surgical drainage of the infected sinus. Evidence also indicates that steroids, when used in addition to antibiotic therapy, may hasten recovery while posing a low risk of worsening infection.

Orbital cellulitis following blowout fractures is generally limited to patients with underlying sinus disease. Prophylactic antibiotics are recommended if CT scans of orbital fractures suggest ongoing sinusitis. The risk of orbital cellulitis is increased if the medial wall is fractured.

Abscess formation may be suggested by progressive proptosis, globe displacement, or failure to show clinical improvement despite appropriate antibiotic therapy. Abscesses usually localize in the subperiosteal space (Fig 4-2), adjacent to the infected sinus, but may extend through the periosteum into the orbital soft tissues. When medical treatment is not successful, further imaging may help clinicians locate the abscess and target the approach for surgical intervention.

However, not all subperiosteal abscesses require surgical drainage. Isolated medial or inferior subperiosteal orbital abscesses in children younger than 9 years with underlying isolated ethmoid sinusitis, intact vision, and only moderate proptosis typically respond to medical therapy. According to the guidelines set forth by Garcia and Harris, management may consist of careful observation *unless any of the following criteria are present:*

- patient aged 9 years or older
- presence of frontal sinusitis
- nonmedial location of subperiosteal abscess (SPA)
- large SPA
- suspicion of anaerobic infection (presence of gas in abscess on CT)
- recurrence of SPA after prior drainage
- evidence of chronic sinusitis (eg, nasal polyps)
- acute optic nerve or retinal compromise
- infection of dental origin (anaerobic infection more likely)

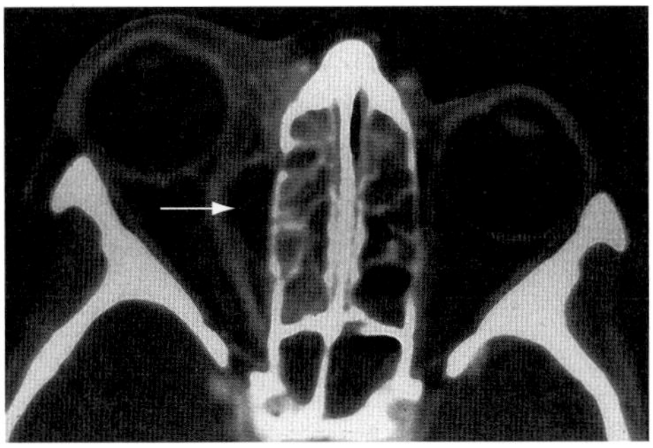

**Figure 4-2** Computed tomography (CT) scan of right orbital subperiosteal abscess *(arrow)* displacing the medial rectus muscle. *(Courtesy of Robert C. Kersten, MD.)*

Surgical drainage coupled with appropriate antibiotic therapy is recommended in older patients and in those with more severe presentation; it usually leads to clinical improvement within 24–48 hours. Concomitant sinus surgery is indicated if sinusitis is present. The refractory nature of orbital abscesses in adolescents and adults is thought to be due to the frequent involvement of multiple pathogens that are drug resistant, particularly anaerobic organisms.

Most patients with orbital cellulitis and abscesses respond to appropriate medical or surgical treatment or to a combination of these. Orbital infections rarely spread posteriorly to the cavernous sinus. Cavernous sinus thrombosis is often heralded by the rapid progression of proptosis, the development of ipsilateral ophthalmoplegia, and the onset of anesthesia in both the first and second divisions of the trigeminal nerve. In rare instances, contralateral ophthalmoplegia has been reported as well. Meningitis and frank brain abscess may develop. A lumbar puncture may reveal acute inflammatory cells and the causative organism on stain and culture. Magnetic resonance imaging (MRI) confirms the diagnosis.

Garcia GH, Harris GJ. Criteria for nonsurgical management of subperiosteal abscess of the orbit: analysis of outcomes 1988–1998. *Ophthalmology.* 2000;107(8):1454–1458.

Harris GJ. Subperiosteal abscess of the orbit: age as a factor in the bacteriology and response to treatment. *Ophthalmology.* 1994;101(3):585–595.

Pushker N, Tejwani LK, Bajaj MS, Khurana S, Velpandian T, Chandra M. Role of oral corticosteroids in orbital cellulitis. *Am J Ophthalmol.* 2013;156(1):178–183. Epub 2013 Apr 24.

## Necrotizing Fasciitis

Necrotizing fasciitis is a severe, potentially vision-threatening or life-threatening bacterial infection involving the subcutaneous soft tissues, particularly the superficial and deep fasciae. Group A β-hemolytic streptococcus is the organism most commonly responsible, but a variety of organisms, including aerobic and anaerobic, gram-positive and gram-negative bacteria, may cause this disorder.

This infection develops rapidly and requires immediate attention because it is potentially fatal. Although most patients are immunocompromised by conditions such as diabetes mellitus or alcoholism, it may also occur in immunocompetent patients. The initial clinical presentation is similar to that of orbital or preseptal cellulitis, with swelling, erythema, and pain, but it may be accompanied by a shocklike syndrome. Because necrotizing fasciitis tends to track along avascular tissue planes, an early sign may be anesthesia over the affected area caused by involvement of deep cutaneous nerves. In addition, disproportionate reports of pain may suggest the possibility of necrotizing fasciitis, as do typical changes in skin color, progressing from rose to blue-gray, with bullae formation and frank cutaneous necrosis. Usually, the course is rapid and the patient requires treatment in an intensive care unit.

Treatment includes early surgical debridement along with IV antibiotics. If the involved pathogen is unknown, broad-spectrum coverage for gram-positive and gram-negative as well as anaerobic organisms is indicated. Clindamycin is of particular value, as it is uniquely effective against the toxins produced by group A streptococcus. To limit the inflammatory damage associated with the toxins, adjunctive corticosteroid therapy after the start of antibiotic therapy has been advocated. Some cases of necrotizing fasciitis limited to the eyelids can be cautiously followed with systemic antibiotic therapy and little or no debridement; this approach should be considered in cases that have clearly defined margins and show no signs of toxic shock.

Patients may experience rapid deterioration, culminating in hypotension, renal failure, and adult respiratory distress syndrome. Clinical series from all body sites report up to a 30% mortality rate, usually due to toxic shock syndrome, but this occurs less commonly in the periocular region.

Lazzeri D, Lazzeri S, Figus M, et al. Periorbital necrotising fasciitis. *Br J Ophthalmol.* 2010; 94(12):1577–1585.

Luksich JA, Holds JB, Hartstein ME. Conservative management of necrotizing fasciitis of the eyelids. *Ophthalmology.* 2002;109(11):2118–2122.

## Orbital Tuberculosis

Though previously recognized mostly in endemic areas of the developing world, tuberculosis has recently reemerged as a public health threat in developed countries as well. Orbital tuberculosis occurs most commonly as a result of hematogenous spread from a pulmonary focus, which is often subclinical. Less often, spread occurs from an adjacent tuberculous sinusitis. Proptosis, motility dysfunction, bone destruction, and chronic draining fistulas may be the presenting findings. In the developed world, tuberculosis is most often associated with human immunodeficiency virus infection and inner-city poverty. The majority of recent orbital cases have been reported in children, and the infection is often mistaken for an orbital malignancy (Fig 4-3). The disease is usually unilateral. Acid-fast bacilli may be difficult to detect in pathologic specimens, which usually show caseation necrosis, epithelioid cells, and Langhans giant cells. Skin testing and fine-needle aspiration biopsy with culture early in the course of the disease may help establish the diagnosis. Antituberculous therapy is usually curative.

Khalil M, Lindley S, Matouk E. Tuberculosis of the orbit. *Ophthalmology.* 1985;92(11): 1624–1627.

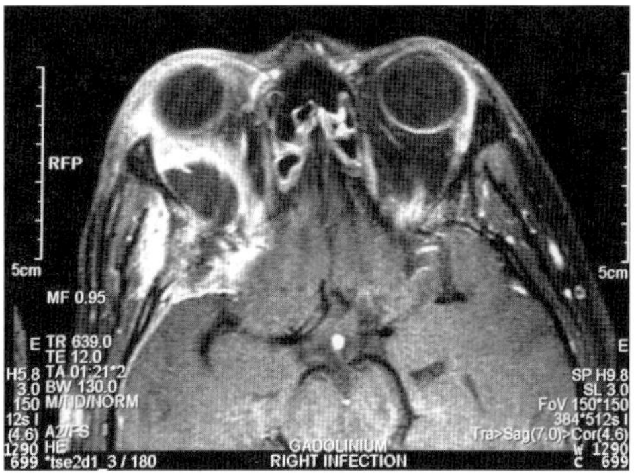


**Figure 4-3** Right orbital mass with intracranial extension secondary to tuberculosis infection, initially diagnosed as a neoplastic lesion. *(Courtesy of Jill Foster, MD.)*

## Zygomycosis

Zygomycosis (also known as *phycomycosis* or *mucormycosis*) is the most common and the most virulent fungal disease involving the orbit. The specific fungal genus involved is usually *Mucor* or *Rhizopus*. These fungi, belonging to the class Zygomycetes, almost always extend into the orbit from an adjacent sinus or the nasal cavity. The fungi invade blood vessel walls, producing thrombosing vasculitis. The resultant tissue necrosis promotes further fungal invasion.

Patients commonly present with proptosis and an orbital apex syndrome (internal and external ophthalmoplegia, ptosis, decreased corneal sensation, and decreased vision). Older adults may be relatively immunosuppressed compared with younger patients and therefore are at risk for these virulent infections.

Predisposing factors include systemic disease with associated metabolic acidosis, diabetes mellitus, malignancies, and treatment with antimetabolites or steroids. Diagnosis is confirmed by a biopsy of the necrotic-appearing tissues in the nasopharynx or the involved sinus or orbit. The histology of zygomycosis shows nonseptate, large branching hyphae that stain with hematoxylin-eosin, unlike most fungi (see the discussion of fungal infections in BCSC Section 5, *Neuro-Ophthalmology*).

Therapeutic measures should be aimed at both systemic control of the underlying metabolic or immunologic abnormality and local surgical debridement. Antifungal therapy should be given via IV administration of amphotericin B or liposomal amphotericin B. Some recent reports in the literature advocate the use of posaconazole or voriconazole in patients who cannot tolerate the adverse effects of amphotericin. Alternatively, other lipid-encapsulated antifungal agents, which permit a higher cumulative dose with a reduced level of toxicity, may be considered. Some authors have proposed adjunctive hyperbaric oxygen therapy. The role of primary exenteration has decreased, but it is unclear whether patient survival (typically poor) has been adversely affected by less-aggressive surgical debridement.

Ferry AP, Abedi S. Diagnosis and management of rhino-orbitocerebral mucormycosis (phycomycosis). A report of 16 personally observed cases. *Ophthalmology.* 1983;90(9):1096–1104.

Kronish JW, Johnson TE, Gilberg SM, Corrent GF, McLeish WM, Scott KR. Orbital infections in patients with human immunodeficiency virus infection. *Ophthalmology.* 1996;103(9): 1483–1492.

Rutar T, Cockerham KP. Periorbital zygomycosis (mucormycosis) treated with posaconazole. *Am J Ophthalmol.* 2006;142(1):187–188.

## Aspergillosis

Fungi in the *Aspergillus* genus can affect the orbit in several distinct clinical entities. *Acute aspergillosis* is a fungal disease characterized by fulminant sinus infection with secondary orbital invasion. Patients present with severe periorbital pain, decreased vision, and proptosis. Diagnosis is confirmed by one or more biopsies. Grocott-Gomori methenamine–silver nitrate stain shows septate branching hyphae of uniform width (see the discussion of fungal infections in BCSC Section 5, *Neuro-Ophthalmology*). Therapy consists of aggressive surgical excision of all infected tissues and administration of amphotericin B, flucytosine, rifampin, voriconazole, caspofungin, or a combination thereof.

*Chronic aspergillosis* is an indolent infection resulting in slow destruction of the sinuses and adjacent structures. Although the prognosis is much better than that for acute fulminant disease, intraorbital and intracranial extension can occur in the chronic invasive form of fungal sinusitis as well and result in significant morbidity.

Chronic, localized noninvasive aspergillosis also involves the sinuses and occurs in immunocompetent patients who may not have a history of atopic disease. Often, there is a history of chronic sinusitis, and proliferation of saprobic organisms results in a tightly packed fungus ball. This type of aspergillosis is characterized by a lack of either inflammation or bone erosion.

*Allergic aspergillosis sinusitis* occurs in immunocompetent patients with nasal polyposis and chronic sinusitis. Patients may have peripheral eosinophilia; elevated total immunoglobulin E (IgE), fungus-specific IgE, and IgG levels; or positive skin test results for fungal antigens. CT scanning reveals thick allergic mucin within the sinus as mottled areas of increased attenuation on nonenhanced images. Bone erosion and remodeling are frequently present but do not signify actual tissue invasion. MRI may be more specific, showing signal void areas on T2-weighted scans. Sinus biopsy results reveal thick, peanut butter–like or green mucus, pathologic study of which reveals numerous eosinophils and eosinophil degradation products, as well as extramucosal fungal hyphae. Endoscopic debridement of the involved sinuses is indicated. Treatment with systemic and topical corticosteroids is also recommended. Up to 17% of patients with allergic fungal sinusitis present first with orbital signs.

Carter KD, Graham SM, Carpenter KM. Ophthalmic manifestations of allergic fungal sinusitis. *Am J Ophthalmol.* 1999;127(2):189–195.

Como JA, Dismukes WE. Oral azole drugs as systemic antifungal therapy. *N Engl J Med.* 1994;330(4):263–272.

Levin LA, Avery R, Shore JW, Woog JJ, Baker AS. The spectrum of orbital aspergillosis: a clinicopathological review. *Surv Ophthalmol.* 1996;41(2):142–154.

### Parasitic Diseases

Parasitic diseases of the orbit are generally limited to developing countries and include trichinosis and echinococcosis. *Trichinosis* is caused by ingestion of the nematode *Trichinella spiralis.* The eyelids and extraocular muscles may be inflamed due to migration of the larvae. *Echinococcosis* is caused by the dog tapeworm *Echinococcus granulosus.* A hydatid cyst containing tapeworm larvae may form in the orbit. Rupture of such a cyst may cause progressive inflammation and a severe immune response. *Taenia solium,* the pork tapeworm, may also encyst and progressively enlarge in the orbital tissues, causing a condition known as *cysticercosis.*

## Noninfectious Inflammation

### Thyroid Eye Disease

Thyroid eye disease (TED; also known as *Graves ophthalmopathy, thyroid-associated orbitopathy, thyroid orbitopathy, thyrotoxic exophthalmos,* and other terms) is an autoimmune inflammatory disorder whose underlying cause continues to be elucidated. The clinical signs, however, are characteristic and include one or more of the following: eyelid retraction, von Graefe sign (lid lag), proptosis, restrictive extraocular myopathy, compressive optic neuropathy, exposure keratopathy, and conjunctival erythema and chemosis (Figs 4-4 through 4-6). TED was originally described as part of the triad that constitutes Graves disease, which includes the aforementioned orbital signs, hyperthyroidism, and pretibial myxedema. Although it is typically associated with Graves hyperthyroidism, TED may also occur with Hashimoto thyroiditis (immune-induced hypothyroidism) or in the absence of thyroid dysfunction. The course of the eye disease does not necessarily parallel the activity of the thyroid gland or the treatment of thyroid abnormalities.

See Key Points 4-1.

## KEY POINTS 4-1

**Thyroid eye disease (TED)** The following list highlights the essential points for the ophthalmologist to remember about TED.

- Eyelid retraction is the most common clinical feature of TED (and TED is the most common cause of eyelid retraction).
- TED is the most common cause of unilateral or bilateral proptosis.
- TED may be markedly asymmetric.
- TED is associated with hyperthyroidism in 90% of patients, but 6% of patients may be euthyroid.
- Severity of TED usually does not parallel serum levels of $T_4$ or $T_3$.
- TED is 6 times as common in women as in men.
- Smoking is associated with increased risk and severity of TED.
- Urgent care may be required for optic neuropathy or severe proptosis with corneal decompensation.
- If surgery is needed, the usual order is orbital decompression, followed by strabismus surgery, followed by eyelid retraction repair (see Chapter 7).

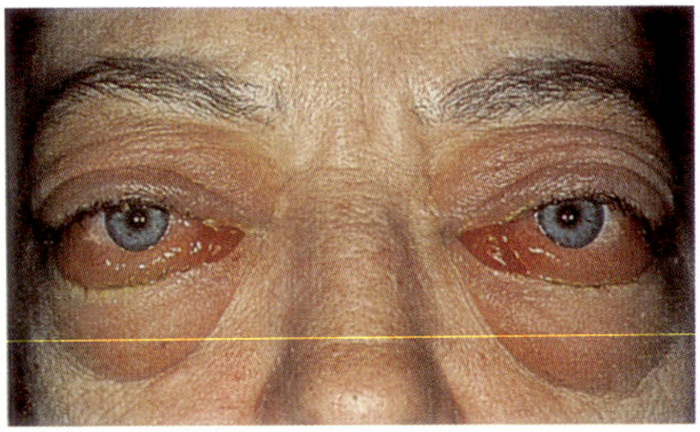

**Figure 4-4** Signs of active inflammation in a patient with thyroid eye disease (TED) include bilateral proptosis, chemosis, and eyelid swelling. *(Courtesy of Jeffrey A. Nerad, MD.)*

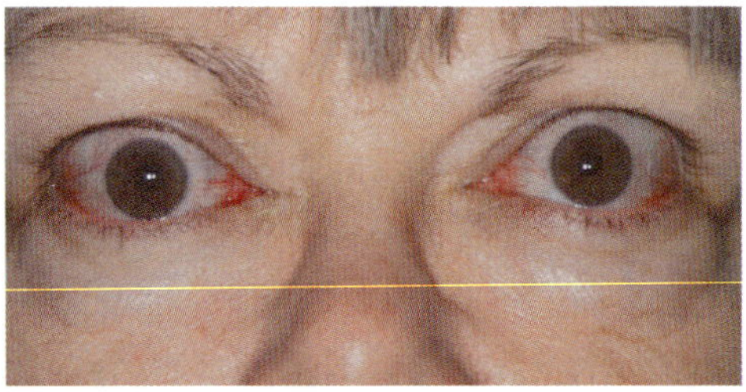

**Figure 4-5** TED, showing bilateral proptosis and upper eyelid retraction. *(Courtesy of Keith D. Carter, MD.)*

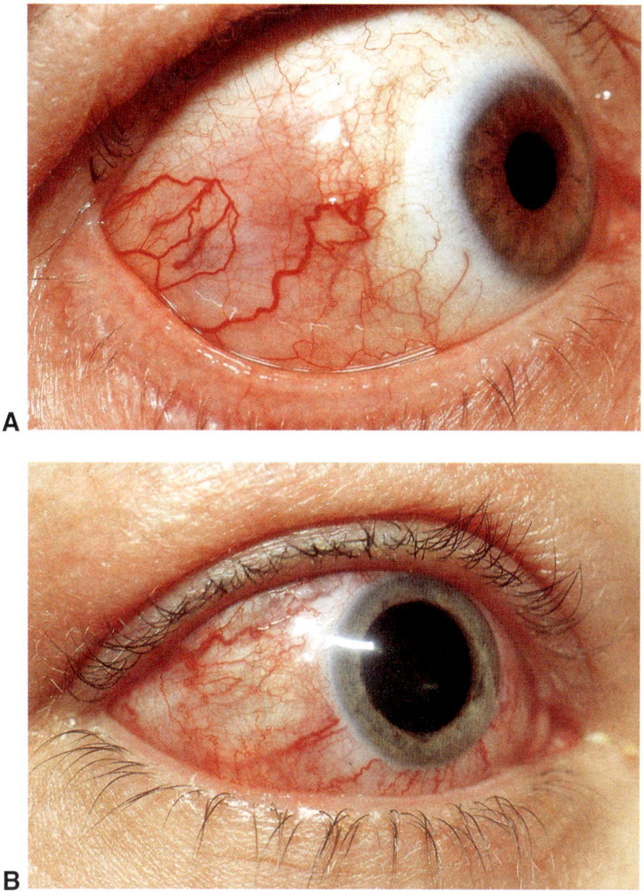


**Figure 4-6** **A,** Conjunctival erythema over the insertions of the rectus muscles is a frequent sign of TED. Typically, there is a clear zone between the anterior extent of the abnormally dilated blood vessels and the corneoscleral limbus. **B,** In contrast, the arterialization of blood vessels that occurs with a direct or indirect carotid-cavernous sinus fistula is usually more diffuse and extends to the limbus, with corkscrew-shaped vessels. *(Courtesy of George B. Bartley, MD.)*

### *Diagnosis*

The diagnosis of TED is made when 2 of the following 3 signs of the disease are present:

1. Concurrent or recently treated immune-related thyroid dysfunction (one or more of the following):
   a. Graves hyperthyroidism
   b. Hashimoto thyroiditis
   c. Presence of circulating thyroid antibodies without a coexisting dysthyroid state (partial consideration given): thyroid-stimulating hormone–receptor (TSH-R) antibodies, thyroid-binding inhibitory immunoglobulins, thyroid-stimulating immunoglobulins, antimicrosomal antibody

2. Typical ocular signs (one or more of the following):
   a. Unilateral or bilateral eyelid retraction with typical temporal flare (with or without lagophthalmos)
   b. Unilateral or bilateral proptosis (as evidenced by comparison with patient's old photos)
   c. Restrictive strabismus in a typical pattern
   d. Compressive optic neuropathy
   e. Fluctuating eyelid edema and/or erythema
   f. Chemosis and/or caruncular edema
3. Radiographic evidence of TED—unilateral or bilateral fusiform enlargement of one or more of the following (Figs 4-7, 4-8):
   a. Inferior rectus muscle
   b. Medial rectus muscle
   c. Superior rectus and/or levator muscle complex
   d. Lateral rectus muscle

If only orbital signs are present, the patient should continue to be observed for other orbital diseases and for the future development of a dysthyroid state.

Gerding MN, van der Meer JW, Broenink M, Bakker O, Wiersinga WM, Prummel MF. Association of thyrotrophin receptor antibodies with the clinical features of Graves' ophthalmopathy. *Clin Endocrinol (Oxf).* 2000;52(3):267–271.

Mourits MP, Prummel MF, Wiersinga WM, Koornneef L. Clinical activity score as a guide in the management of patients with Graves' ophthalmopathy. *Clin Endocrinol (Oxf).* 1997;47(1):9–14.

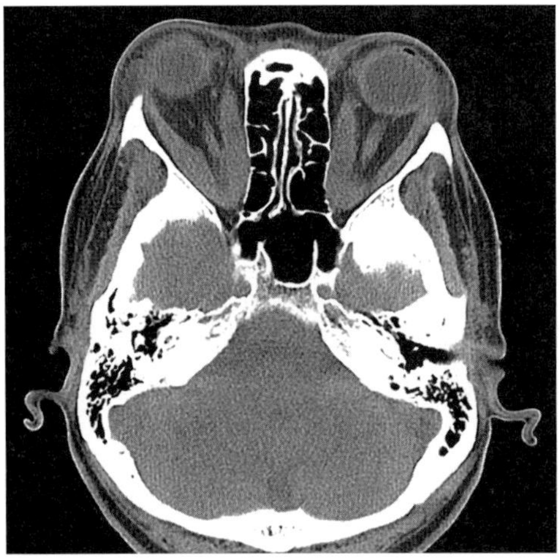

**Figure 4-7** TED. Axial orbital CT scan shows characteristic fusiform extraocular muscle enlargement that spares the tendons. *(Courtesy of Keith D. Carter, MD.)*

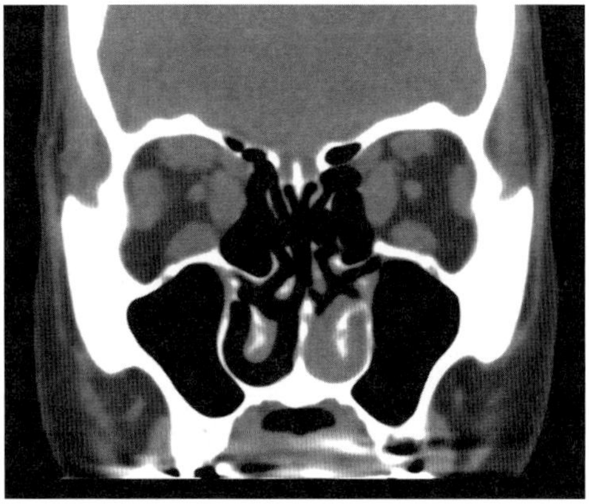

**Figure 4-8** Coronal orbital CT scan shows bilateral enlargement of extraocular muscles in TED. *(Courtesy of Keith D. Carter, MD.)*

### Pathogenesis

Over the last decade, the focus of research has shifted away from the extraocular muscles and/or myocytes to the orbital fibroblasts as the primary target of the inflammatory process associated with TED. Of particular importance is the recognition that unlike fibroblasts from other parts of the body, orbital fibroblasts express CD40 receptors, which are generally found on B cells. Orbital fibroblasts—through the expression of characteristic surface receptors, gangliosides, and proinflammatory genes—play an active role in modulating the inflammatory process. When engaged by T-cell–bound CD154, several fibroblast proinflammatory genes are upregulated, including interleukin-6 (IL-6), IL-8, and prostaglandin $E_2$. In turn, synthesis of hyaluronan and glycosaminoglycan (GAG) is increased. The upregulation of GAG synthesis is known to be essential in the pathology of TED, and it occurs at a rate that is 100 times as great in orbital fibroblasts derived from patients with TED as in abdominal fibroblasts in the same patients. This cascade of upregulation is dampened by the addition of therapeutic levels of corticosteroids.

Orbital fibroblasts are embryologically derived from the neural crest and, as such, possess developmental plasticity. A subpopulation of orbital fibroblasts appears capable of undergoing adipocyte differentiation. It is believed that this response to the inflammatory matrix is responsible for the fatty hypertrophy that predominates in some patients, particularly those younger than 40 years.

Recent studies have also identified a circulating immunoglobulin (IgG) that recognizes and activates the insulin-like growth factor I receptor expressed on the surface of numerous cell types, including fibroblasts. These autoantibodies have been found in a majority of patients with Graves disease and may contribute to orbital pathogenesis by stimulating orbital fibroblasts to secrete GAGs, cytokines, and chemoattractants. These latter signaling families may contribute to orbital inflammation and congestion. Manipulation of this pathway by available biologic agents (eg, rituximab and monoclonal antibodies against tumor necrosis factor α—infliximab, adalimumab, and etanercept) may show promise as a therapeutic strategy for treating patients with TED.

Kazim M, Goldberg RA, Smith TJ. Insights into the pathogenesis of thyroid-associated orbitopathy: evolving rationale for therapy. *Arch Ophthalmol.* 2002;120(3):380–386.

Minakaran N, Ezra DG. Rituximab for thyroid-associated ophthalmopathy. *Cochrane Database Syst Rev.* 2013;5:CD009226.

Naik V, Khadavi N, Naik MN, et al. Biologic therapeutics in thyroid-associated ophthalmopathy: translating disease mechanism into therapy. *Thyroid.* 2008;18(9):967–971.

Ponto KA, Kanitz M, Olivo PD, Pitz S, Pfeiffer N, Kahaly GJ. Clinical relevance of thyroid-stimulating immunoglobulins in Graves' ophthalmopathy. *Ophthalmology.* 2011;118(11): 2279–2285.

Tsui S, Naik V, Hoa N, et al. Evidence for an association between thyroid-stimulating hormone and insulin-like growth factor 1 receptors: a tale of two antigens implicated in Graves' disease. *J Immunol.* 2008;181(6):4397–4405.

### Epidemiology

A 1996 epidemiologic study of white patients in the United States with TED determined that the overall age-adjusted incidence rate for women was 16 cases per 100,000 population per year, whereas the rate for men was 3 cases per 100,000 population per year. TED affects women approximately 6 times as frequently as men (accounting for 86% versus 14% of cases, respectively). The peak incidence rates occurred in the age groups 40–44 years and 60–64 years in women and 45–49 years and 65–69 years in men. The median age at the time of diagnosis of TED was 43 years (range, 8–88 years). Development of TED is up to 7 times as likely among smokers as among nonsmokers.

### *Clinical features*

Among patients with TED, approximately 90% have Graves hyperthyroidism, 6% are euthyroid, 3% have Hashimoto thyroiditis, and 1% have primary hypothyroidism. There is a close temporal relationship between the development of hyperthyroidism and the development of TED: in about 20% of patients, the diagnoses are made at the same time; in approximately 60% of patients, the eye disease occurs within 1 year of onset of the thyroid disease. For patients who have no history of abnormal thyroid function or regulation at the time of diagnosis of TED, the risk for development of thyroid disease is approximately 25% within 1 year and 50% within 5 years. Although hyperthyroidism is present or will develop in most patients with TED, TED is present or will develop in only about 30% of patients with autoimmune hyperthyroidism.

Eyelid retraction is the most common ophthalmic feature of TED, being present either unilaterally or bilaterally in more than 90% of patients at some point in their clinical course (see Chapter 11, Fig 11-18A). Exophthalmos of one or both eyes affects approximately 60% of patients, restrictive extraocular myopathy is apparent in about 40% of patients, and optic nerve dysfunction occurs in one or both eyes in approximately 5% of patients with TED. Only 5% of patients have the complete constellation of classic findings: eyelid retraction, exophthalmos, optic nerve dysfunction, extraocular muscle involvement, and hyperthyroidism.

Upper eyelid retraction, either unilateral or bilateral, is documented in approximately 75% of patients at the time of diagnosis of TED. Lid lag in downgaze also is a frequent early sign, being present either unilaterally or bilaterally in 50% of patients at the initial examination. The most frequent ocular symptom when TED is first confirmed is dull, deep orbital pain or discomfort, which affects 30% of patients. Some degree of diplopia is reported by approximately 17% of patients, lacrimation or photophobia by 15%–20% of patients, and blurred vision by 7% of patients. Decreased vision attributable to optic neuropathy is present in less than 2% of eyes at the time of diagnosis of TED.

Pretibial myxedema and acropachy (soft-tissue swelling and periosteal changes affecting the distal extremities, principally fingers and toes) accompany TED in approximately 4% and 1% of patients, respectively, and are associated with a poor prognosis for the orbitopathy. Myasthenia gravis occurs in less than 1% of patients.

Bartley GB, Fatourechi V, Kadrmas EF, et al. Clinical features of Graves' ophthalmopathy in an incidence cohort. *Am J Ophthalmol.* 1996;121(3):284–290.

Holds JB, Buchanan AG. Thyroid eye disease. *Focal Points: Clinical Modules for Ophthalmologists.* San Francisco: American Academy of Ophthalmology; 2010, module 10.

### *Treatment and prognosis*

TED is a self-limiting disease that on average lasts 1 year in nonsmokers and between 2 and 3 years in smokers. After the active disease plateaus, a quiescent burnt-out phase ensues. Reactivation of inflammation occurs in approximately 5%–10% of patients over their lifetime.

Treatment of patients with TED follows a stepwise and graded approach based on patient-reported symptoms, clinical examination, and ancillary testing (Tables 4-3, 4-4). Several studies have proposed clinical scoring systems such as NO SPECS, Clinical Activity Score (CAS), and VISA classification as assessment tools for guiding the evaluation and treatment of patients with TED; however, no system prevails as the gold standard.

**Table 4-3 Evaluation of Thyroid Eye Disease**

| |
|---|
| **Clinical examination** |
| Corrected distance visual acuity |
| Color vision |
| Pupillary examination |
| Ocular motility |
| Hertel exophthalmometry |
| Intraocular pressure (in primary gaze and upgaze) |
| Adnexal examination |
| Slit-lamp examination |
| Dilated fundus examination |
| **Laboratory studies** |
| $T_3$, free $T_4$, TPO, TRAb, TSH, TSI |
| **Imaging studies** |
| Orbital ultrasonography (assessment of extraocular muscle size and reflectivity) |
| Orbital computed tomography scan or magnetic resonance imaging (including coronal imaging) |

TPO = thyroid peroxidase; TRAb = thyroid-stimulating hormone receptor antibody; TSH = thyroid-stimulating hormone; TSI = thyroid-stimulating immunoglobulins.

**Table 4-4 Management of Thyroid Eye Disease**

| |
|---|
| **Mild disease** |
| Observation |
| Patient education and lifestyle changes |
| Smoking cessation |
| Salt restriction |
| Elevation of head of bed |
| Use of sunglasses |
| Ocular surface lubrication |
| Establishment of a euthyroid state |
| Oral selenium |
| **Moderate disease** |
| Topical cyclosporine |
| Eyelid taping at night |
| Moisture goggles or chambers |
| Prism glasses or selective ocular patching |
| Moderate-dose oral steroid therapy |
| **Severe disease** |
| High-dose intravenous steroid therapy |
| Surgical orbital decompression (followed by strabismus surgery and/or eyelid surgery) |
| Periocular radiotherapy |
| **Refractory disease** |
| Steroid-sparing immunomodulators (rituximab, others) |

Most patients with TED require only supportive care, including use of topical ocular lubricants; in some cases, topical cyclosporine has helped reduce ocular surface irritation. Patients may also find certain lifestyle changes helpful. For example, eating a reduced-salt diet limits water retention and orbital edema, and sleeping with the head of the bed elevated specifically reduces fluid retention within the orbit. Wearing wraparound sunglasses relieves symptoms of dry eye and photophobia. If diplopia is present, use of temporary prism lenses helps maintain binocular fusion during the active phase of the disease. Preliminary work has shown that blocking the CD20 receptor on B lymphocytes with rituximab affects the clinical course of TED by reducing inflammation and proptosis; however, a recent Cochrane review suggests that there is not currently enough evidence to support the use of rituximab in treating TED.

If orbital inflammation is severe, intervention may be necessary to prevent or ameliorate corneal exposure, globe subluxation, or optic neuropathy. Therapy usually is directed toward either decreasing orbital congestion and inflammation (through use of periocular corticosteroids or, if response is inadequate, by administration of systemic corticosteroids or periocular radiotherapy) or expanding the orbital bony volume (by surgical orbital decompression).

Establishing a euthyroid state is an important part of the care of patients with TED. Hyperthyroidism is most commonly treated with antithyroid drugs. If the patient does not tolerate the medications or if the medications fail to restore a persistent euthyroid state, the clinician usually tries radioactive iodine (RAI) as the next treatment modality. In some studies, TED has been demonstrated to worsen after RAI treatment, presumably because of the release of TSH-R antigens, which incite an enhanced immune response. In addition, hypothyroidism occurring after RAI treatment may exacerbate TED via stimulation of TSH-R. Hyperthyroid patients with severe, active TED; those with elevated $T_3$ levels; and smokers appear to be at greatest risk for exacerbation of eye disease after RAI treatment. Consequently, some patients are treated concurrently with oral corticosteroids. Although this may be a reasonable strategy for high-risk patients, the regular use of moderate-dose prednisone for 3 months, during which time the thyroid gland involutes, is not indicated for the average patient. Block-and-replace therapy with iodine 131, methimazole, and thyroxine may prevent exacerbation of eye findings by limiting posttreatment TSH spikes. Patients with severe TED (rapidly progressive and congestive, with compressive optic neuropathy) may, as an alternative to RAI, benefit from thyroidectomy, which renders them hypothyroid without extended antigen release.

Approximately 20% of patients with TED undergo surgical treatment. In one review, 13% of patients underwent eyelid surgery; 9%, strabismus surgery; and 7%, orbital decompression. Only 2% required all 3 types of surgery. Men and older patients are more likely to have TED severe enough to require surgical intervention. Surgery should be delayed until the disease has stabilized, unless urgent intervention is required to reverse vision loss due to compressive optic neuropathy or corneal exposure unresponsive to maximal medical measures. Elective orbital decompression, strabismus surgery, and eyelid retraction repair are usually not considered until a euthyroid state has been maintained and the ophthalmic signs have been confirmed to be stable for 6–9 months.

Acute-phase TED, which features compressive optic neuropathy and flare-ups deemed clinically significant based on scoring systems (eg, VISA, CAS), can be effectively treated with IV corticosteroids. The usual starting dose is 500 mg to 1 g methylprednisolone weekly for 6–12 weeks. Hepatic function should be checked before initial administration and monitored throughout treatment because of this agent's reported association with fatal hepatotoxicity. If oral corticosteroids are used, the usual starting dose is 1 mg/kg of prednisone. This dose is maintained for 2–4 weeks until a clinical response is apparent. The dose is then reduced as rapidly as can be tolerated by the patient, based on the clinical response of optic nerve function. Although they are effective at reversing optic nerve compression, high-dose corticosteroids are poorly tolerated and are associated with an extensive list of potential systemic adverse effects, which limit their long-term use. Thus, some authors have advocated the adjunctive use of orbital radiotherapy (2000 cGy). The mechanism for radiotherapy's effect on the orbit is not well understood, but beyond temporary lymphocyte sterilization, there is evidence that this dose induces terminal differentiation of fibroblasts and kills tissue-bound monocytes, which play an important role in antigen presentation.

A number of studies have demonstrated the effectiveness of orbital radiotherapy in the treatment of compressive optic neuropathy. However, the literature lacks consensus on this topic. It is important to note that radiation therapy carries the rare risk of exacerbating retinopathy, particularly in patients with diabetes mellitus or other risk factors for ischemic retinopathy.

Although it has historically been used to treat optic neuropathy, severe orbital congestion, and advanced proptosis, orbital decompression has been used increasingly to restore normal globe position in patients without sight-threatening ophthalmopathy. In the stable phase of disease, the surgical plan for decompression should be graded to achieve the greatest return to the premorbid state at the least possible risk. Preoperative review of the patient's old photos allows the surgeon to determine the amount of decompressive effect desired. The preoperative CT scan details the relative contributions of extraocular muscle enlargement and fat expansion to the proptosis (see Figs 4-7, 4-8). Typically, there is a difference in the phenotype of the orbital involvement based on the patient's age. Patients younger than 40 years show enlargement of the orbital fat compartment, whereas those older than 40 typically show more significant extraocular muscle enlargement. This difference determines the effectiveness of bone versus fat decompression surgery. Orbital decompression may alter extraocular motility; if orbital decompression is indicated, the orbital surgery should precede strabismus surgery. See Chapter 7 for further discussion of orbital decompression.

If intractable diplopia persists in primary gaze or in the reading position, prisms or strabismus surgery may be helpful in restoring single vision. In addition, procedures such as levator recession and/or müllerectomy to correct eyelid retraction may decrease corneal exposure and help improve appearance. Because extraocular muscle surgery may affect eyelid retraction, strabismus surgery should precede eyelid surgery.

Alternatively, botulinum toxin may be employed in rare instances to temporarily paralyze a tight extraocular muscle in restrictive strabismus or to weaken the levator palpebrae superioris muscle to treat eyelid retraction.

A long-term follow-up study of patients in an incidence cohort demonstrated that vision loss from optic neuropathy was uncommon and that persistent diplopia usually could be treated with prism spectacles. Subjectively, however, more than 50% of patients thought that their eyes looked abnormal, and 38% of patients were dissatisfied with the appearance of their eyes. Thus, although few patients experience long-term functional impairment from TED, the psychological and aesthetic sequelae of the disease are considerable.

Bartalena L, Marcocci C, Bogazzi F, et al. Relation between therapy for hyperthyroidism and the course of Graves' ophthalmopathy. *N Engl J Med.* 1998;338(2):73–78.

Bartley GB, Fatourechi V, Kadrmas EF, et al. Long-term follow-up of Graves ophthalmopathy in an incidence cohort. *Ophthalmology.* 1996;103(6):958–962.

Bradley EA, Gower EW, Bradley DJ, et al. Orbital radiation for Graves ophthalmopathy: a report by the American Academy of Ophthalmology. *Ophthalmology.* 2008;115(2):398–409.

Dolman PJ, Rootman J. VISA classification for Graves orbitopathy. *Ophthal Plast Reconstr Surg.* 2006;22(5):319–324.

Marocci C, Kahaly GJ, Krassas GE, et al; European Group on Graves' Orbitopathy. Selenium and the course of mild Graves' orbitopathy. *N Engl J Med.* 2011;364(20):1920–1931.

Minakaran N, Ezra DG. Rituximab for thyroid-associated ophthalmopathy. *Cochrane Database Syst Rev.* 2013;5:CD009226. Epub 2013 May 31.

Morgenstern KE, Evanchan J, Foster JA, et al. Botulinum toxin type A for dysthyroid upper eyelid retraction. *Ophthal Plast Reconstr Surg.* 2004;20(3):181–185.

Mourits MP, van Kempen-Harteveld ML, Garcia MB, Koppeschaar HP, Tick L, Terwee CB. Radiotherapy for Graves' orbitopathy: randomised placebo-controlled study. *Lancet.* 2000; 355(9214):1505–1509.

Thornton J, Kelly SP, Harrison RA, Edwards R. Cigarette smoking and thyroid eye disease: a systematic review. *Eye (Lond).* 2007;21(9):1135–1145.

Trokel S, Kazim M, Moore S. Orbital fat removal. Decompression for Graves orbitopathy. *Ophthalmology.* 1993;100(5):674–682.

Verity DH, Rose GE. Acute thyroid eye disease (TED): principles of medical and surgical management. *Eye (Lond).* 2013;27(3):308–319. Epub 2013 Feb 15.

## IgG4 Disease

Recently, another immune-mediated entity associated with orbitopathy has been described. IgG4 disease is a multiorgan disease with mass-forming lesions. It is characterized by the infiltration of IgG4-expressing plasma cells with inflammatory T lymphocytes in various organs, producing elevation in the levels of serum IgG4 and an acute-phase response. The disease is associated with dacryoadenitis, xanthogranuloma, orbital amyloidosis, and nonspecific orbital inflammation. IgG4 disease responds well to treatment with steroids.

Karamchandani JR, Younes SF, Warnke RA, Natkunam Y. IgG4-related systemic sclerosing disease of the ocular adnexa: a potential mimic of ocular lymphoma. *Am J Clin Pathol.* 2012;137(5):699–711.

## Vasculitis

The vasculitides are inflammatory conditions in which the vessel walls are infiltrated by inflammatory cells. These lesions represent a type III hypersensitivity reaction to circulating immune complexes and usually lead to significant ocular or orbital morbidity. They are often associated with systemic vasculitis. The following discussion focuses mainly on the orbital manifestations of the vasculitides. See also BCSC Section 1, *Update on General Medicine*; Section 5, *Neuro-Ophthalmology*; and Section 9, *Intraocular Inflammation and Uveitis.*

### Giant cell arteritis

Although the orbital vessels are inflamed in giant cell arteritis (GCA; also known as *temporal arteritis*), it is not typically thought of as an orbital disorder. The vasculitis affects the aorta and branches of the external and internal carotid arteries and vertebral arteries but usually spares the intracranial carotid branches, which lack an elastic lamina. Symptoms of vision loss are caused by central retinal artery occlusion or ischemic optic neuropathy, and diplopia may result from ischemic dysfunction of other cranial nerves. Symptoms of headache, scalp tenderness, jaw claudication, or malaise are often present. The erythrocyte sedimentation rate (ESR) is markedly elevated in 90% of patients, and diagnostic confidence is increased if the C-reactive protein level and the platelet count are elevated. Temporal artery biopsy usually provides a definitive diagnosis, but bilateral biopsies are sometimes necessary because of intervals of normal tissue between affected segments. GCA should be managed as an ophthalmic emergency. Failure to diagnose and treat GCA immediately after loss of vision in one eye is particularly tragic because timely treatment with corticosteroids usually prevents an attack in the second eye. Generalized orbital ischemia resulting from temporal arteritis is a rare manifestation of the disease.

Goodwin JA. Temporal arteritis. *Focal Points: Clinical Modules for Ophthalmologists.* San Francisco: American Academy of Ophthalmology; 1992, module 2.

### Granulomatosis with polyangiitis

Granulomatosis with polyangiitis (GPA), formerly known as Wegener granulomatosis, is characterized by necrotizing granulomatous vasculitis, lesions of the upper and lower respiratory tract, necrotizing glomerulonephritis, and a small-vessel vasculitis that can affect any organ system, including the orbit. Clinically, the full-blown syndrome includes sinus mucosal involvement with bone erosion, tracheobronchial necrotic lesions, cavitary lung lesions, and glomerulonephritis (Fig 4-9). The orbit and nasolacrimal drainage system may be involved by extension from the surrounding sinuses. Up to 25% of patients with GPA have associated scleritis. Limited forms of the disease have been described in which the renal component is absent or in which there is solitary orbital involvement by a granulomatous and lymphocytic vasculitis. Such isolated orbital involvement may be unilateral or bilateral; may lack frank necrotizing vasculitis on histologic examination; and, in the absence of respiratory tract and renal findings, may be difficult to diagnose.

Characteristic pathologic findings consist of the triad of vasculitis, granulomatous inflammation (with or without giant cells), and tissue necrosis. Often, only 1 or 2 of these 3 are present on extrapulmonary biopsies. Antineutrophil cytoplasmic antibody (ANCA) titers measured by serum immunofluorescence have been shown to be associated with certain systemic vasculitides. The ANCA test distinguishes 2 types of immunofluorescence patterns. Diffuse granular fluorescence within the cytoplasm (c-ANCA) is highly specific for GPA. This pattern is caused by autoantibodies directed against proteinase-3, which can

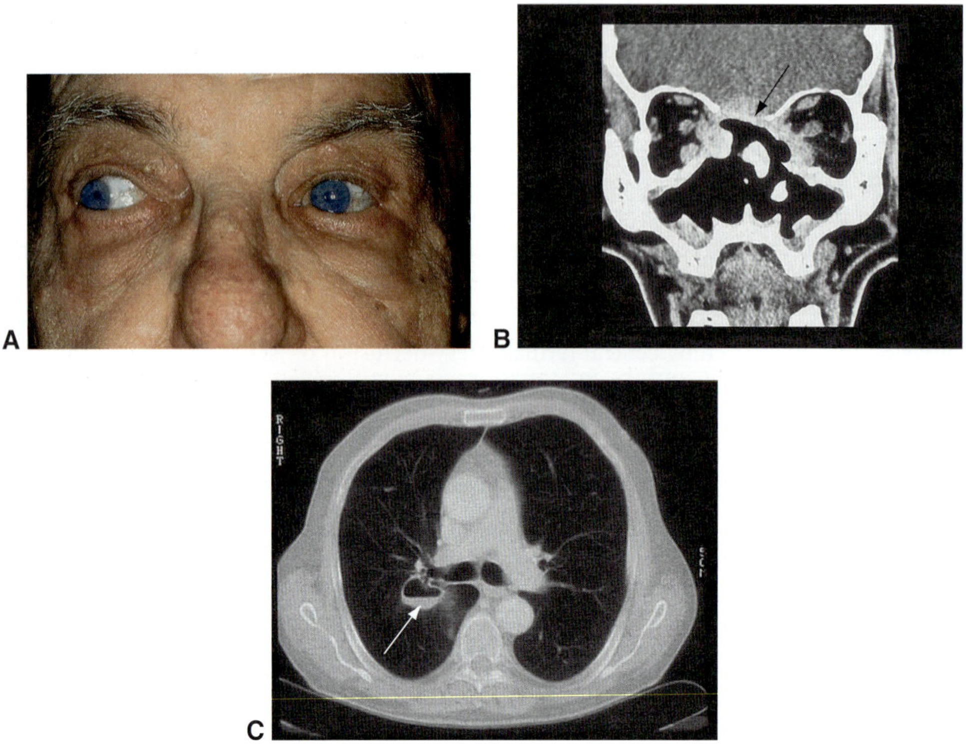

**Figure 4-9** Granulomatosis with polyangiitis (GPA), formerly known as Wegener granulomatosis. **A,** Restrictive strabismus of the left eye due to inflammatory tissue extending into the medial aspects of the orbit. **B,** Coronal CT scan showing extensive destruction of the nasal and sinus cavities with inflammatory tissue extending into orbits and brain *(arrow)*. **C,** CT of chest showing cavitary lung lesions *(arrow)*. *(Courtesy of Jeffrey A. Nerad, MD.)*

also be detected by enzyme-linked immunosorbent assay (ELISA). Fluorescence surrounding the nucleus (p-ANCA) is an artifact of ethanol fixation and can be caused by autoantibodies against many different target antigens. This finding is therefore nonspecific and needs to be confirmed by ELISA for ANCA reacting with myeloperoxidase (MPO-ANCA). MPO-ANCA testing has a high specificity for small-vessel vasculitis. Absolute levels of ANCA do not define disease severity or activity, but changing titers can give a general idea of disease activity or response to therapy. The c-ANCA findings may be negative early in the course of the disease, especially in the absence of multisystem involvement.

GPA may proceed to a fulminant, life-threatening course. Treatment relies on immunosuppression, usually with cyclophosphamide, and should be coordinated with a rheumatologist. Treatment with corticosteroids alone is associated with a significantly higher rate of mortality. Long-term treatment with TMP-SMX appears to suppress disease activity in some patients.

### *Polyarteritis nodosa*

Like giant cell arteritis, polyarteritis nodosa is a vasculitis that may affect orbital vessels but does not usually cause orbital disease. Instead, the ophthalmic manifestations are the result of retinal and choroidal infarction. In this multisystem disease, small-sized and medium-sized arteries are affected by inflammation characterized by the presence of neutrophils and eosinophils, with necrosis of the muscularis layer.

## Sarcoidosis

Sarcoidosis is a multisystem disease of unknown origin. It occurs most commonly in persons of African or Scandinavian descent. The lungs are most commonly involved, but the orbit may be affected. Histologically, the lesions are composed of noncaseating collections of epithelioid histiocytes in a granulomatous pattern. A mononuclear inflammation often appears at the periphery of the granuloma. The lacrimal gland is the site most frequently affected within the orbit, and the inflammation is typically bilateral. Gallium scanning of the lacrimal glands is nonspecific but has been reported to show lacrimal gland involvement in 80% of patients with systemic sarcoidosis, although only 7% of patients have clinically detectable enlargement of the lacrimal glands. Other orbital soft tissues, including the extraocular muscles and optic nerve, are very rarely involved. Infrequently, sinus involvement with associated lytic bone lesions invades into the adjacent orbit.

A biopsy specimen of the affected lacrimal gland or of a suspicious conjunctival lesion may establish the diagnosis. Random conjunctival biopsies have a low yield. Chest radiography or CT to detect hilar adenopathy or pulmonary infiltrates, blood tests for angiotensin-converting enzyme, and measurement of serum lysozyme and serum calcium levels may be used to establish the diagnosis of sarcoidosis. Because gallium scanning is nonspecific, bronchoscopy with washings and biopsy may be needed to confirm the diagnosis.

Isolated orbital lesions demonstrating noncaseating granulomas can occur without associated systemic disease. This condition is called orbital sarcoidosis.

See BCSC Section 5, *Neuro-Ophthalmology,* and Section 9, *Intraocular Inflammation and Uveitis,* for more extensive discussion and clinical photographs of sarcoidosis.

## Nonspecific Orbital Inflammation

Nonspecific orbital inflammation (NSOI) is defined as a benign inflammatory process of the orbit characterized by a polymorphous lymphoid infiltrate with varying degrees of fibrosis, without a known local or systemic cause. It is a diagnosis of exclusion that should be used only after all specific causes of inflammation have been eliminated. It has previously been called *orbital pseudotumor, idiopathic orbital inflammation,* or *idiopathic orbital inflammatory syndrome.*

The pathogenesis of NSOI remains controversial. However, it is generally believed to be an immune-mediated process because it is often associated with systemic immunologic disorders including Crohn disease, systemic lupus erythematosus, rheumatoid arthritis, diabetes mellitus, myasthenia gravis, and ankylosing spondylitis. In addition, NSOI typically has a rapid and favorable response to systemic corticosteroid treatment, as well as to other immunosuppressive agents, indicating a cell-mediated component.

The symptoms and clinical findings in NSOI may vary widely but are dictated by the degree and anatomical location of the inflammation. NSOI tends to occur in 5 orbital locations or patterns. In order of frequency, the most common are the extraocular muscles *(myositis)*, the lacrimal gland *(dacryoadenitis)*, the anterior orbit (eg, *scleritis*), the orbital apex, or diffuse inflammation throughout the orbit. Although NSOI is usually limited to the orbit, it may also extend into the adjacent sinuses or intracranial space.

Although symptoms depend on the location of the involved tissue, deep-rooted, boring pain is a typical feature. Extraocular muscle restriction, proptosis, conjunctival inflammation, and chemosis are common, as are eyelid erythema and soft-tissue swelling. Pain associated with ocular movement suggests myositis. Vision may be impaired if the optic nerve or posterior sclera is involved. In dacryoadenitis, CT reveals diffuse enlargement of the lacrimal gland (the most common target area in this type). CT, MRI, and ultrasonography reveal thickening of the extraocular muscles if the inflammatory response has a myositic component. The extraocular muscle tendons of insertion may be thickened in up to 50% of patients with NSOI; in contrast, TED typically spares the muscle insertions. An inflammatory infiltrate of the retrobulbar fat pad is commonly seen, and contrast enhancement of the sclera may be caused by tenonitis (producing the *ring sign*). B-scan ultrasonography often shows an acoustically hollow area corresponding to an edematous Tenon capsule. Peripheral blood eosinophilia, elevated ESR and antinuclear antibody levels, and mild cerebrospinal fluid pleocytosis are often present.

These typical clinical presentations, combined with orbital imaging, strongly suggest the diagnosis of NSOI (Fig 4-10). Prompt response to systemic steroids supports the

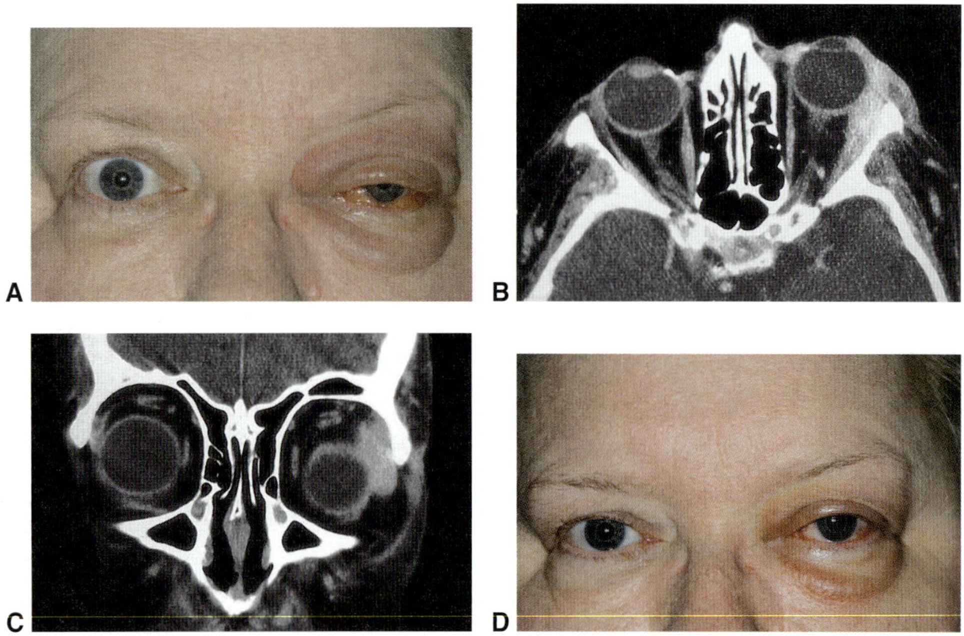


**Figure 4-10** **A,** Acute onset of inflammation of the left eyelid, proptosis, pain, and left lateral rectus paresis. **B,** Axial CT scan showing left-eye proptosis and hazy inflammatory swelling of lateral rectus and lacrimal gland, suggestive of the diagnosis of nonspecific orbital inflammation. **C,** Coronal CT scan showing inflammatory process adjacent to the lateral rectus. **D,** Marked improvement of inflammatory changes following a 48-hour course of oral prednisone. *(Parts A and D courtesy of Keith D. Carter, MD; parts B and C courtesy of Robert C. Kersten, MD.)*

diagnosis, but the physician must remember that the inflammation associated with other orbital processes (eg, metastases, lymphoma, ruptured dermoid cysts, infections) may also improve with systemic steroid administration. A thorough systemic evaluation should be undertaken if there is any uncertainty regarding the diagnosis.

Not all patients with NSOI present with the classic signs and symptoms. There may be atypical pain, limited inflammatory signs, or presence of a fibrotic variant called *sclerosing NSOI*. Such lesions more commonly require biopsy for diagnosis. Simultaneous bilateral orbital inflammation in adults suggests the possibility of systemic vasculitis. In children, however, approximately one-third of cases of NSOI are bilateral and are rarely associated with systemic disorders, although half of the children have headache, fever, vomiting, abdominal pain, and lethargy. Uveitis, elevated ESR, and eosinophilia may also be more common in children.

Histologically, NSOI is characterized by a pleomorphic cellular infiltrate consisting of lymphocytes, plasma cells, and eosinophils with variable degrees of reactive fibrosis. The fibrosis becomes more marked as the process becomes more chronic, and early or acute cases are usually more responsive to steroids than are the advanced stages associated with fibrosis. The sclerosing subtype demonstrates a predominance of fibrosis with sparse cellular inflammation. Historically, hypercellular lymphoid proliferations were often grouped with the pseudotumors; however, more recent consensus confirms that such proliferations are different clinical and histologic entities from NSOI.

Mottow-Lippa L, Jakobiec FA, Smith M. Idiopathic inflammatory orbital pseudotumor in childhood. II. Results of diagnostic tests and biopsies. *Ophthalmology.* 1981;88(6):565–574.

### *Treatment*

Once other diagnoses have been excluded, initial therapy for NSOI consists of systemic corticosteroids. Initial daily adult dosage is typically 1 mg/kg of prednisone. Acute cases generally respond rapidly, with an abrupt resolution of the associated pain. Steroids can be tapered as soon as the clinical response is complete, but this tapering should proceed more slowly below about 40 mg/day and very slowly below 20 mg/day, based on the clinical response. Rapid reduction of systemic steroids may allow a recurrence of inflammatory symptoms and signs. Some investigators believe that the use of pulse-dosed IV dexamethasone followed by oral prednisone may produce clinical improvement when oral prednisone alone fails to control the inflammation.

Because other pathologic orbital processes may be masked by steroids, an incomplete therapeutic response or recurrent disease suggests the need for orbital biopsy, which can provide histologic confirmation and exclude specific inflammatory diseases. Thus, other investigators advise biopsy before empiric steroids are begun to avoid delayed or missed diagnoses. Biopsy allows identification of specific disease and possible systemic implications and thereby enables the clinician to develop a better-targeted treatment plan. In one study, 50% of biopsied inflammatory lacrimal gland lesions were associated with systemic disease, including GPA, sclerosing inflammation, Sjögren syndrome, sarcoidal reactions, and autoimmune disease.

Given the low morbidity of the procedure and the high incidence of systemic disease involving the lacrimal gland, biopsy is recommended for isolated inflammation of the lacrimal gland. Many advocate biopsy of almost all infiltrative lesions, except for 2 clinical scenarios: orbital myositis and orbital apex syndrome. In these situations, characteristic clinical and radiographic findings may strongly support the presumed diagnosis, and the risk of biopsy may outweigh the risk of a missed diagnosis. However, cases of recurrent or nonresponsive orbital myositis or orbital apex syndrome warrant a biopsy.

*Sclerosing NSOI* responds poorly to steroids and to low-dose (2000 cGy) radiotherapy and typically requires more aggressive immunosuppression with cyclosporine, methotrexate, or cyclophosphamide.

Mombaerts I, Goldschmeding R, Schlingemann RO, Koornneef L. What is orbital pseudotumor? *Surv Ophthalmol.* 1996;41(1):66–78.

Rootman J. *Orbital Disease: Present Status and Future Challenges.* Boca Raton, FL: Taylor & Francis; 2005:1–13.

Rootman J, McCarthy M, White V, Harris G, Kennerdell J. Idiopathic sclerosing inflammation of the orbit: a distinct clinicopathologic entity. *Ophthalmology.* 1994;101(3):570–584.

CHAPTER 5

# Orbital Neoplasms and Malformations

## Vascular Tumors, Malformations, and Fistulas

### Infantile (Capillary) Hemangioma

Infantile (capillary) hemangiomas are common primary benign tumors of the orbit in children (Fig 5-1). These lesions may be present at birth or appear in the first few weeks of life. Hemangiomas enlarge dramatically over the first 6–12 months of life and then begin to involute at some point after the first year of life; 75% of lesions resolve during the first 3–7 years of life. Female sex, low birth weight, prematurity, and maternal chorionic villus sampling are associated with infantile hemangiomas.

Congenital infantile hemangiomas may be superficial—in which case they involve the skin and appear as a bright red, soft mass with a dimpled texture—or they may be subcutaneous and bluish. Hemangiomas located deeper within the orbit may present as a progressively enlarging mass without any overlying skin change. Magnetic resonance imaging (MRI) may be used to help distinguish infantile hemangiomas from other vascular malformations by demonstrating characteristic fine intralesional vascular channels and high blood flow.

In the periocular area, infantile hemangiomas have a propensity for the superonasal quadrant of the orbit and the medial upper eyelid (see also Congenital Eyelid Lesions in Chapter 10). They may be associated with hemangiomas on other parts of the body; lesions that involve the neck can compromise the airway and lead to respiratory obstruction, and multiple large visceral lesions can produce thrombocytopenia *(Kasabach-Merritt syndrome).*

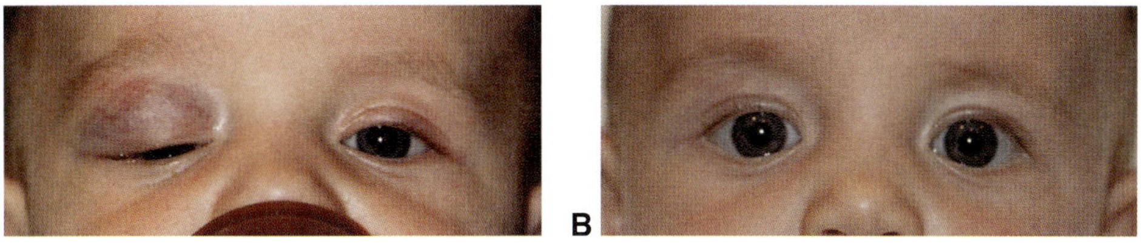

A B

**Figure 5-1** **A,** Infantile (capillary) hemangioma of the right upper eyelid. **B,** Marked regression of infantile hemangioma 6 weeks after propranolol therapy was initiated. *(Courtesy of William R. Katowitz, MD.)*

### *Management*

The main ocular complications of infantile hemangiomas are amblyopia, strabismus, and anisometropia. Disruption of vision or severe disfigurement may require therapy, but treatment may be deferred until it is clear that the natural course of the lesion will not lead to the desired result.

Most lesions regress spontaneously; therefore, observation, refractive correction, and amblyopia therapy are the first line of management. For infantile hemangiomas requiring therapy, the management paradigm has changed. New treatments using β-blockers, including oral propranolol and topical timolol gel, are used as initial therapy. Topical timolol gel may be initiated for superficial tumors, with limited systemic adverse effects. Oral propranolol, used for larger and deeper lesions, appears to have fewer adverse effects than systemic steroids. Hypoglycemia and cardiovascular adverse effects are possible. For lesions unresponsive to or showing limited improvement with β-blockers, traditional treatment with steroids, administered either topically, by local injection, or orally are used (see Congenital Eyelid Lesions in Chapter 10). Adverse effects of steroid injection include skin necrosis, subcutaneous fat atrophy, systemic growth retardation, and retinal embolic vision loss. Surgical excision with meticulous hemostasis may be considered for nodular lesions that are smaller, subcutaneous, or refractory to steroids. Radiation therapy has also been used, but it can cause cataract formation, bony hypoplasia, and future malignancy. Pulsed-dye laser therapy may be used to treat superficial components of the hemangioma. Sclerosing solutions are not recommended because of the severe scarring that results.

Chambers CB, Katowitz WR, Katowitz JA, Binenbaum G. A controlled study of topical 0.25% timolol maleate gel for the treatment of cutaneous infantile capillary hemangiomas. *Ophthal Plast Reconstr Surg.* 2012;28(2):103–106.

Fridman G, Grieser E, Hill R, Khuddus N, Bersani T, Slonim C. Propranolol for the treatment of orbital infantile hemangiomas. *Ophthal Plast Reconstr Surg.* 2011;27(3):190–194.

## Cavernous Hemangioma

Cavernous hemangiomas are the most common benign neoplasm of the orbit in adults (Fig 5-2). Women are affected more often than men. The principal finding is slowly progressive proptosis (see Fig 5-2A), but growth may accelerate during pregnancy. Other findings may include retinal striae, hyperopia, optic nerve compression, increased intraocular pressure (IOP), and strabismus. Orbital imaging shows a homogeneously enhancing, well-encapsulated mass that, on MRI, demonstrates small intralesional vascular channels containing slowly flowing blood. Chronic lesions may contain radiodense phleboliths. Arteriography and venography usually are not useful in diagnosis because the lesion has very limited communication with the systemic circulation.

Histologically, the lesions are encapsulated and are composed of large cavernous spaces containing red blood cells. The walls of the spaces contain smooth muscle.

### *Management*

Treatment consists of surgical excision if the lesion compromises ocular function, causes significant proptosis, or demonstrates significant growth. The surgical approach is dictated

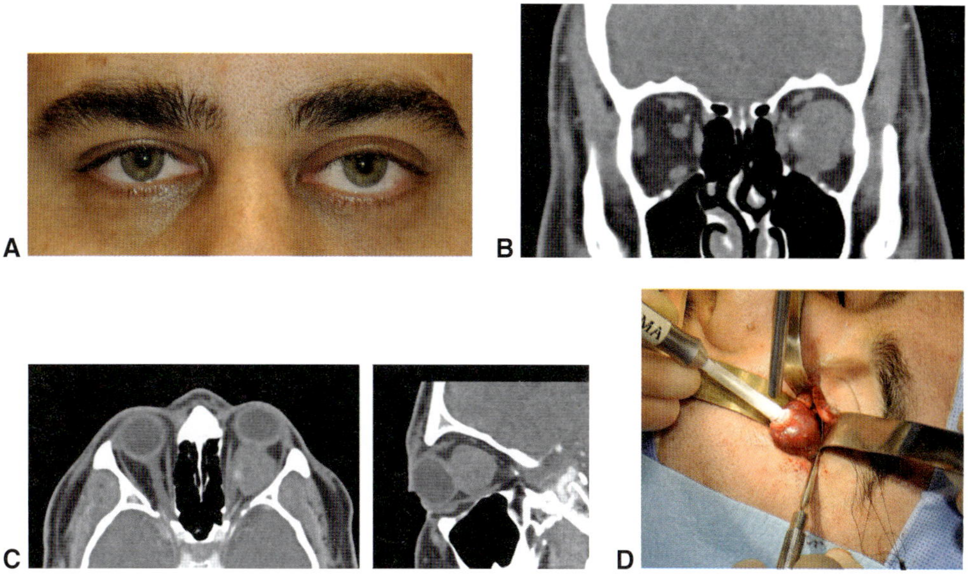

**Figure 5-2** **A,** Left cavernous hemangioma showing proptosis. **B,** Coronal computed tomography (CT) scans showing a well-circumscribed cavernous hemangioma within the muscle cone. **C,** Axial *(left)* and sagittal *(right)* CT scans showing the mass. **D,** Intraoperative traction with a cryoprobe allows complete removal of the mass. *(Courtesy of Bobby S. Korn, MD, PhD.)*

by the location of the lesion. Because of their relative isolation from the surrounding tissues, cavernous hemangiomas have surgical planes that allow easier separation of these tumors from normal orbital tissues, thus making them easier to remove than many other orbital tumors. Coronal imaging is important in determining the position of the cavernous hemangioma relative to the optic nerve. These tumors rarely involute spontaneously.

### Hemangiopericytoma

Hemangiopericytomas are uncommon encapsulated, hypervascular, hypercellular lesions that appear in midlife. These lesions resemble cavernous hemangiomas on both computed tomography (CT) and MRI, but they appear bluish intraoperatively. Hemangiopericytomas are composed of plump pericytes that surround a rich capillary network. Histologically, these lesions are unique in that microscopically "benign" lesions may recur and metastasize, whereas microscopically "malignant" lesions may remain localized. There is no correlation between the mitotic rate and the clinical behavior. Treatment consists of complete excision because they may recur, undergo malignant degeneration, or metastasize.

### Lymphatic Malformation

Lymphatic malformations (LMs; previously called *lymphangiomas*) (Fig 5-3A) are believed to represent vascular dysgenesis. They result from a disruption of the initially pluripotent vascular anlage, which leads to aberrant development and congenital malformation. In the orbit, they usually become apparent in the first or second decade of life; they may also

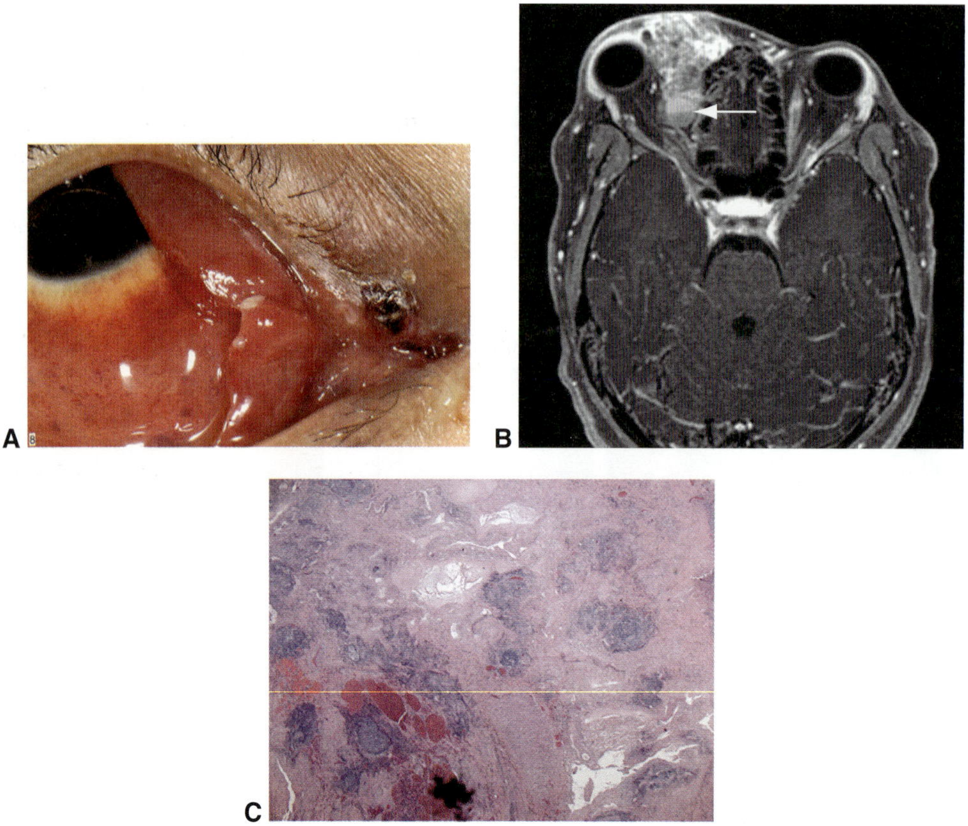

**Figure 5-3** **A,** Lymphatic malformation. **B,** Postcontrast axial T1-weighted magnetic resonance image (MRI) with fat suppression. Note the cyst with fluid level *(arrow)*. **C,** Hematoxylin and eosin stain showing germinal centers and lymph-filled channels. *(Courtesy of Alon Kahana, MD, PhD.)*

occur in the conjunctiva, eyelids, oropharynx, or sinuses. LMs often contain both venous and lymphatic components. They may enlarge during upper respiratory tract infections, probably because of the response of the lymphoid tissues within the lesion. They may also present with sudden proptosis caused by spontaneous intralesional hemorrhage that can be diagnosed on MRI (Fig 5-3B).

Histologically, LMs are characterized by large, serum-filled channels lined by flat endothelial cells that have immunostaining patterns consistent with lymphatic capillaries (Fig 5-3C). Because their endothelial cells do not proliferate, they are not neoplasms. Scattered follicles of lymphoid tissues are found in the interstitium. These lesions have an infiltrative pattern and are not encapsulated.

The natural history of LMs varies and is unpredictable. Some are localized and progress slowly, whereas others may diffusely infiltrate orbital structures and inexorably enlarge. Sudden hemorrhage from interstitial capillaries may present as abrupt proptosis or as a mass lesion. MRI may show pathognomonic features (multiple grapelike cystic lesions with fluid–fluid layering of the serum and red blood cells), confirming the diagnosis (see Fig 5-3B).

### *Management*

Historically, surgical intervention was deferred unless vision was affected. Because of the infiltrating nature of LMs, surgical resection was frustrating; subtotal resection was generally necessary to avoid sacrificing important structures. Recently, intralesional sclerosing agents have been successful in treating the larger cystic components of these lesions and reducing tumor bulk. The cyst is drained, and its extent is evaluated with contrast media. Then sodium morrhuate is introduced and withdrawn, and the cyst is rinsed. Absolute alcohol or other sclerosing agents are then introduced, withdrawn, and rinsed. More than one treatment may be required. Retained sclerosing foams of doxycycline and bleomycin have been successful in treating the microcysts. The lower incidence of adverse effects associated with sclerosing treatments has presented new opportunities for intervention.

When acute hemorrhage occurs and is complicated by significant proptosis, optic neuropathy, or corneal ulceration, ultrasound-guided aspiration of blood through a hollow-bore needle or by open surgical exploration can be attempted. Mild hematomas may resolve spontaneously.

Noncontiguous intracranial vascular malformations have been reported to occur in up to 25% of patients with orbital LMs. These lesions have a low rate of spontaneous hemorrhage and are not treated prophylactically.

Harris GJ. Orbital vascular malformations: a consensus statement on terminology and its clinical implications. Orbital Society. *Am J Ophthalmol.* 1999;127(4):453–455.

Harris GJ, Sakol PJ, Bonavolontà G, De Conciliis C. An analysis of thirty cases of orbital lymphangioma: pathophysiologic considerations and management recommendations. *Ophthalmology.* 1990;97(12):1583–1592.

Hill RH III, Shiels WE II, Foster JA, Czyz CN, Everman KR, Cahill KV. Percutaneous drainage and ablation as first line therapy for macrocystic and microcystic orbital lymphatic malformations. *Ophthal Plast Reconstr Surg.* 2012;28(2):119–125.

Rootman J, Hay E, Graeb D, Miller R. Orbital-adnexal lymphangiomas: a spectrum of hemodynamically isolated vascular hamartomas. *Ophthalmology.* 1986;93(12):1558–1570.

## Venous Malformation

Venous malformations of the orbit (also known as *orbital varices*) are low-flow vascular lesions resulting from vascular dysgenesis. Patients may exhibit enophthalmos at rest, when the lesion is not engorged. Proptosis that increases when the patient's head is dependent or after a Valsalva maneuver suggests the presence of a venous malformation. The diagnosis can be confirmed via contrast-enhanced rapid spiral CT during a Valsalva maneuver (or other means of decreasing venous return); cases show characteristic enlargement of the engorged veins. Phleboliths may be present on imaging.

Treatment is usually conservative. Biopsy should be avoided because of the risk of hemorrhage. Surgery is reserved for relief of significant pain or for cases in which the venous malformation causes vision-threatening compressive optic neuropathy. Complete surgical excision is difficult, as these lesions often intertwine with normal orbital structures and directly communicate with the abundant venous reservoir in the cavernous sinus. Intraoperative embolization of the lesion may aid surgical removal. Embolization with coils inserted through a distal venous cutdown has also been reported to diminish symptoms.

## Arteriovenous Malformation

Arteriovenous malformations (AVMs) are high-flow developmental anomalies that, like venous malformations, result from vascular dysgenesis. They are composed of abnormally formed anastomosing arteries and veins without an intervening capillary bed. Dilated corkscrew episcleral vessels may be prominent. After these lesions are studied via arteriography, they may be treated with selective occlusion of the feeding vessels, followed by surgical excision of the malformations. However, exsanguinating arterial hemorrhage may occur with surgical intervention.

## Arteriovenous Fistula

Arteriovenous fistulas are acquired lesions characterized by abnormal direct communication between an artery and a vein; blood flow does not pass through an intervening capillary bed. An arteriovenous fistula (Figs 5-4, 5-5) may be caused by trauma or degeneration. There are 2 forms of acquired arterial diversion that affect the cavernous sinus—direct carotid-cavernous sinus fistulas and indirect, or "dural," carotid-cavernous sinus fistulas. *Direct carotid-cavernous fistulas* are characterized by a connection between the internal carotid artery and the cavernous sinus and typically occur after a trauma that causes a tear or hole in a branch artery of the internal carotid within the cavernous sinus. They may also occur as a result of iatrogenic intervention, for example, during neurosurgical or neuroradiologic procedures. Direct carotid-cavernous fistulas have a high rate of

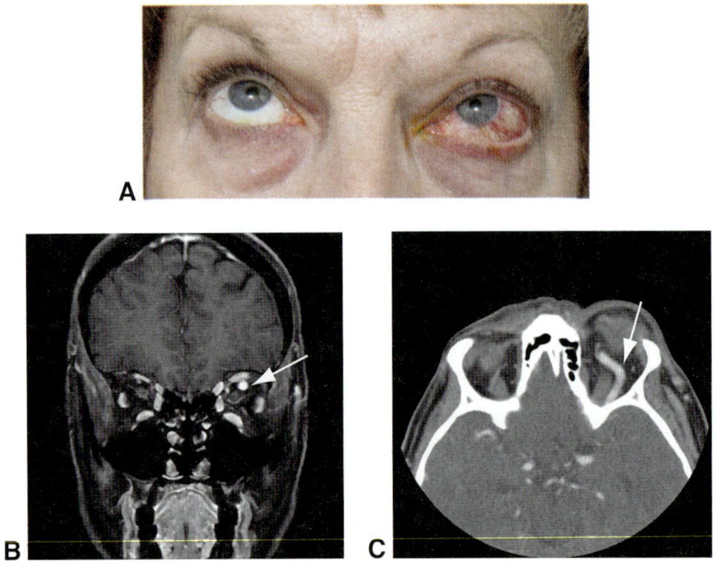


**Figure 5-4** **A,** Carotid-cavernous fistula of the left eye with proptosis due to congested orbital tissue and arterialization of episcleral and conjunctival vessels. **B,** MRI, coronal view (different patient), showing the dilated superior ophthalmic vein *(arrow)*. Note the enlarged superior rectus levator complex. **C,** CT angiogram. Intracranial arteries and the superior ophthalmic vein fill at the same time because the vein is arterialized. Blood is seen in the vein during the arterial phase *(arrow)*. *(Courtesy of Wayne Cornblath, MD.)*

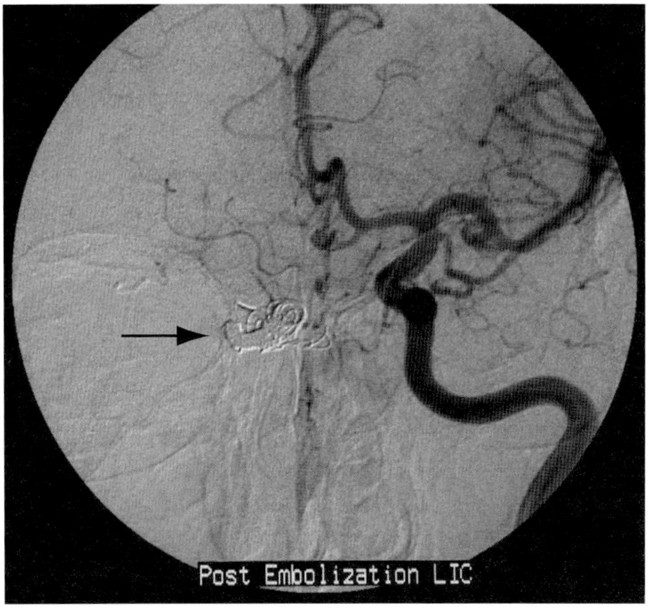


**Figure 5-5** Angiogram of a carotid-cavernous fistula after embolization. The coils in the fistula can be seen *(arrow)*. *(Courtesy of Morris E. Hartstein, MD.)*

blood flow and produce characteristic tortuous epibulbar vessels and a bruit that may be audible to the examiner and the patient. Pulsatile proptosis may also be present. Ischemic ocular damage results from diversion of arterialized blood into the venous system, which causes venous outflow obstruction. This in turn results in elevated IOP, choroidal effusions, blood in the Schlemm canal, and nongranulomatous anterior uveitis. Ocular motility abnormalities can occur from either congestion within the orbit or increased pressure in the cavernous sinus. The latter can cause compression of cranial nerves III, IV, or, most commonly, VI, with associated extraocular muscle palsies. CT scans may show diffuse enlargement of some or all of the extraocular muscles resulting from venous engorgement and a characteristically enlarged superior ophthalmic vein.

*Indirect,* or *dural, carotid-cavernous fistulas* are characterized by a connection between meningeal branches of the internal or external carotid artery or both and the cavernous sinus. These fistulas form most often as a degenerative process in older patients with systemic hypertension, vascular disease, and/or atherosclerosis. Because dural fistulas generally have lower rates of blood flow than direct carotid-cavernous fistulas, their onset can be insidious, with only mild orbital congestion, proptosis, and pain. Arterialization of the conjunctival veins causes chronic red eye. Increased episcleral venous pressure results in asymmetric elevation of IOP on the ipsilateral side, and patients with chronic fistulas are at risk for glaucomatous optic disc damage.

Magnetic resonance angiography (MRA) may be ordered to help diagnose arteriovenous fistulas. While MRA has a lower side effect profile, it is not as sensitive as conventional angiography; the x-ray angiogram thus remains the gold standard for diagnosis. Stroke is a rare but possible adverse effect of angiography.

Treatment of an arteriovenous fistula is determined by balancing the severity of symptoms and the risks associated with intervention. Intervention is typically an endovascular treatment (coils or glue) to block the fistula. As high-flow lesions, direct carotid-cavernous fistulas usually require intervention. Small dural carotid-cavernous fistulas often close spontaneously and may initially be observed. Data suggest that patients with dural carotid-cavernous fistulas are at higher risk for intracranial hemorrhage because of the arterialization of the venous system; therefore, some investigators have recommended more aggressive management of these lesions. Transvenous access is used to reach dural fistulas for treatment, while direct carotid-cavernous fistulas are still treated primarily via a transarterial approach. Occasionally, a transvenous approach by transcutaneous canalization of the superior ophthalmic vein is employed for embolization, which may require an orbitotomy to directly access the vein.

See BCSC Section 5, *Neuro-Ophthalmology,* for additional discussion of carotid-cavernous sinus fistulas.

Barrow DL, Spector RH, Braun IF, Landman JA, Tindall SC, Tindall GT. Classification and treatment of spontaneous carotid-cavernous sinus fistulas. *J Neurosurg.* 1985;62(2): 248–256.

Meyers PM, Halbach VV, Dowd CF, et al. Dural carotid cavernous fistula: definitive endovascular management and long-term follow-up. *Am J Ophthalmol.* 2002;134(1):85–92.

### Orbital Hemorrhage

An orbital hemorrhage may result from trauma, surgery, or spontaneous bleeding from vascular malformations. In rare instances, a spontaneous hemorrhage may be caused by a sudden increase in venous pressure (eg, due to a Valsalva maneuver). A spontaneous orbital hemorrhage almost always occurs in the superior subperiosteal space. It should be allowed to resorb unless there is associated visual compromise, in which case urgent drainage is indicated. Also see the section Orbital Hemorrhage in Chapter 6.

Atalla ML, McNab AA, Sullivan TJ, Sloan B. Nontraumatic subperiosteal orbital hemorrhage. *Ophthalmology.* 2001;108(1):183–189.

## Neural Tumors

The neural tumors include optic nerve gliomas, neurofibromas, meningiomas, and schwannomas.

### Optic Nerve Glioma

Optic nerve gliomas are uncommon, usually benign tumors that occur predominantly in children in the first decade of life (Fig 5-6).

Up to half of optic nerve gliomas are associated with neurofibromatosis. The chief clinical feature is gradual, painless, unilateral axial proptosis associated with vision loss and an afferent pupillary defect. Other ocular findings may include optic atrophy, optic disc swelling, nystagmus, and strabismus. The chiasm is involved in roughly half of cases

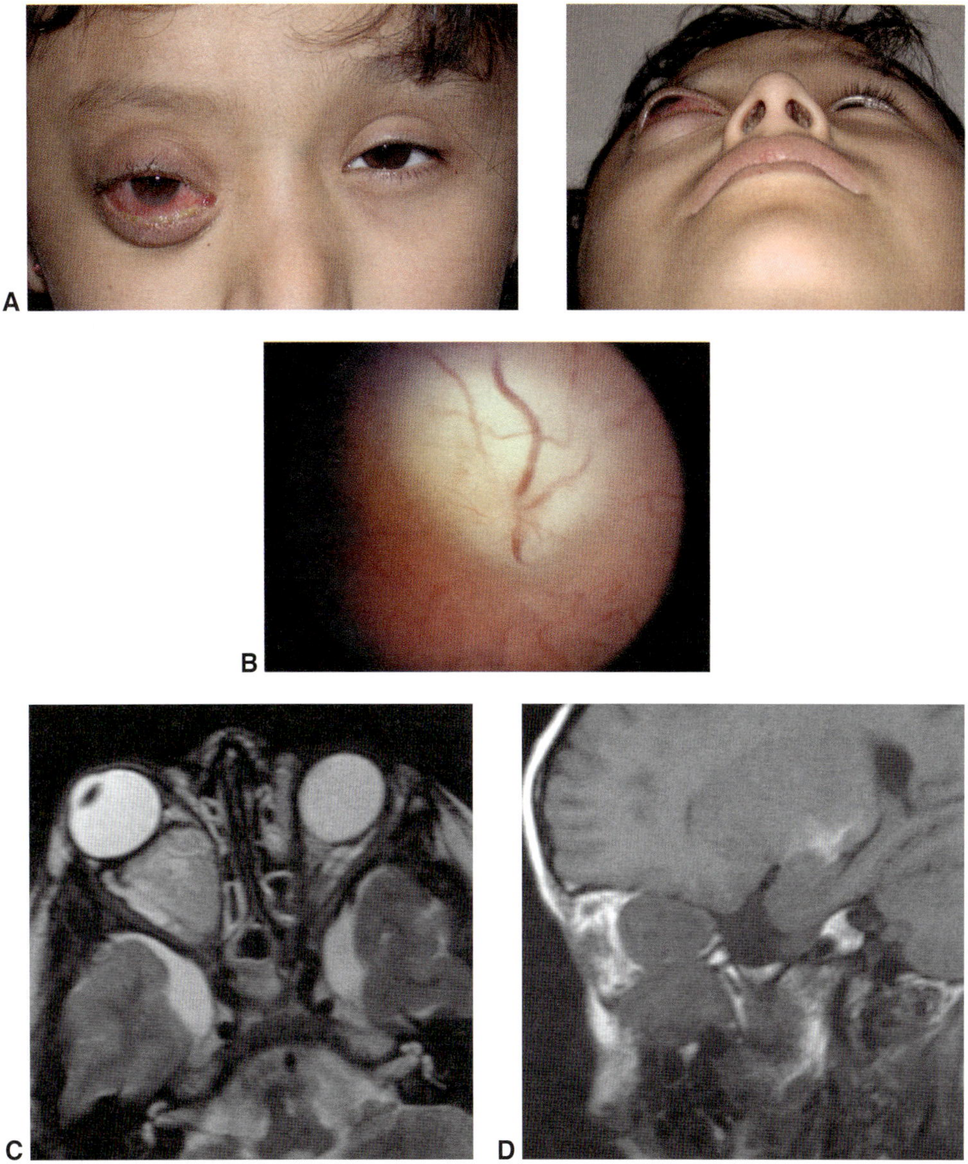

**Figure 5-6** **A,** Right optic nerve glioma. This child had severe proptosis and exposure and light perception vision. **B,** Funduscopic view. Note swollen disc with obscured disc margins. **C,** Axial T2-weighted MRI showing glioma of the optic nerve extending into the optic canal. **D,** Sagittal MRI showing a heterogeneous mass in the apex of the orbit. *(Parts A, C, and D courtesy of Raymond Douglas, MD; part B courtesy of Roger A. Dailey, MD.)*

of optic nerve glioma. Intracranial involvement may be associated with intracranial hypertension as well as decreased function of the hypothalamus and pituitary gland.

Gross pathology of resected tumors reveals a smooth, fusiform intradural lesion. Microscopically, benign tumors in children are considered to be juvenile pilocytic (hairlike) astrocytomas. Other histologic findings include arachnoid hyperplasia, mucosubstance, and Rosenthal fibers (see the discussion of the pathologic features of glioma in BCSC Section 4, *Ophthalmic Pathology and Intraocular Tumors*). Optic gliomas arising in patients with neurofibromatosis often proliferate in the subarachnoid space. Those occurring in patients without neurofibromatosis usually expand within the optic nerve substance without invading the dura mater.

Optic nerve gliomas can usually be diagnosed by means of orbital imaging. CT and MRI typically show fusiform enlargement of the optic nerve, often with stereotypical kinking of the nerve. MRI may also show cystic degeneration, if present, and may be more accurate in defining the extent of an optic canal lesion and intracranial disease.

It is usually unnecessary to perform a biopsy of a suspected lesion, as neuroimaging is frequently diagnostic. Moreover, biopsy tissue obtained from too peripheral a portion of the optic nerve may capture reactive meningeal hyperplasia adjacent to the optic nerve glioma and lead to the misdiagnosis of fibrous meningioma, and biopsy of the optic nerve itself may produce additional loss of visual field or vision.

*Malignant optic nerve gliomas (glioblastomas)* are very rare and tend to affect adult males. Initial signs and symptoms of malignant gliomas include severe retro-orbital pain, unilateral or bilateral vision loss, and, typically, massive swelling and hemorrhage of the optic nerve head (disc pallor may also be observed with posterior lesions). Despite treatment, including high-dose radiotherapy and chemotherapy, these tumors usually result in death within 6–12 months.

### Management

The treatment of optic nerve gliomas is controversial. Although most cases remain stable or progress very slowly, leading some authors to consider them benign hamartomas, the occasional case behaves aggressively. There are rare reports of spontaneous regression of optic nerve and visual pathway gliomas. Cystic enlargement of the lesions associated with sudden vision loss can occur even without true cellular growth. A treatment plan must be carefully individualized for each patient. The following options may be considered.

**Observation only** Presumed optic nerve glioma, particularly with good vision on the involved side, may be carefully followed if the radiographic evidence is characteristic of this type of tumor and if the glioma is confined to the orbit. Follow-up examinations and appropriate radiographic studies, preferably MRI, must be performed at regular intervals. Many patients maintain good vision and never require surgery.

**Surgical excision** Rapid intraorbital tumor growth may prompt surgical resection in an effort to isolate the tumor from the optic chiasm and thus prevent chiasmal invasion. The surgeon should use a transcranial approach to obtain tumor-free surgical margins. Additional surgical indications for excision of tumors confined to the orbit include proptosis with corneal exposure and cosmetic compromise that is unacceptable to the patient. Removal through an intracranial approach may also be indicated at the time of initial diagnosis or after a short period of observation if the tumor involves the prechiasmal intracranial portion of the optic nerve. Complete excision is possible if the tumor ends 2–3 mm anterior to the chiasm.

**Chemotherapy** Combination chemotherapy using actinomycin D, vincristine, etoposide, and other agents has also been reported to be effective in patients with progressive chiasmal-hypothalamic gliomas. Chemotherapy may delay the need for radiation therapy and thus enhance long-term intellectual development and preservation of endocrine function in children. However, chemotherapy may also carry long-term risks of bloodborne cancers.

**Radiation therapy** Radiation therapy is considered if the tumor cannot be resected (usually chiasmal or optic tract lesions) and if symptoms (particularly neurologic) progress after chemotherapy. Postoperative radiation of the chiasm and optic tract may also be considered if good radiographic studies document subsequent growth of the tumor within the chiasm or if chiasmal and optic tract involvement is extensive. Because of debilitating adverse effects (including intellectual disability, growth retardation, and secondary tumors within the radiation field), radiation is generally held as a last resort for children who have not completed growth and development.

In summary, any treatment plan must be carefully individualized. Therapeutic decisions must be based on the tumor's growth characteristics, the extent of optic nerve and chiasmal involvement as determined by clinical and radiographic evaluation, the vision of the involved and uninvolved eye, the presence or absence of concomitant neurologic or systemic disease, and the history of previous treatment. (See additional discussion of optic nerve glioma in BCSC Section 5, *Neuro-Ophthalmology.*)

Dutton JJ. Gliomas of the anterior visual pathway. *Surv Ophthalmol.* 1994;38(5):427–452.

Glass LR, Canoll P, Lignelli A, Ligon AH, Kazim M. Optic nerve glioma: case series with review of clinical, radiologic, molecular, and histopathologic characteristics. *Ophthal Plast Reconstr Surg.* 2014;30(5):372–376.

Nair AG, Pathak RS, Iyer VR, Gandhi RA. Optic nerve glioma: an update. *Int Ophthalmol.* 2014;34(4):999–1005.

Pepin SM, Lessell S. Anterior visual pathway gliomas: the last 30 years. *Semin Ophthalmol.* 2006;21(3):117–124.

## Neurofibroma

Neurofibromas are tumors composed chiefly of proliferating Schwann cells within the nerve sheaths (Figs 5-7, 5-8). Axons, endoneural fibroblasts, and mucin are also noted histologically. *Plexiform neurofibromas* consist of diffuse proliferations of Schwann cells within nerve sheaths, and they usually occur in neurofibromatosis 1 (NF1). They are well vascularized and infiltrative lesions, making complete surgical excision difficult. *Discrete*

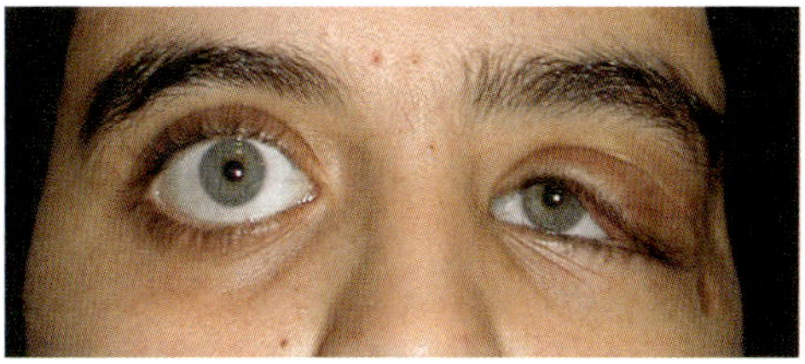

**Figure 5-7** Neurofibromatosis of the left upper eyelid with classic plexiform infiltration and S-shaped configuration of the eyelid. *(Courtesy of Jill Foster, MD.)*

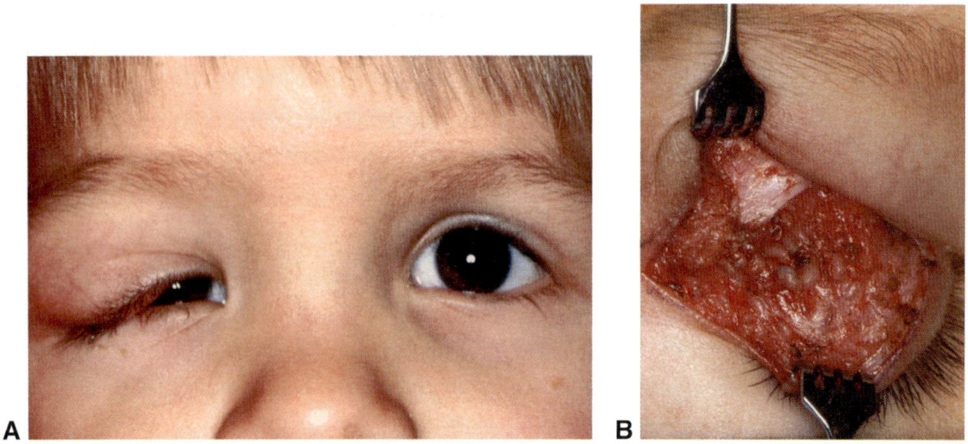


**Figure 5-8** **A,** Ptosis of the right upper eyelid, with S-shaped deformity characteristic of plexiform neurofibroma infiltration. **B,** Plexiform neurofibroma excision during ptosis surgery. On percutaneous palpation, the subcutaneous fibrous neoplastic cords have a "bag of worms" consistency. *(Courtesy of Roberta E. Gausas, MD.)*

*neurofibromas* are less common than the plexiform type, and they can usually be excised surgically without recurrence. In either instance, surgery is limited to tumors that compromise vision or produce disfigurement.

### *Neurofibromatosis 1*

Patients with neurofibromas are evaluated for neurofibromatosis. Also known as *von Recklinghausen disease,* NF1 is inherited through an autosomal dominant gene with incomplete penetrance. Because NF1 is characterized by the presence of hamartomas involving the skin, eye, central nervous system, and viscera, it is classified as a phakomatosis. Neurofibromatosis 1 is the most common phakomatous disorder. Significant orbital features that can be seen in NF1 include plexiform neurofibromas involving the lateral aspect of the upper eyelid and causing an S-shaped contour of the eyelid margin (see Figs 5-7, 5-8), pulsating proptosis secondary to sphenoid bone dysplasia, and optic nerve glioma. See BCSC Section 6, *Pediatric Ophthalmology and Strabismus,* for further discussion of neurofibromatosis and other phakomatoses.

Bechtold D, Hove HD, Prause JU, Heegaard S, Toft PB. Plexiform neurofibroma of the eye region occurring in patients without neurofibromatosis type 1. *Ophthal Plast Reconstr Surg.* 2012;28(6):413–415.

Lee V, Ragge NK, Collin JR. Orbitotemporal neurofibromatosis. Clinical features and surgical management. *Ophthalmology.* 2004;111(2):382–388.

## Meningioma

Meningiomas are invasive tumors that arise from the arachnoid villi. Orbital meningiomas usually originate intracranially along the sphenoid wing with secondary extension into the orbit through the bone, the superior orbital fissure, or the optic canal (Fig 5-9),

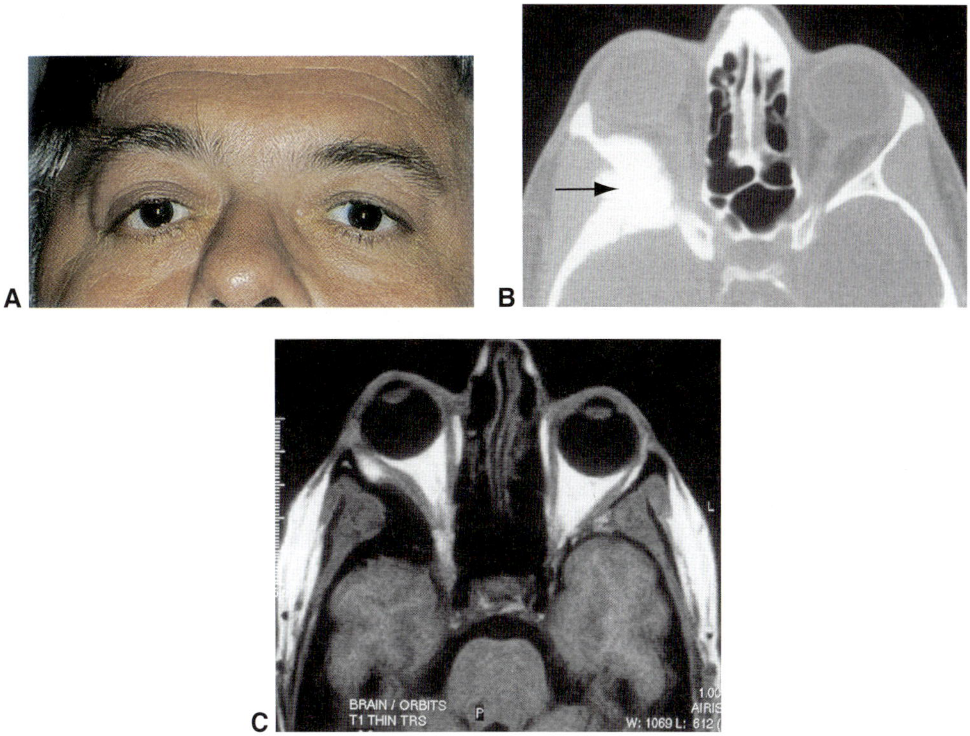


**Figure 5-9** **A,** Right proptosis and fullness of the right temple secondary to sphenoid wing meningioma. **B,** CT scan of another orbital meningioma arising from the sphenoid wing *(arrow)*. **C,** T1-weighted MRI. Note hyperostosis of the sphenoid bone. *(Part A courtesy of Jeffrey A. Nerad, MD; parts B and C courtesy of Roberta E. Gausas, MD.)*

or they may arise primarily in the orbital portion of the optic nerve sheath (Fig 5-10). Ophthalmic manifestations are related to the location of the primary tumor. Meningiomas arising near the sella and optic nerve cause early visual field defects and papilledema or optic atrophy. Tumors arising near the pterion (posterior end of the parietosphenoid fissure, at the lateral portion of the sphenoid bone) often produce a temporal fossa mass and may be associated with proptosis or nonaxial displacement of the globe. Eyelid edema (especially of the lower eyelid) and chemosis are common. Interestingly, while primary optic nerve sheath meningiomas can, in rare cases, produce axial proptosis with preserved vision, depending on their anatomical location, meningiomas can produce early profound vision loss without any proptosis.

Sphenoid wing meningiomas produce hyperostosis of the involved bone (see Fig 5-9C) and hyperplasia of associated soft tissues. When contrast enhancement is used, MRI helps define the extent of meningiomas along the dura. The presence of a dural tail (reactive thickening of the dura adjacent to the meningioma) helps distinguish a meningioma from fibrous dysplasia.

Primary orbital meningiomas usually originate in the arachnoid of the optic nerve sheath. They occur most commonly in women in their third or fourth decade of life.

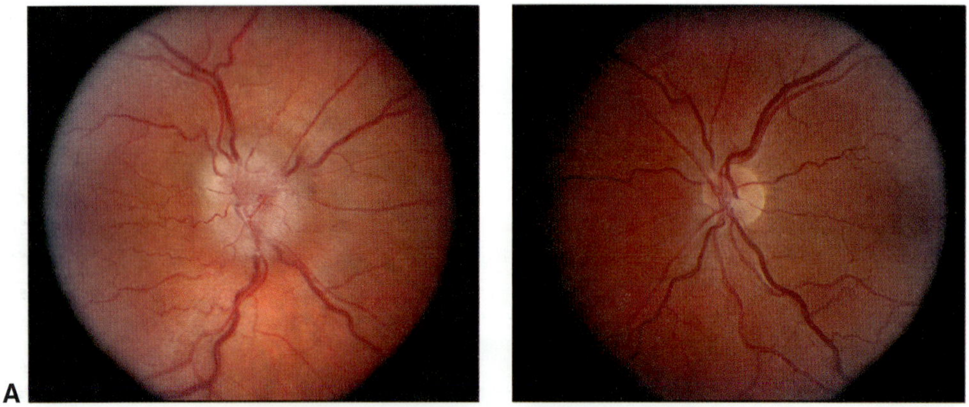

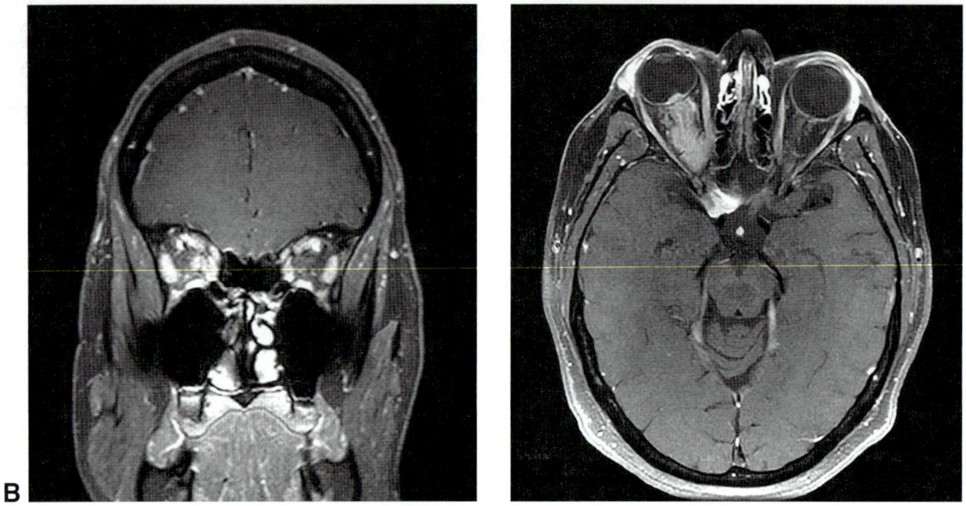

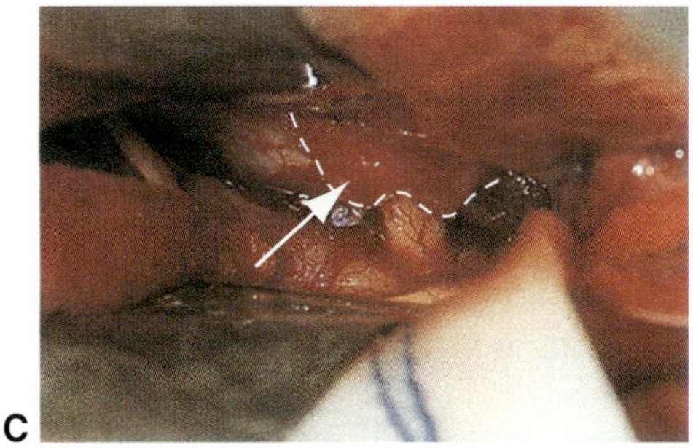

**Figure 5-10** **A,** Swollen right optic nerve with tortuous arteries and dilated veins *(left)* and normal left optic nerve *(right)*. **B,** Coronal *(left)* and axial *(right)* T1-weighted, gadolinium-enhanced MRI scans showing optic nerve sheath meningioma. Note tram tracks and enlargement of the optic nerve sheath. **C,** The meningioma is exposed through a craniotomy and superior orbitotomy. The intraoperative view shows the intracranial prechiasmal optic nerve. Note the cuff *(arrow, dashes)* of the meningioma wrapping around the optic nerve and extending out from the optic canal. *(Parts A and B courtesy of Wayne Cornblath, MD; part C courtesy of Jeffrey A. Nerad, MD.)*

Symptoms usually include a gradual, painless, unilateral loss of vision. Examination typically shows decreased vision and a relative afferent pupillary defect. Proptosis and ophthalmoplegia may also be present. The optic nerve head may appear normal, atrophic, or swollen, and optociliary shunt vessels may be visible. Occasionally, optic nerve sheath meningiomas occur bilaterally or meningiomas occur ectopically in the orbit; these are associated with neurofibromatosis.

Imaging characteristics are usually sufficient to allow diagnosis of optic nerve sheath meningiomas. Both CT and MRI show diffuse tubular enlargement of the optic nerve with contrast enhancement. In some cases, CT can show calcification within the meningioma, referred to as *tram-tracking* (see Fig 5-10B). MRI reveals a fine pattern of enhancing striations emanating from the lesion in a longitudinal fashion. These striations represent the infiltrative nature of what otherwise appears to be an encapsulated lesion. As with the sphenoid wing meningiomas, MRI can show dural extension through the optic canal into the intracranial space.

Malignant meningioma is rare and results in rapid tumor growth that is not responsive to surgical resection, radiotherapy, or chemotherapy. Histologically, malignant meningiomas are indistinguishable from the more common benign group.

### Management

*Sphenoid wing meningiomas* are typically observed until they cause functional deficits, such as profound proptosis, compressive optic neuropathy, motility impairment, or cerebral edema. Treatment includes resection of the tumor through a combined approach to the intracranial and orbital component. Complete surgical resection is not always a practical goal because of tumor extent beyond the surgical field. Rather, the goal of surgery is to reverse the volume-induced compressive effects of the lesion. Postoperative radiotherapy may be used to reduce the risk of further growth and spread of the residual tumor, or patients can be followed up clinically and with serial MRI scans.

Treatment of *optic nerve sheath meningiomas* in the orbit must also be individualized. Both the extent of vision loss and the presence of intracranial extension are important factors in treatment planning. Observation is indicated if vision is minimally affected and no intracranial extension is present. If the tumor is confined to the orbit and vision loss is significant or progressive, radiation therapy should be considered. Fractionated stereotactic radiotherapy often results in stabilization or improvement of visual function. If the patient is observed or treated with radiation, periodic MRI examination is used to carefully monitor for possible posterior or intracranial extension. With rare exceptions, attempts to surgically excise optic nerve sheath meningiomas result in irreversible vision loss due to compromise of the optic nerve blood supply. Thus, surgery is reserved for patients with severe vision loss and profound proptosis. In such cases, the optic nerve is excised with the tumor, from the back of the globe to the chiasm, if preoperative MRI suggests the opportunity for complete resection.

Bloch O, Sun M, Kaur G, Barani IJ, Parsa AT. Fractionated radiotherapy for optic nerve sheath meningiomas. *J Clin Neurosci.* 2012;19(9):1210–1215.

Dutton JJ. Optic nerve sheath meningiomas. *Surv Ophthalmol.* 1992;37(3):167–183.

Lesser RL, Knisely JP, Wang SL, Yu JB, Kupersmith MJ. Long-term response to fractionated radiotherapy of presumed optic nerve sheath meningioma. *Br J Ophthalmol.* 2010;94(5): 559–563.

Shapey J, Sabin HI, Danesh-Meyer HV, Kaye AH. Diagnosis and management of optic nerve sheath meningiomas. *J Clin Neurosci.* 2013;20(8):1045–1056.

### Schwannoma

Schwannomas, sometimes known as *neurilemomas,* are proliferations of Schwann cells that are encapsulated by perineurium. These tumors have a characteristic biphasic pattern of solid areas with nuclear palisading *(Antoni A pattern)* and myxoid areas *(Antoni B pattern).* These tumors are usually well encapsulated and can be excised with relative ease. Hypercellular schwannomas sometimes recur even after what is thought to be complete removal, but they seldom undergo malignant transformation.

## Mesenchymal Tumors

### Rhabdomyosarcoma

Rhabdomyosarcoma is the most common primary orbital malignancy of childhood (Fig 5-11). The average age of onset is 5–7 years. The classic clinical picture is that of a child with sudden onset and rapid progression of unilateral proptosis. However, patients in their early teens may experience a less dramatic course, with gradually progressive proptosis lasting from weeks to more than a month. There is often a marked adnexal response with edema and discoloration of the eyelids. Ptosis and strabismus may also be present. A mass may be palpable, particularly in the superonasal quadrant of the eyelid. However, the tumor may be retrobulbar, may involve any quadrant of the orbit, and may in rare cases arise from the conjunctiva. The patient sometimes has an unrelated history of trauma to the orbital area, which can lead to a delay in diagnosis and treatment.

If a rhabdomyosarcoma is suspected, the workup should proceed urgently. CT and MRI can be used to define the location and extent of the tumor. A biopsy should be undertaken, usually through an anterior orbitotomy. It is often possible to completely remove a rhabdomyosarcoma if it has a pseudocapsule. If this is not practical, there is some

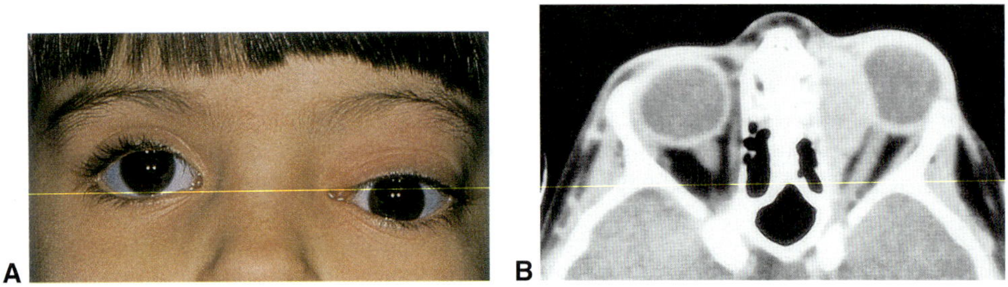

**Figure 5-11** **A,** Young child with rapid onset of axial proptosis and lateral and downward displacement of the left eye. **B,** CT scan showing a medial orbital mass, confirmed by biopsy to be rhabdomyosarcoma. *(Courtesy of Jeffrey A. Nerad, MD.)*

indication that the smaller the volume of residual tumor, the more effective is the combination of adjuvant radiation and chemotherapy in achieving a cure. In diffusely infiltrating tumors, a large biopsy specimen should be obtained so that adequate material is available for frozen sections, permanent light-microscopy sections, electron microscopy, and immunohistochemistry. Cross-striations are often not visible on light microscopy and may be more readily apparent on electron microscopy.

The physician should palpate the cervical and preauricular lymph nodes of the patient with orbital rhabdomyosarcoma to evaluate for regional metastases. Chest radiography, bone marrow aspiration and biopsy, and lumbar puncture should be performed to search for more distant metastases. Sampling of the bone marrow and the cerebrospinal fluid is best performed, if possible, with the patient under anesthesia at the time of the initial orbital biopsy.

Rhabdomyosarcomas arise from undifferentiated pluripotential mesenchymal elements in the orbital soft tissues and not from the extraocular muscles. They may be grouped into the following 4 categories:

- *Embryonal.* This is by far the most common type, accounting for more than 80% of cases. The embryonal form has a predilection for the superonasal quadrant of the orbit. The tumor is composed of loose fascicles of undifferentiated spindle cells, only a minority of which show cross-striations in immature rhabdomyosarcomas on trichrome staining. Embryonal rhabdomyosarcomas are associated with a good (94%) 5-year survival rate.
- *Alveolar.* This form has a predilection for the inferior orbit and accounts for 9% of orbital rhabdomyosarcomas. The tumor displays regular compartments composed of fibrovascular strands in which rounded rhabdomyoblasts either line up along the connective tissue strands or float freely in the alveolar spaces. This is the most malignant form of rhabdomyosarcoma; the 5-year survival rate for alveolar subtype is 65% (National Cancer Institute clinical trial IRS-III).
- *Pleomorphic.* Pleomorphic rhabdomyosarcoma is the least common and most differentiated form. In this type, many of the cells are straplike or rounded, and cross-striations are easily visualized with trichrome stain. The pleomorphic variety has the best prognosis (5-year survival rate of 97%).
- *Botryoid.* This rare variant of embryonal rhabdomyosarcoma appears grapelike. It is not found in the orbit as a primary tumor; rather, the botryoid variant occurs as a secondary invader from the paranasal sinuses or from the conjunctiva.

### Management

Before 1965, the standard treatment of orbital rhabdomyosarcoma was orbital exenteration, and the survival rate was poor. Since 1965, radiation therapy and systemic chemotherapy have become the mainstays of primary treatment, based on the guidelines set forth by the Intergroup Rhabdomyosarcoma Study Group. Exenteration is reserved for recurrent cases. The total dose of local radiation varies from 4500 to 6000 cGy, given over a period of 6 weeks. The goal of systemic chemotherapy is to eliminate microscopic cellular metastases. With radiation and chemotherapy, survival rates are better than 90% if the orbital tumor has not invaded or extended beyond the bony orbital walls. Adverse effects of radiation are common in children and include cataract, radiation dermatitis, and bony hypoplasia if orbital development has not been completed.

See also BCSC Section 6, *Pediatric Ophthalmology and Strabismus.*

Ognjanovic S, Linabery AM, Charbonneau B, Ross JA. Trends in childhood rhabdomyosarcoma incidence and survival in the United States, 1975–2005. *Cancer.* 2009;115(18): 4218–4226.

Raney RB, Walterhouse DO, Meza JL, et al. Results of the Intergroup Rhabdomyosarcoma Study Group D9602 protocol, using vincristine and dactinomycin with or without cyclophosphamide and radiation therapy, for newly diagnosed patients with low-risk embryonal rhabdomyosarcoma: a report from the Soft Tissue Sarcoma Committee of the Children's Oncology Group. *J Clin Oncol.* 2011;29(10):1312–1318.

Shields CL, Shields JA, Honavar SG, Demirci H. Clinical spectrum of primary ophthalmic rhabdomyosarcoma. *Ophthalmology.* 2001;108(12):2284–2292.

## Miscellaneous Mesenchymal Tumors

Tumors of fibrous connective tissue, cartilage, and bone are uncommon lesions that may involve the orbit. A number of these mesenchymal tumors were likely incorrectly classified before the availability of immunohistochemical staining, which has allowed them to be differentiated and classified accurately.

*Fibrous histiocytoma* is the most common of these tumors. It is characteristically very firm and displaces normal structures. Both fibroblastic and histiocytic cells in a storiform (matlike) pattern are found in these locally aggressive tumors. Fewer than 10% have metastatic potential. This tumor is sometimes difficult to distinguish, clinically and histologically, from hemangiopericytoma.

*Solitary fibrous tumor* is composed of spindle-shaped cells that are strongly CD34-positive on immunohistochemical studies. It can occur anywhere in the orbit. It may recur, undergo malignant degeneration, and metastasize if incompletely excised.

*Fibrous dysplasia* (Fig 5-12) is a benign developmental disorder of bone that may involve a single region or be polyostotic. CT shows hyperostotic bone, and MRI shows the lack of dural enhancement that distinguishes this condition from meningioma. When associated with cutaneous pigmentation and endocrine disorders, the condition is known as *Albright syndrome.* Resection or debulking is performed when the lesion results in disfigurement or vision loss due to stricture of the optic canal.

*Osteomas* are benign tumors that can involve any of the periorbital sinuses. CT scans show dense hyperostosis with well-defined margins. The lesions can produce proptosis, compressive optic neuropathy, and orbital cellulitis secondary to obstructive sinusitis. Most are incidental, slow-growing lesions that require no treatment. Complete excision is advised when the tumor is symptomatic.

Malignant mesenchymal tumors such as *liposarcoma, fibrosarcoma, chondrosarcoma,* and *osteosarcoma* rarely appear in the orbit. When chondrosarcomas and osteosarcomas are present, they usually destroy normal bone and have characteristic calcifications visible in radiographs and CT scans. Children with a history of bilateral retinoblastoma are at higher risk for osteosarcoma, chondrosarcoma, or fibrosarcoma, even if they have not been treated with therapeutic radiation.

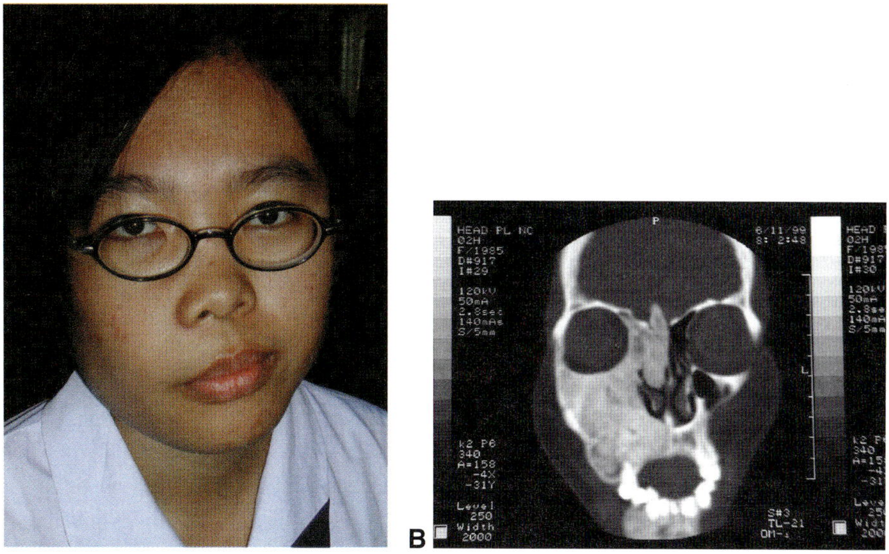

**Figure 5-12** Fibrous dysplasia. **A,** Facial asymmetry. **B,** CT scan shows characteristic hyperostosis of involved facial bones. *(Courtesy of Jerry Popham, MD.)*

Katz BJ, Nerad JA. Ophthalmic manifestations of fibrous dysplasia: a disease of children and adults. *Ophthalmology.* 1998;105(12):2207–2215.

## Lymphoproliferative Disorders

### Lymphoid Hyperplasia and Lymphoma

Lymphoproliferative lesions of the ocular adnexa constitute a heterogeneous group of neoplasms that are defined by clinical, histologic, immunologic, molecular, and genetic characteristics. Lymphoproliferative neoplasms account for more than 20% of all orbital tumors.

Most orbital lymphoproliferative lesions are non-Hodgkin lymphomas. In the United States, the incidence of non-Hodgkin lymphoma of all anatomical sites has been increasing at a rate of 3%–4% per year (representing a 50% increase over the last 20 years), and non-Hodgkin lymphoma is now the fourth most common malignancy among men and women. The incidence of orbital lymphomas has been increasing at an even greater rate. Workers with long-term exposure to bioactive solvents and reagents are at increased risk for non-Hodgkin lymphoma, as are older adults and patients with chronic autoimmune diseases.

#### *Identification and classification of lymphoproliferative disorders*

Classification of non-Hodgkin lymphomas continues to evolve and is largely based on nodal architecture. Extranodal sites, including the orbit, have been included in the Revised European-American Lymphoma (REAL) classification. However, orbital extranodal disease appears to represent a biological continuum and to behave unpredictably. Often, extraorbital lymphoma develops in patients with orbital lymphoid infiltrates that appear benign histologically, whereas other patients with malignant lymphoma of the ocular adnexa may respond satisfactorily to local therapy without subsequent systemic involvement. Currently, 70%–80% of orbital lymphoproliferative lesions are designated as malignant lymphomas on the basis of monoclonal cell-surface markers, whereas 90% are found to be malignant on the basis of molecular genetic studies. The significance of this discrepancy is not yet clear, as polymerase chain reaction studies have shown that, over time, some conjunctival lymphoid lesions fluctuate between being monoclonal and polyclonal.

Most orbital lymphomas are derived from B cells. T-cell lymphoma is rare and more lethal. B-cell lymphoma is divided into Hodgkin and non-Hodgkin tumors, with the former rarely metastasizing to the orbit. Malignant non-Hodgkin B-cell lymphoma accounts for more than 90% of orbital lymphoproliferative disease. The 4 most common types of orbital lymphomas, based on the REAL classification, are as follows:

1. *Mucosa-associated lymphoid tissue (MALT) lymphomas* account for 40%–60% of orbital lymphomas. MALT lesions were originally described as occurring in the gastrointestinal tract, where approximately 50% of MALT lymphomas arise. Studies have suggested that proliferation of early MALT tumors may be antigen driven. Therapy directed at the antigen (eg, against *Helicobacter pylori* in gastric lymphomas) may result in regression of early lesions. There is evidence to suggest that some conjunctival MALT lymphomas are associated with chronic chlamydial infection. In contrast to MALT lymphomas occurring in other areas of the body, those in the ocular adnexa do not appear to be preferentially associated with mucosal tissue (ie, conjunctiva, lacrimal gland).

   Although MALT lymphomas have a low grade of malignancy, long-term follow-up has demonstrated that systemic disease develops in at least 50% of patients at 10 years. MALT lymphomas undergo spontaneous remission in 5%–15% of cases. They undergo histologic transformation to a higher-grade lesion, usually of a large cell type, in 15%–20% of cases. Such transformation usually occurs after several years and is not related to therapy.
2. *Chronic lymphocytic lymphoma (CLL)* also represents a low-grade lesion of small, mature-appearing lymphocytes.
3. *Follicular center lymphoma* represents a low-grade lesion with follicular centers.
4. *High-grade lymphomas* include large cell lymphoma, lymphoblastic lymphoma, and Burkitt lymphoma.

See also BCSC Section 4, *Ophthalmic Pathology and Intraocular Tumors.*

### Clinical presentation

The typical lymphoproliferative lesion presents as a gradually progressive, painless mass. These tumors are often located anteriorly in the orbit (Fig 5-13) or beneath the conjunctiva, where they may show the typical salmon-patch appearance (Fig 5-14). Lymphoproliferative lesions, whether benign or malignant, usually mold to surrounding orbital structures rather than invade them; consequently, disturbances of extraocular motility or visual function are unusual. Reactive lymphoid hyperplasias and low-grade lymphomas often have a history of slow expansion over a period of months to years. Orbital imaging reveals a

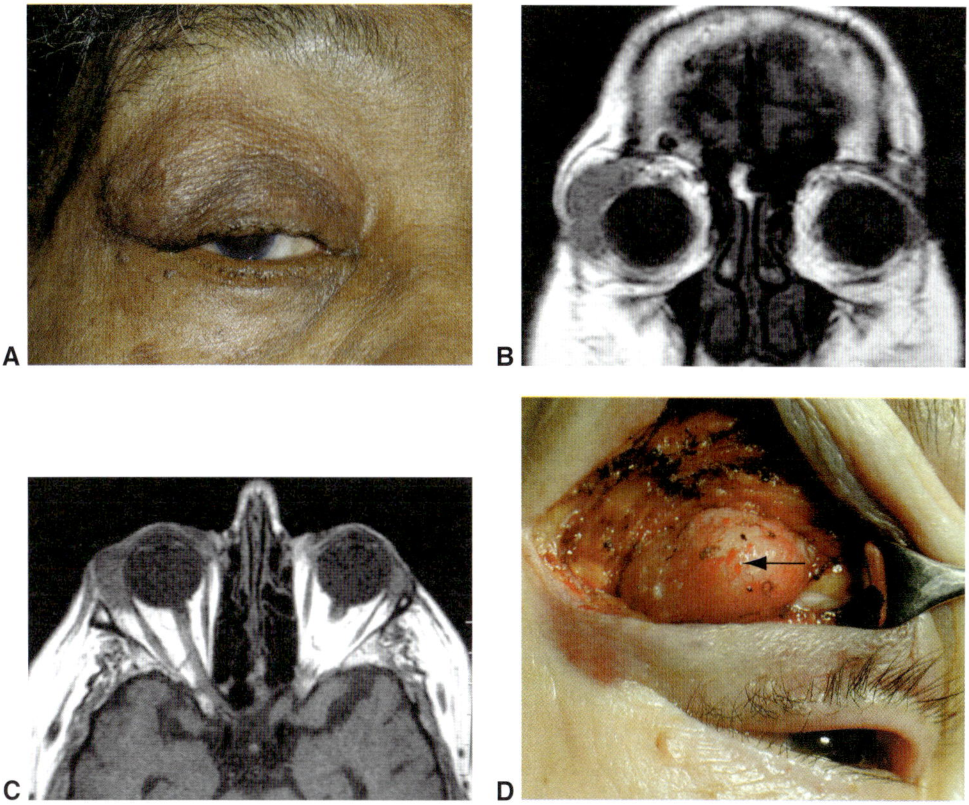


**Figure 5-13** **A,** Right upper eyelid ptosis and fullness with a palpable mass beneath the orbital rim. **B,** Coronal MRI demonstrating right lacrimal gland enlargement with infiltration of anterior orbital tissues. **C,** Axial MRI showing characteristic molding of the lesion to adjacent structures. **D,** Incisional biopsy of the abnormal infiltration of the lacrimal gland reveals orbital lymphoma *(arrow)*. *(Courtesy of Roberta E. Gausas, MD.)*

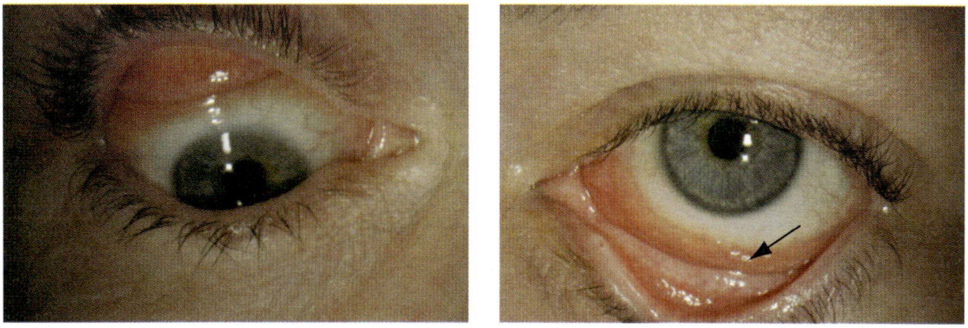

**Figure 5-14** Subconjunctival salmon-patch lesion in the upper and lower fornix *(arrow)* characteristic of conjunctival and anterior orbital lymphoma. *(Courtesy of Christine C. Nelson, MD.)*

characteristic puttylike molding of the tumor to normal structures. Bone erosion or infiltration is usually not seen except with high-grade malignant lymphomas. Up to 50% of orbital lymphoproliferative lesions arise in the lacrimal fossa. Lymphomas in the retrobulbar fat may appear more infiltrative. Approximately 17% of orbital lymphoid lesions occur bilaterally, but this does not necessarily indicate the presence of extraorbital disease.

### *Diagnosis*

For all lymphoproliferative lesions, an open biopsy is preferred to allow retrieval of an adequate tissue specimen, which is used to establish a diagnosis and to characterize the lesion's morphologic, immunologic, cytogenetic, and molecular properties under the REAL classification. A portion of the tissue should be placed in a suitable fixative for light microscopy. The majority of the specimen should be sent fresh to a molecular diagnostics laboratory for possible flow cytometry and polymerase chain reaction analysis. Alternatively, fine-needle aspiration biopsy can provide adequate sample volume to establish all but the morphologic characteristics of the lesion. Conjunctival biopsy for follicular conjunctivitis can sometimes reveal a lymphoproliferative lesion.

Both reactive hyperplasia and malignant lymphoma are hypercellular proliferations with sparse or absent stromal components. Histologically, light microscopy may reveal a continuum from reactive hyperplasia to low-grade lymphoma to higher-grade malignancy. Within this spectrum, it may be difficult to characterize a given lesion by light microscopy alone. In such cases, immunopathology and molecular diagnostic studies have been proposed to aid further categorization.

Malignant lymphomas are thought to represent clonal expansions of abnormal precursor cells. Immunologic identification of cell-surface markers on lymphocytes can be used to classify tumors as containing B cells or T cells and as being either monoclonal or polyclonal in origin. Specific monoclonal antibodies directed against surface light-chain ($\kappa$ or $\lambda$) immunoglobulins are used to study cells in smears, histologic sections, or cell suspensions to determine whether the cells represent monoclonal (ie, malignant) proliferations.

Newer techniques of molecular analysis allow more precise identification of tumor clonality by extracting, amplifying, and hybridizing tumor DNA with radioactively labeled nucleotide probes. DNA hybridization is more sensitive than cell-surface marker typing in detecting clonality, but this technique is also more time-consuming and expensive. DNA genetic studies have shown that most lymphoproliferative lesions that appear to be immunologically polyclonal actually harbor small monoclonal proliferations of B lymphocytes. The finding of monoclonality, established by either immunophenotype or molecular genetics, does not predict which tumors will ultimately result in systemic disease.

Approximately 90% of orbital lymphoproliferative disease is monoclonal and 10% is polyclonal by molecular genetic studies, but both types of lesions may involve prior, concurrent, or future systemic spread. This occurs in more than half of periocular lymphomas: 20%–30% of periocular lymphoproliferative lesions have a history of previous or concomitant systemic disease and an additional 30% develop it over 5 years. The anatomical site of origin offers some prediction of the risk of the presence or development of systemic non-Hodgkin lymphoma. The risk is lowest for conjunctival lesions, greater for orbital lesions, and highest for lesions arising in the eyelid. Lymphoid lesions developing in the lacrimal fossa may carry a greater risk of systemic disease than those occurring elsewhere in the orbit. Bilateral periocular involvement markedly increases the risk of systemic disease, but such involvement is not definitive evidence of systemic disease. It is also clear that the risk of systemic disease is increased for decades after the original lesion is diagnosed, regardless of the initial lesion's location in the orbit or its clonality.

#### *Management*

Because the various lymphoproliferative lesions show great overlap in terms of clinical behavior, all patients with hypercellular lymphoid lesions (whether monoclonal or polyclonal) should be examined by an oncologist. Depending on the histologic type of the lesion, the examination may include a general physical examination, a complete blood count, a bone marrow biopsy, a liver and spleen scan, a chest radiograph, and serum immunoprotein electrophoresis. The oncologist may also recommend CT of the thorax and abdomen to check for mediastinal and retroperitoneal lymph node involvement. The patient should be reexamined periodically because systemic lymphoma may occur many years after the presentation of an isolated orbital lymphoid neoplasm.

Although systemic corticosteroids are useful in the treatment of nonspecific orbital inflammation, they are not recommended in the treatment of lymphoproliferative lesions. Radiotherapy is the treatment of choice for patients with localized ocular adnexal lymphoproliferative disease. A dose of 2000–3000 cGy is typically administered. This regimen achieves local control in virtually all cases and, if the lesion is isolated, may prevent systemic spread. A surgical cure usually cannot be achieved because of the infiltrative nature of lymphoid tumors.

The treatment of low-grade lymphoid lesions that have already undergone systemic dissemination is somewhat controversial because indolent lymphomas are generally refractory to chemotherapy and are associated with long-term survival, even if untreated. Many oncologists take a watchful waiting approach and treat only symptomatic disease. Lymphomas that are more aggressive require radiation, aggressive chemotherapy, or both; up to one-third of these lesions can be cured.

Rasmussen PK, Coupland SE, Finger PT, et al. Ocular adnexal follicular lymphoma: a multicenter international study. *JAMA Ophthalmol.* 2014;132(7):851–858.

Sullivan TJ, Whitehead K, Williamson R, et al. Lymphoproliferative disease of the ocular adnexa: a clinical and pathologic study with statistical analysis of 69 patients. *Ophthal Plast Reconstr Surg.* 2005;21(3):177–188.

Watkins LM, Carter KD, Nerad JA. Ocular adnexal lymphoma of the extraocular muscles: case series from the University of Iowa and review of the literature. *Ophthal Plast Reconstr Surg.* 2011;27(6):471–476.

White WL, Ferry JA, Harris NL, Grove AS Jr. Ocular adnexal lymphoma: a clinicopathologic study with identification of lymphomas of mucosa-associated lymphoid tissue type. *Ophthalmology.* 1995;102(12):1994–2006.

### Plasma Cell Tumors

Lesions composed predominantly of mature plasma cells may be plasmacytomas or localized plasma cell–rich pseudotumors. Multiple myeloma should be ruled out, particularly if there is bone destruction or any immaturity or mitotic activity among the plasmacytic elements. Some lesions are composed of lymphocytes and lymphoplasmacytoid cells with the combined properties of both lymphocytes and plasma cells. Plasma cell tumors display the same spectrum of clinical involvement as do lymphoproliferative lesions but are much less common.

## Histiocytic Disorders

*Langerhans cell histiocytosis* (formerly, *histiocytosis X*) is a collection of rare disorders of the mononuclear phagocytic system. These disorders are thought to result from abnormal immune regulation. All subtypes are characterized by an accumulation of proliferating dendritic histiocytes. The disease occurs most commonly in children, with a peak incidence between 5 and 10 years of age, and varies in severity from benign lesions with spontaneous resolution to chronic dissemination resulting in death. Older names representing the various manifestations of histiocytic disorders (*eosinophilic granuloma of bone, Hand-Schüller-Christian disease,* and *Letterer-Siwe disease*) are being displaced by the terms *unifocal* and *multifocal eosinophilic granuloma of bone* and *diffuse soft tissue histiocytosis.*

The most frequent presentation in the orbit is a lytic defect, usually affecting the superotemporal orbit or sphenoid wing and causing relapsing episodes of orbital inflammation, which are often initially misinterpreted as infectious orbital cellulitis. Ultimately, the mass may cause proptosis. Younger children more often present with significant overlying soft-tissue inflammation; they are also more likely to have evidence of multifocal or systemic involvement. Even if the initial workup shows no evidence of systemic dissemination, younger patients require regular observation for detection of subsequent multiorgan involvement.

Histiocytic disorders have a reported survival rate of only 50% in patients presenting under 2 years of age; if the disease develops after age 2, the survival rate rises to 87%. Treatment of localized orbital disease consists of confirmatory biopsy with debulking, which may be followed by intralesional steroid injection or low-dose radiation therapy. Spontaneous remission has also been reported. Although destruction of the orbital bone may be extensive at the time of presentation, the bone usually reossifies completely. Children with systemic disease are treated aggressively with chemotherapy.

Woo KI, Harris GJ. Eosinophilic granuloma of the orbit: understanding the paradox of aggressive destruction responsive to minimal intervention. *Ophthal Plast Reconstr Surg.* 2003; 19(6):429–439.

## Xanthogranuloma

Adult xanthogranuloma of the adnexa and orbit is often associated with systemic manifestations. These manifestations are the basis for classification into the following 4 syndromes, presented in their order of frequency:

1. necrobiotic xanthogranuloma (NBX)
2. adult-onset asthma with periocular xanthogranuloma (AAPOX)
3. Erdheim-Chester disease (ECD)
4. adult-onset xanthogranuloma (AOX)

NBX is characterized by the presence of subcutaneous lesions in the eyelids and anterior orbit; the lesions may also occur throughout the body. Although skin lesions are seen in all of these syndromes, the lesions in NBX have a propensity to ulcerate and fibrose. Frequent systemic findings include paraproteinemia and multiple myeloma.

AAPOX is a syndrome that includes periocular xanthogranuloma, asthma, lymphadenopathy, and, often, increased immunoglobulin G levels.

ECD, the most devastating of the adult xanthogranulomas, is characterized by dense, progressive, recalcitrant fibrosclerosis of the orbit and internal organs, including the mediastinum, the pericardium, and the pleural, perinephric, and retroperitoneal spaces. Whereas xanthogranuloma of the orbit and adnexa tends to be anterior in NBX, AAPOX, and AOX, it is often diffuse in ECD and leads to vision loss. Bone involvement is common and death frequent, despite aggressive therapies.

AOX is an isolated xanthogranulomatous lesion without systemic involvement. *Juvenile xanthogranuloma* is a separate non-Langerhans histiocytic disorder that occurs as a self-limited, corticosteroid-sensitive, and usually focal subcutaneous disease of childhood. See BCSC Section 6, *Pediatric Ophthalmology and Strabismus,* for additional discussion of juvenile xanthogranuloma.

Sivak-Callcott JA, Rootman J, Rasmussen SL, et al. Adult xanthogranulomatous disease of the orbit and ocular adnexa: new immunohistochemical findings and clinical review. *Br J Ophthalmol.* 2006;90(5):602–608.

## Lacrimal Gland Tumors

Most lacrimal gland masses represent nonspecific inflammation (dacryoadenitis). They present with acute inflammatory signs and usually respond to anti-inflammatory medication (see the section Nonspecific Orbital Inflammation in Chapter 4). Of those lacrimal gland tumefactions not presenting with inflammatory signs and symptoms, the majority represent lymphoproliferative disorders (discussed previously): up to 50% of orbital lymphomas develop in the lacrimal fossa. Only a minority of lacrimal fossa lesions are epithelial neoplasms of the lacrimal gland.

Imaging is helpful in evaluating lesions in the lacrimal gland region. Inflammatory and lymphoid proliferations within the lacrimal gland tend to cause it to expand diffusely and appear elongated, whereas epithelial neoplasms tend to appear as isolated globular masses. Inflammatory and lymphoproliferative lesions usually mold around the globe, whereas epithelial neoplasms tend to displace and indent it. The bone of the lacrimal fossa is remodeled in response to a slowly growing benign epithelial lesion of the lacrimal gland, whereas there is typically no bony change due to a lymphoproliferative lesion.

### Epithelial Tumors of the Lacrimal Gland

Approximately 50% of epithelial tumors are benign mixed tumors (pleomorphic adenomas), and about 50% are carcinomas. Approximately half of the carcinomas are adenoid cystic carcinomas, and the remainder are malignant mixed tumors, primary adenocarcinomas, mucoepidermoid carcinomas, or squamous carcinomas.

### *Pleomorphic adenoma*

*Pleomorphic adenoma (benign mixed tumor)* is the most common epithelial tumor of the lacrimal gland (Fig 5-15). This tumor usually occurs in adults during the fourth or fifth decade of life and affects slightly more men than women. Patients present with a progressive, painless downward and inward displacement of the globe with axial proptosis. Symptoms are usually present for more than 12 months.

A firm, lobular mass may be palpated near the superolateral orbital rim, and orbital imaging often reveals enlargement or expansion of the lacrimal fossa. On imaging, the lesion appears well circumscribed but may have a slightly nodular configuration.

Microscopically, benign mixed tumors have a varied cellular structure consisting primarily of a proliferation of benign epithelial cells and a stroma composed of spindle-shaped cells with occasional cartilaginous, mucinous, or even osteoid degeneration or metaplasia. This variability accounts for the designation *mixed tumor.* The lesion is circumscribed by a pseudocapsule.

**Management** Treatment is complete removal of the tumor with its pseudocapsule and a surrounding margin of orbital tissue. Surgery should be performed without a preliminary

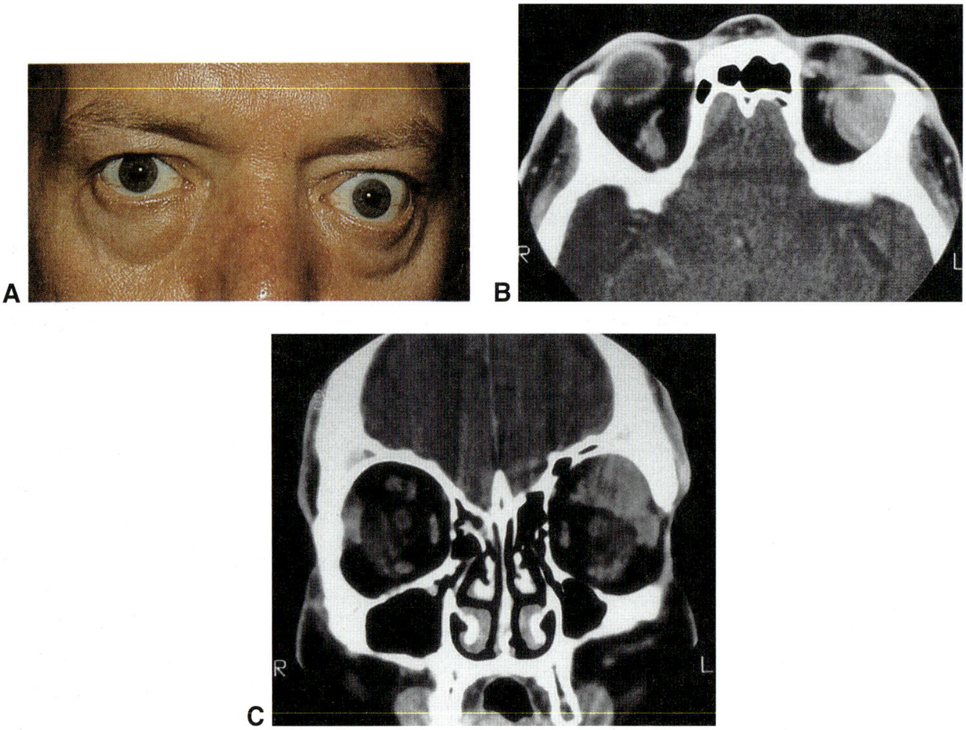


**Figure 5-15** **A,** Proptosis and downward displacement of the left eye in a man with thyroid eye disease and a benign mixed tumor of the lacrimal gland. **B,** Axial CT scan showing a tumor in the lacrimal fossa. No bony remodeling is present in this case. **C,** Coronal CT scan showing a rounded mass in the lacrimal gland consistent with benign mixed tumor. *(Courtesy of Robert C. Kersten, MD.)*

biopsy: in an early study, the recurrence rate was 32% when the capsule of the pleomorphic adenoma was incised for direct biopsy. In recurrences, the risk of malignant degeneration is 10% per decade.

Chawla B, Kashyap S, Sen S, et al. Clinicopathologic review of epithelial tumors of the lacrimal gland. *Ophthal Plast Reconstr Surg.* 2013;29(6):440–445.

Rose GE, Wright JE. Pleomorphic adenoma of the lacrimal gland. *Br J Ophthalmol.* 1992; 76(7):395–400.

#### *Adenoid cystic carcinoma*

Also known as *cylindroma,* adenoid cystic carcinoma is the most common malignant tumor of the lacrimal gland. This highly malignant tumor may cause pain because of perineural invasion and bone destruction. The relatively rapid course, with a history of generally less than 1 year, and early onset of pain help differentiate this malignant tumor from benign mixed tumor, which tends to show progressive proptosis for more than a year and is painless. The tumor usually extends into the posterior orbit because of its capacity to infiltrate and its lack of true encapsulation. Recurrence after resection is problematic.

Microscopically, this tumor is made of disarmingly benign-appearing cells that grow in tubules, solid nests, or a Swiss-cheese pattern. The basaloid morphology is associated with worse survival than the cribriform variant. Infiltration of the orbital tissues, including perineural invasion, is often seen in microscopic sections.

#### *Malignant mixed tumor*

These lesions are histologically similar to benign mixed tumors, but they have areas of malignant change, usually poorly differentiated adenocarcinomas. They typically arise from a long-standing primary benign mixed tumor or from a benign mixed tumor that has recurred following initial incomplete excision or violation of the pseudocapsule (see the section “Pleomorphic adenoma”). A change in growth rate is a hallmark of malignant degeneration.

#### *Management of malignant lacrimal gland tumors*

Suspicion of a malignant lacrimal gland tumor warrants biopsy with permanent histologic confirmation. Exenteration and radical orbitectomy with removal of the roof, lateral wall, and floor along with the overlying soft tissues and anterior portion of the temporalis muscle have failed to produce improvement in long-term survival rates. High-dose radiation therapy (conventional electrons, photons, and neutrons have all been used), in conjunction with surgical debulking, may be offered as an alternative. Intracarotid chemotherapy followed by exenteration has also been advocated; however, the duration of follow-up is not yet adequate to prove the efficacy of this treatment. Despite these measures, perineural extension into the cavernous sinus often occurs, and the typical clinical course is that of multiple painful recurrences with ultimate mortality from intracranial extension or, less commonly, from systemic metastases (which are managed by local resection), usually occurring a decade or more after the initial presentation.

Bernardini FP, Devoto MH, Croxatto JO. Epithelial tumors of the lacrimal gland: an update. *Curr Opin Ophthalmol.* 2008;19(5):409–413.
Esmaeli B, Golio D, Kies M, DeMonte F. Surgical management of locally advanced adenoid cystic carcinoma of the lacrimal gland. *Ophthal Plast Reconstr Surg.* 2006;22(5):366–370.

### Nonepithelial Tumors of the Lacrimal Gland

Most of the nonepithelial lesions of the lacrimal gland represent lymphoid proliferation or inflammations. Up to 50% of orbital lymphoproliferative lesions occur in the lacrimal gland. Inflammatory conditions such as nonspecific orbital inflammation and sarcoidosis are covered in Chapter 4. Lymphoepithelial lesions may also occur either in Sjögren syndrome or as a localized lacrimal gland and salivary gland lesion *(Mikulicz syndrome).*

Benign lymphocytic infiltrates may be seen in patients, particularly women, who have bilateral swelling of the lacrimal gland, producing a dry eye syndrome. This condition can occur insidiously or following a symptomatic episode of lacrimal gland inflammation. The enlargement of the lacrimal glands may not be clinically apparent. Biopsy specimens of the affected glands show a spectrum of lymphocytic infiltration, from scattered patches of lymphocytes to lymphocytic replacement of the lacrimal gland parenchyma, with preservation of the inner duct cells, which are surrounded by proliferating myoepithelial cells *(epimyoepithelial islands).* This combination of lymphocytes and epimyoepithelial islands has led some authors to designate this manifestation as a lymphoepithelial lesion. Some patients with lymphocytic infiltrates may also have systemic rheumatoid arthritis and, therefore, have classic Sjögren syndrome. These lesions may develop into low-grade B-cell lymphoma (see the discussion in the section Lymphoproliferative Disorders). Associated dry eye symptoms may improve with the use of topical cyclosporine.

Kubota T, Moritani S, Ichihara S. Clinicopathologic and immunohistochemical features of primary ductal adenocarcinoma of lacrimal gland: five new cases and review of literature. *Graefes Arch Clin E Ophthalmol.* 2013;251(8):2071–2076.
Shields JA, Shields CL, Epstein JA, Scartozzi R, Eagle RC Jr. Review: primary epithelial malignancies of the lacrimal gland: the 2003 Ramon L. Font lecture. *Ophthal Plast Reconstr Surg.* 2004;20(1):10–21.
von Holstein SL, Coupland SE, Briscoe D, Le Tourneau C, Heegaard S. Epithelial tumours of the lacrimal gland: a clinical, histopathological, surgical and oncological survey. *Acta Ophthalmol.* 2013;91(3):195–206.

## Secondary Orbital Conditions

Secondary orbital tumors are those that extend into the orbit from contiguous structures, such as the globe, the eyelids, the sinuses, or the brain.

### Globe and Eyelid Origin

Tumors and inflammations from within the eye (especially from choroidal melanomas and retinoblastomas) or from the eyelid (eg, sebaceous gland carcinoma, squamous cell carcinoma, and basal cell carcinoma) can invade the orbit. Primary eyelid tumors are discussed in Chapter 10. Retinoblastoma, choroidal melanoma, and other ocular neoplasms are covered in BCSC Section 4, *Ophthalmic Pathology and Intraocular Tumors,* and Section 6, *Pediatric Ophthalmology and Strabismus.*

Gill HS, Moscato EE, Chang AL, Soon S, Silkiss RZ. Vismodegib for periocular and orbital basal cell carcinoma. *JAMA Ophthalmol.* 2013;131(12):1591–1594.

Yin VT, Pfeiffer ML, Esmaeli B. Targeted therapy for orbital and periocular basal cell carcinoma and squamous cell carcinoma. *Ophthal Plast Reconstr Surg.* 2013;29(2):87–92.

## Sinus Disease Affecting the Orbit

Tumors from the nose or the paranasal sinuses may secondarily invade the orbit. Proptosis and globe displacement are common. The diagnosis is made by imaging, which is ordered to include the base of the sinuses for proper evaluation.

*Mucoceles* and *mucopyoceles* of the sinuses (Fig 5-16) are cystic structures with pseudostratified ciliated columnar (respiratory) epithelium resulting from obstruction of the sinus excretory ducts. These lesions may invade the orbit by expansion and erosion of the bones of the orbital walls. In the case of mucoceles, the cysts are usually filled with thick mucoid secretions; in the case of pyoceles, they are filled with pus. Most mucoceles arise from the frontal or ethmoid sinuses. Surgical treatment includes evacuation of the mucocele and reestablishment of drainage of the affected sinus or obliteration of the sinus by mucosal stripping and packing with bone or fat.

Another orbital condition that is the result of sinus outflow pathology is *silent sinus syndrome* (Fig 5-17). Chronic subclinical sinusitis presumably causes thinning of the bone of the involved sinus, leading to enophthalmos due to collapse of the orbital floor. This

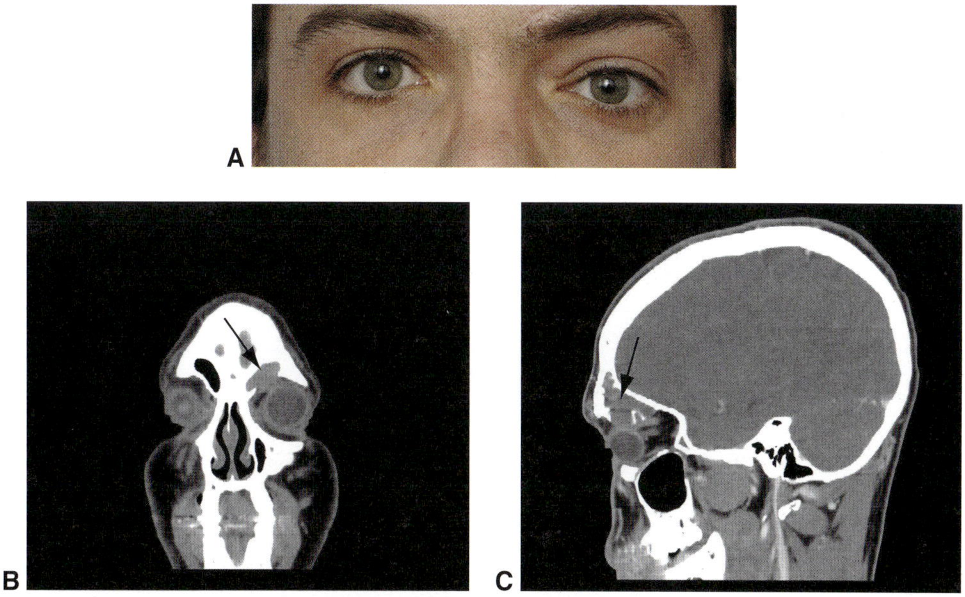


**Figure 5-16** **A,** Adult patient with left chronic sinusitis and downward displacement of the globe. Coronal **(B)** and sagittal **(C)** CT scans showing a left frontal sinus mucocele that demonstrates expansion into the superior orbit *(arrows)*. *(Courtesy of Christine C. Nelson, MD.)*

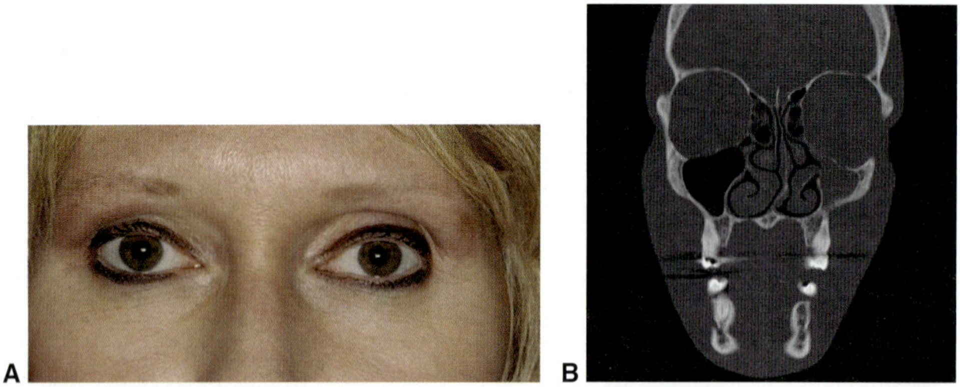

**Figure 5-17** **A,** Silent sinus syndrome on the left with spontaneous enophthalmos, deep superior sulcus, and upper eyelid retraction. **B,** Coronal CT scan of a hypoplastic, opacified left maxillary sinus with reduced volume and displacement of the orbital floor. *(Courtesy of Christine C. Nelson, MD.)*

collapse may occur in association with a recent significant change in atmospheric pressure, as occurs, for example, during airplane travel or scuba diving. The upper eyelid may appear relatively retracted, and there may be transient diplopia. Treatment includes restoration of normal sinus drainage and reconstruction of the orbital floor.

*Squamous cell carcinoma* and *adenocarcinoma* of the sinuses may secondarily invade the orbit (Fig 5-18). These malignancies usually arise within the maxillary sinuses,

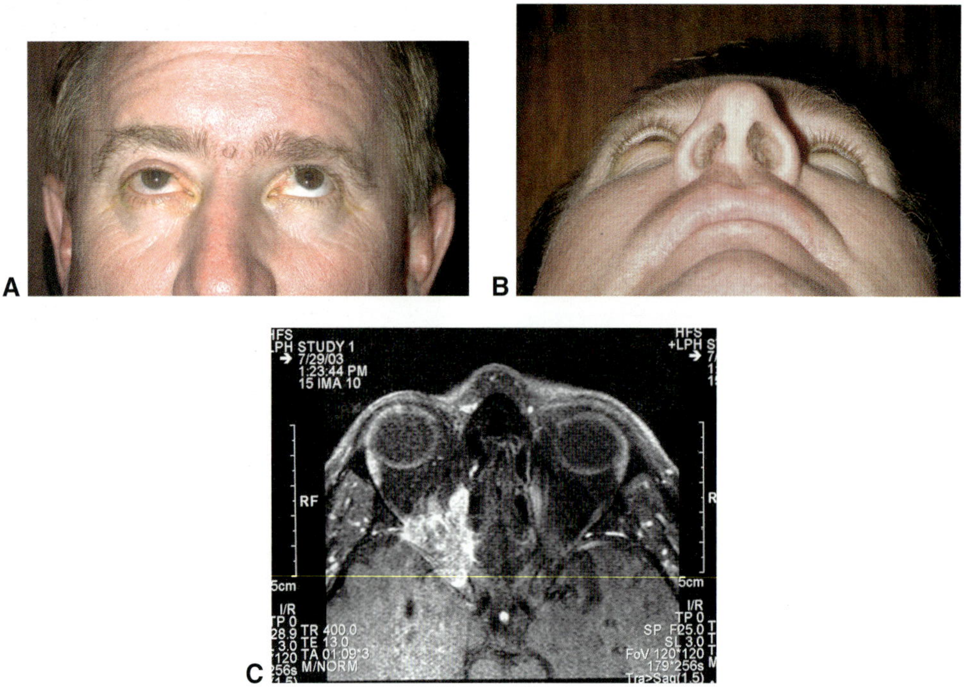


**Figure 5-18** **A,** Squamous cell carcinoma of the sinuses invading the orbit. Note the alteration in motility and limitation of upgaze. **B,** Worm's-eye view shows exophthalmos. **C,** MRI scan showing spread of sinus squamous cell carcinoma to the posterior orbit. *(Courtesy of Jill Foster, MD.)*

followed by the nasopharynx or the oropharynx. Nasal obstruction, epistaxis, or epiphora may be associated with the growth of such tumors. Treatment is usually a combination of surgical excision and radiation therapy and often includes exenteration if the periorbita is traversed by tumor.

Nonepithelial tumors that can invade the orbit from the sinuses, nose, and facial bones include a wide variety of benign and malignant lesions. Among the most common of these are osteomas (Fig 5-19), fibrous dysplasia, and miscellaneous sarcomas.

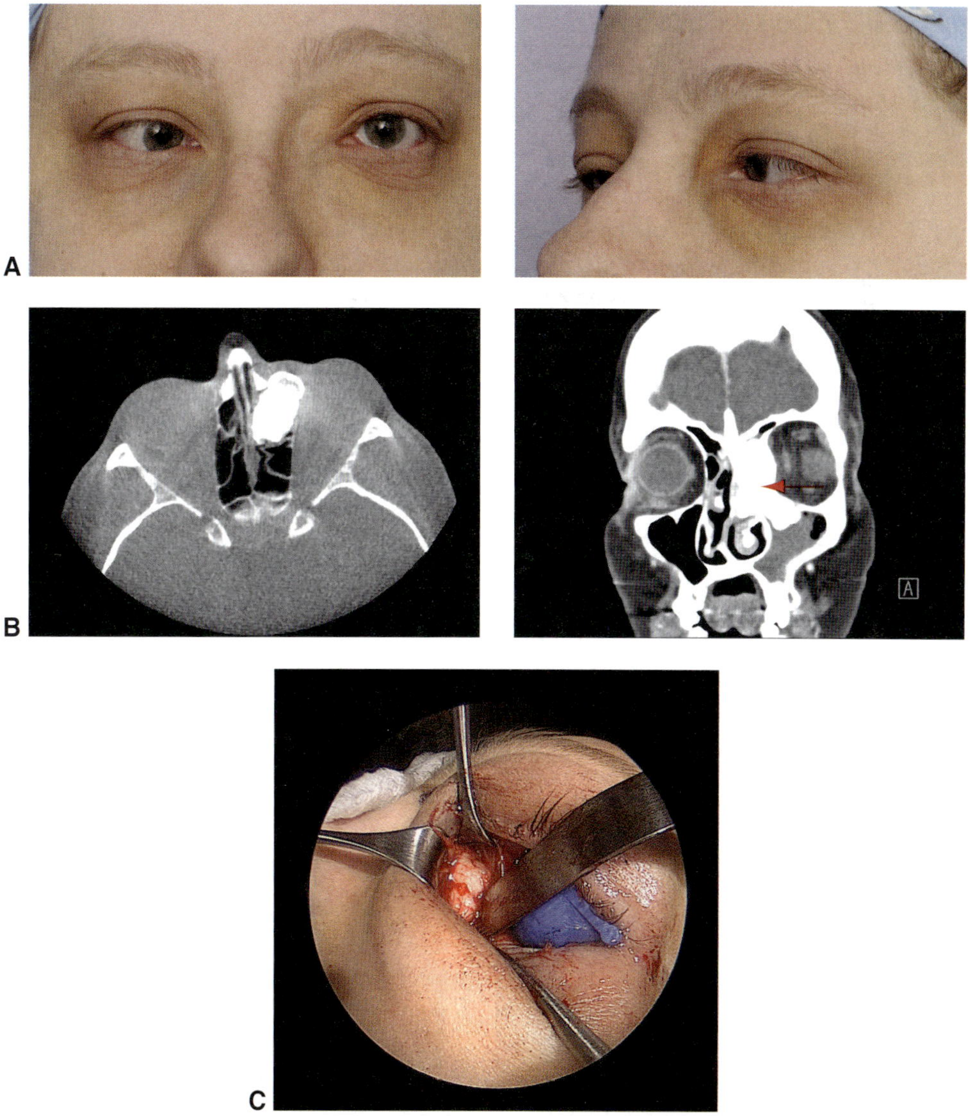

**Figure 5-19** **A,** Osteoma of the left medial canthus causing proptosis, restriction of the left medial rectus muscle, and a palpable hard mass. **B,** CT scan showing axial *(left)* and coronal *(right)* views of the extensive osteoma *(arrow)* of the left medial wall and floor. **C,** Intraoperative resection of the osteoma. *(Courtesy of Christine C. Nelson, MD.)*

Johnson LN, Krohel GB, Yeon EB, Parnes SM. Sinus tumors invading the orbit. *Ophthalmology.* 1984;91(3):209–217.

Soparkar CN, Patrinely JR, Cuaycong MJ, et al. The silent sinus syndrome: a cause of spontaneous enophthalmos. *Ophthalmology.* 1994;101(4):772–778.

Wei LA, Ramey NA, Durairaj VD, et al. Orbital osteoma: clinical features and management options. *Ophthal Plast Reconstr Surg.* 2014;30(2):168–174.

## Metastatic Tumors

### Metastatic Tumors in Children

In children, distant tumors metastasize to the orbit more frequently than to the globe (in contrast to adults, who more frequently have metastases to the choroid).

#### *Neuroblastoma*

Metastatic orbital neuroblastoma typically produces an abrupt ecchymotic proptosis that may be bilateral. A deposition of blood in the eyelids may lead to the mistaken impression of injury (Fig 5-20). Horner syndrome may also be evident in some cases. Commonly, bone destruction is apparent on CT, particularly in the lateral orbital wall or sphenoid marrow. Metastases typically occur late in the course of the disease, when the primary tumor can be detected readily in the abdomen, mediastinum, or neck. Treatment is primarily chemotherapy; radiotherapy is reserved for cases of impending vision loss due to compressive optic neuropathy. The survival rate is related to the patient's age at diagnosis. Patients diagnosed before 1 year of age have a 90% survival rate. Only 10% of those diagnosed at an older age survive. Congenital neuroblastoma of the cervical ganglia may produce an ipsilateral Horner syndrome with heterochromia.

Miller NR, Newman NJ, Biousse V, Kerrison JB, eds. *Walsh & Hoyt's Clinical Neuro-Ophthalmology.* 6th ed. Philadelphia: Lippincott Williams & Wilkins; 2005.

#### *Leukemia*

In advanced stages, leukemia may produce unilateral or bilateral proptosis. *Acute lymphoblastic leukemia* is the type of leukemia most likely to metastasize to the orbit. A primary leukemic orbital mass, called *granulocytic sarcoma* or *chloroma,* is a rare variant of

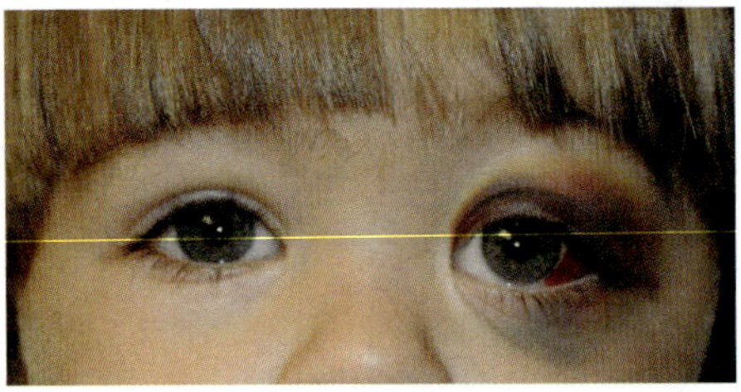

A

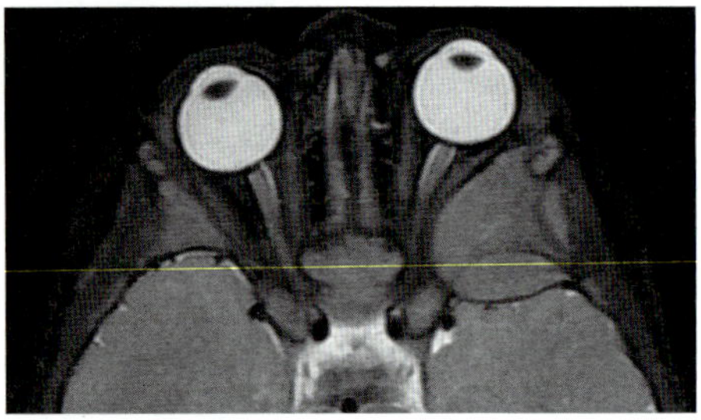

B

**Figure 5-20** **A,** Child with metastatic left orbital neuroblastoma. **B,** MRI shows a large infiltrating lesion of the left sphenoid wing extending into the orbital soft tissues and the temporal fossa. *(Courtesy of Bobby S. Korn, MD, PhD.)*

myelogenous leukemia. Least common are metastases to the subarachnoid space of the optic nerve. These cases present with sudden vision loss and swelling of the optic nerve. They constitute an emergency and are treated with orbital radiotherapy. Typically, orbital lesions present in advance of blood or bone marrow signs of leukemia, which almost invariably follow within several months. Special stains for cytoplasmic esterase in the cells (Leder stain) indicate that these are granulocytic precursor cells. Chances for survival are improved if chemotherapy is instituted before the discovery of leukemic involvement in bone marrow or peripheral blood.

Aggarwal E, Mulay K, Honavar SG. Orbital extra-medullary granulocytic sarcoma: clinicopathologic correlation with immunohistochemical features. *Surv Ophthalmol.* 2014;59(2):232–235.

Ple-plakon PA, Demirci H, Cheng JX, Elner VM. Orbital myeloid sarcoma in an adult with acute myeloid leukemia, FAB M1 and 12p-deletion. *Ophthal Plast Reconstr Surg.* 2013;29(3):e73–e75.

Stockl FA, Dolmetsch AM, Saornil MA, Font RL, Burnier MN Jr. Orbital granulocytic sarcoma. *Br J Ophthalmol.* 1997;81(12):1084–1088.

## Metastatic Tumors in Adults

Although virtually any carcinoma of the internal organs and cutaneous melanoma can metastasize to the orbit, breast and lung tumors account for most orbital metastases. The presence of pain, proptosis, inflammation, bone destruction, and early ophthalmoplegia suggests the possibility of metastatic carcinoma.

Some 75% of patients have a history of a known primary tumor, but in 25% the orbital metastasis is the presenting sign. The extraocular muscles are frequently involved because of their abundant blood supply. The second most common site is the bone marrow space of the sphenoid bone because of the relatively high volume of low-flow blood in this site (Fig 5-21). Lytic destruction of this part of the lateral orbital wall is highly suggestive of metastatic disease. Elevation of serum carcinoembryonic antigen levels also may suggest a metastatic process. Fine-needle aspiration biopsy can be performed in the office and may obviate the need for orbitotomy and open biopsy.

A
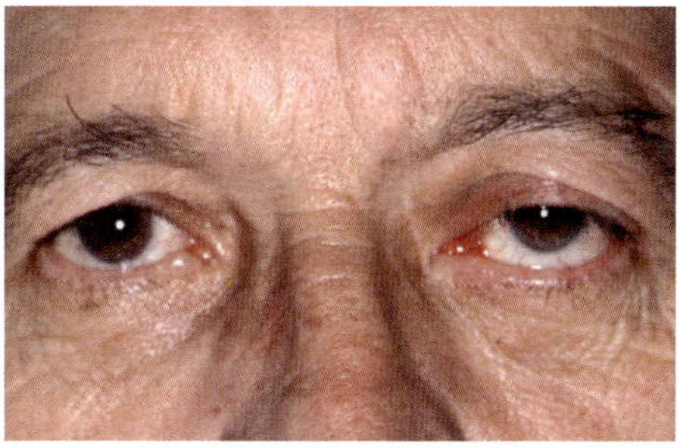
B
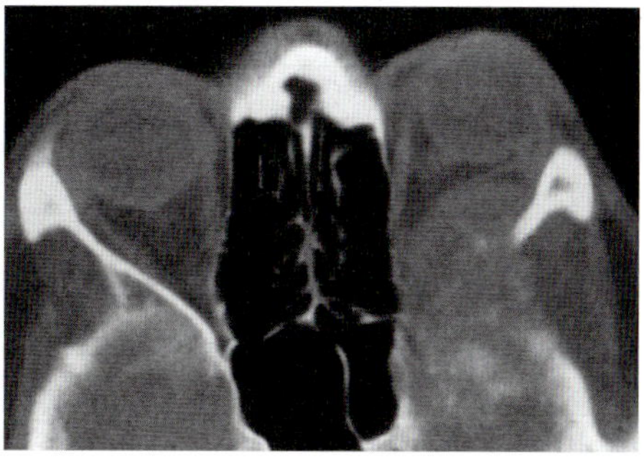

**Figure 5-21** **A,** Left proptosis and orbital congestion in an older man with prostate carcinoma. **B,** CT scan showing a left posterior orbital mass with adjacent bony destruction, confirmed by biopsy to be metastatic prostate cancer. *(Courtesy of Roberta E. Gausas, MD.)*

### Breast carcinoma

The most common primary source of orbital metastases in women is breast cancer. Metastases may occur many years after the breast has been removed; thus, a history should always include inquiries about previous cancer surgery. Breast metastasis to the orbit may elicit a fibrous response that causes enophthalmos and possibly restriction of ocular motility (Fig 5-22).

Some patients with breast cancer respond favorably to hormonal therapy. This response usually correlates with the presence of estrogen and other hormone receptors found in the tumor tissue. If metastatic breast cancer is found at the time of orbital exploration, fresh tissue should be submitted for estrogen receptor assay even if this test was previously performed because estrogen receptor content may differ between the primary and the metastatic lesions. Hormone therapy is most likely to help patients whose tumors are receptor-positive.

### Bronchogenic carcinoma

The most frequent origin of orbital metastasis in men is bronchogenic carcinoma. The primary lesion may be quite small, and CT of suspicious lung lesions may be performed in patients suspected of having orbital metastases.

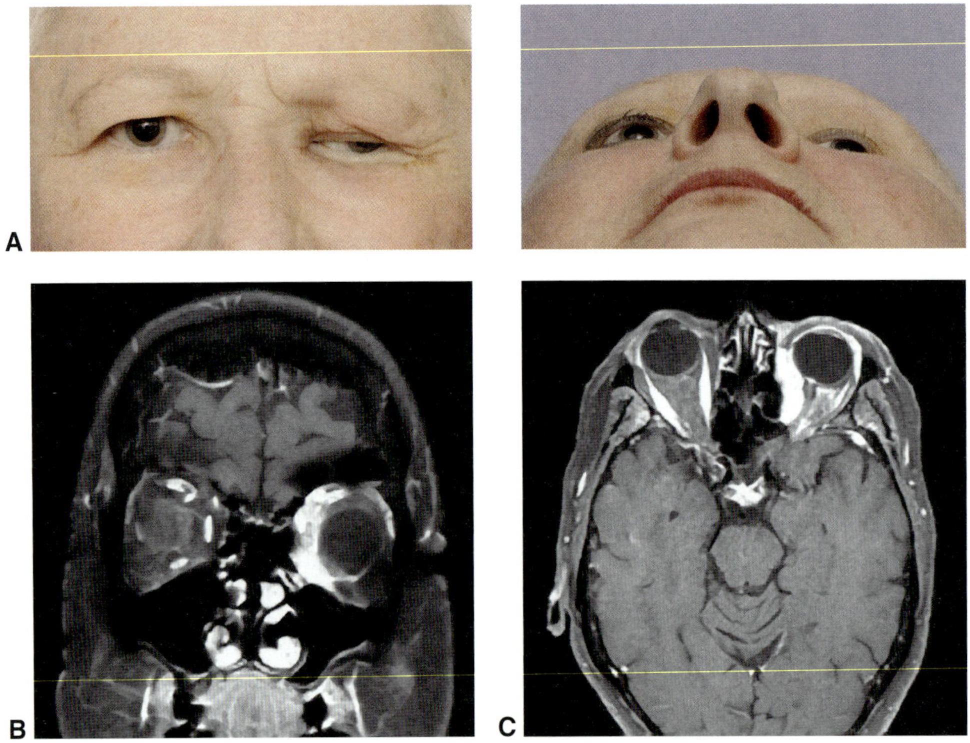

**Figure 5-22** **A,** Left enophthalmos secondary to breast carcinoma metastasis to the orbit. Coronal **(B)** and axial **(C)** MRI images showing medial infiltration of the orbit. *(Courtesy of Hakan Demirci, MD.)*

#### *Prostate carcinoma*

Metastatic prostate carcinoma can produce a clinical picture resembling that of acute nonspecific orbital inflammation. Typically, a lytic bone lesion is identified on imaging.

### Management of Orbital Metastases

The treatment of metastatic tumors of the orbit is usually palliative, consisting of local radiation therapy. Some metastatic tumors, such as carcinoids and renal cell carcinomas, may be candidates for wide excision of the orbital lesion because some patients may survive for many years following resection of isolated metastases from these primary tumors. Consultation with the patient's oncologist should identify candidates who might benefit from wide excision.

Garrity JA, Henderson JW, Cameron JD. *Henderson's Orbital Tumors.* 4th ed. Philadelphia: Lippincott Williams & Wilkins; 2007.

Rootman J, ed. *Diseases of the Orbit: A Multidisciplinary Approach.* 2nd ed. Philadelphia: Lippincott Williams & Wilkins; 2002.

CHAPTER 6

# Orbital Trauma

Orbital trauma can damage the facial bones and adjacent soft tissues. Fractures may be associated with injuries to orbital contents, intracranial structures, and paranasal sinuses. Orbital hemorrhage and foreign bodies may also result in damage to the orbit. Ophthalmic manifestations of orbital trauma may include decreased vision, intraocular injury, strabismus, and eyelid or globe malposition.

Because of the high incidence of concomitant intraocular injury, an ocular examination should be performed on patients who have sustained orbital trauma. Ocular damage accompanying orbital trauma may include hyphema, angle recession, corneoscleral laceration, retinal tear, retinal dialysis, retinal edema, and vitreous hemorrhage.

## Midfacial (Le Fort) Fractures

Le Fort fractures involve the maxilla and are often complex and asymmetric (Figs 6-1, 6-2). By definition, Le Fort fractures must extend posteriorly through the pterygoid plates. These fractures may be divided into 3 categories, although clinically they often do not conform precisely to these groupings.

- *Le Fort I* is a low transverse maxillary fracture above the teeth with no orbital involvement.
- *Le Fort II* fractures generally have a pyramidal configuration and involve the nasal, lacrimal, and maxillary bones as well as the medial orbital floor.
- *Le Fort III* fractures cause craniofacial disjunction in which the entire facial skeleton is completely detached from the base of the skull and suspended only by soft tissues. The orbital floor and medial and lateral orbital walls are involved.

Treatment may include dental stabilization with arch bars and open reduction of the fracture with rigid fixation using titanium plating systems.

## Orbital Fractures

### Zygomatic Fractures

Zygomaticomaxillary complex (ZMC) fractures are referred to as *quadripod fractures* (Fig 6-3) because the zygoma is usually fractured at 4 of its articulations with the adjacent

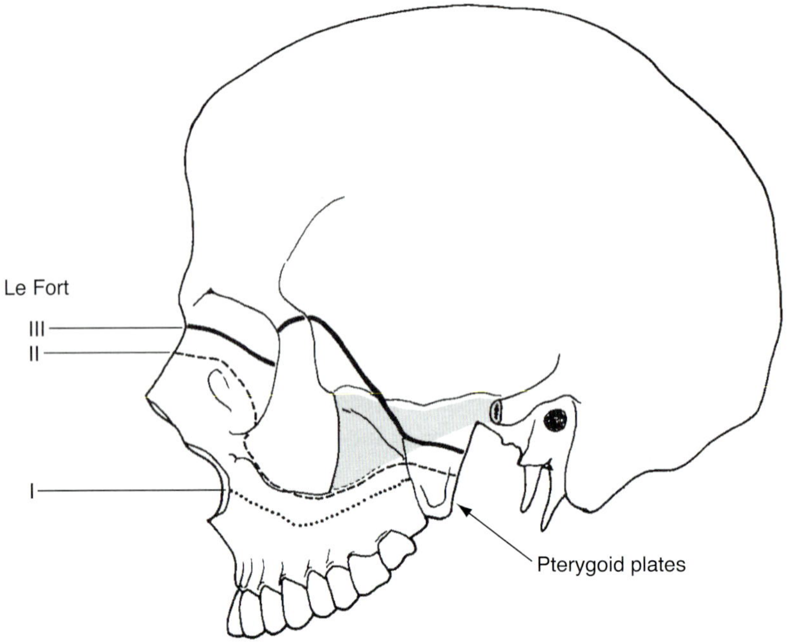


**Figure 6-1** Le Fort fractures (lateral view). Note that all the fractures extend posteriorly through the pterygoid plates *(arrow)*. *(Modified with permission from Converse JM, ed.* Reconstructive Plastic Surgery: Principles and Procedures in Correction, Reconstruction, and Transplantation. *2nd ed. Philadelphia: Saunders; 1977:2.)*

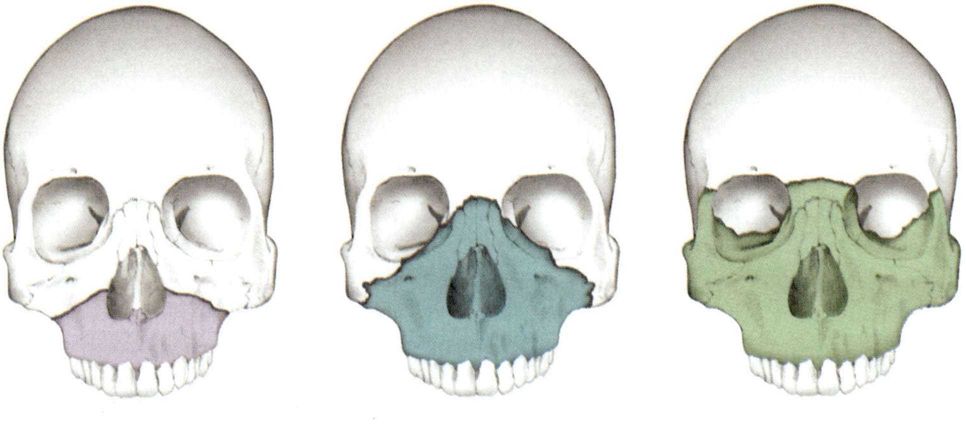


**Figure 6-2** Le Fort's classification of midfacial fractures. Le Fort I, horizontal fracture of the maxilla, also known as Guérin fracture. Le Fort II, pyramidal fracture of the maxilla. Le Fort III, craniofacial dysjunction. *(Modified with permission from Converse JM, ed.* Reconstructive Plastic Surgery: Principles and Procedures in Correction, Reconstruction, and Transplantation. *2nd ed. Philadelphia: Saunders; 1977:2. Illustration by Cyndie C. H. Wooley.)*

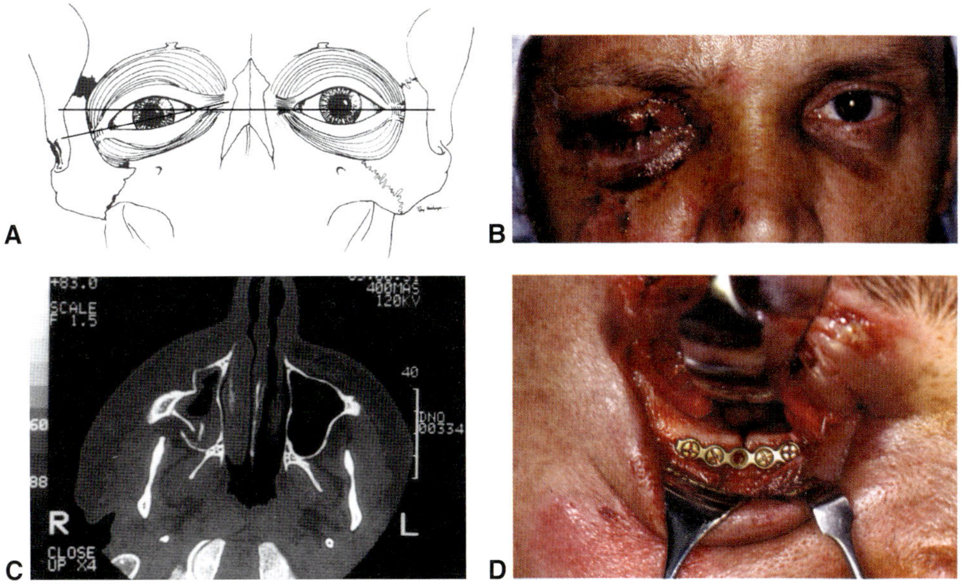


**Figure 6-3** **A,** Zygomaticomaxillary complex (ZMC) fracture (anterior view). Downward displacement of the globe and lateral canthus as a result of frontozygomatic separation and downward displacement of the zygoma and the floor of the orbit. **B,** Globe ptosis and lateral canthal dystopia due to depressed ZMC fracture. **C,** Axial computed tomography (CT) scan showing depression of malar prominence and telescoping of bone fragment into the maxillary sinus. **D,** Intraoperative view showing rigid plate fixation of orbital rim fracture in prior patient. *(Part A modified with permission from Converse JM, ed.* Reconstructive Plastic Surgery: Principles and Procedures in Correction, Reconstruction, and Transplantation. *2nd ed. Philadelphia: Saunders; 1977:2. Parts B, C, and D courtesy of John B. Holds, MD.)*

bones (frontozygomatic suture, inferior orbital rim, zygomatic arch, and lateral wall of the maxillary sinus). ZMC fractures involve the orbital floor to varying degrees. If the zygoma is not significantly displaced, treatment may not be necessary. ZMC fractures can cause globe displacement, cosmetic deformity, diplopia, and trismus (limitation of mandibular opening) due to fracture impingement on the coronoid process of the mandible.

When treatment is indicated, the best results are obtained with open reduction of the fracture and rigid plate fixation (see Fig 6-3). Exact realignment and stabilization of the lateral maxillary buttress and the lateral orbital wall are essential for accurate fracture reduction and can be achieved through a sublabial or buccal sulcus incision. If the lateral maxillary buttress is only mildly displaced, complete reduction and fixation can be accomplished through an eyelid incision.

Chang EL, Hatton MP, Bernardino CR, Rubin PA. Simplified repair of zygomatic fractures through a transconjunctival approach. *Ophthalmology.* 2005;112(7):1302–1309.

## Orbital Apex Fractures

Orbital apex fractures usually occur in association with other fractures of the face, orbit, or skull and may involve the optic canal, superior orbital fissure, and structures that pass through them. Possible associated complications include damage to the optic nerve, with decreased vision; cerebrospinal fluid leak; and carotid-cavernous sinus fistula. Indirect traumatic optic neuropathy usually results from stretching, tearing, twisting, or bruising of the fixed canalicular portion of the nerve as the cranial skeleton suffers sudden deceleration. In most patients, thin-section computed tomography (CT) through the orbital apex and anterior clinoid processes shows fractures at or adjacent to the optic canal. The management of neurogenic vision loss after blunt head trauma is discussed later in this chapter in the section Traumatic Vision Loss With Clear Media.

## Orbital Roof Fractures

Orbital roof fractures are usually caused by blunt trauma or missile injuries. In older patients, frontal trauma is partially absorbed by the frontal sinus, which diffuses the force and prevents extension of the fracture along the orbital roof. Roof fractures are more common in young children because the frontal sinus has not yet pneumatized and also because the ratio of the cranial vault to the midface is greater in children than in adults, making frontal impact more likely with a fall. The brain and cribriform plate may be involved. Complications of orbital roof fractures include intracranial injuries, cerebrospinal fluid rhinorrhea, pneumocephalus, subperiosteal hematoma, ptosis, and extraocular muscle imbalance. In roof fractures, the entrapment of extraocular muscles is rare, with most early diplopia resulting from hematoma, edema, or contusion of the orbital structures. In severely comminuted fractures, pulsating exophthalmos may occur as a delayed complication. Young children may develop nondisplaced linear roof fractures after fairly minor trauma, which may present with delayed ecchymosis of the upper eyelid. Most roof fractures do not require repair. Indications for surgery are generally neurosurgical, and treatment often involves a team approach with a neurosurgeon and an orbital surgeon.

Hink EM, Wei LA, Durairaj VD. Clinical features and treatment of pediatric orbit fractures. *Ophthal Plast Reconstr Surg.* 2014;30(2):124–131.

## Medial Orbital Fractures

Naso-orbital-ethmoidal (NOE) fractures (Fig 6-4) usually result from the face striking solid surfaces. These fractures commonly involve the frontal process of the maxilla, the lacrimal bone, and the ethmoid bones along the medial wall of the orbit. Patients characteristically have a depressed bridge of the nose and traumatic telecanthus. These fractures are categorized as types I–III, with type I being a central fragment of bone attached to canthal tendon, type II having comminuted fracture of the central fragment, and type III having a comminuted tendon attachment or avulsed tendon.

Complications include cerebral and ocular damage, severe epistaxis due to avulsion of the anterior ethmoidal artery, orbital hematoma, cerebrospinal fluid rhinorrhea, damage to the lacrimal drainage system, lateral displacement of the medial canthus, and associated fractures of the medial orbital wall and floor. Treatment includes repair of the nasal

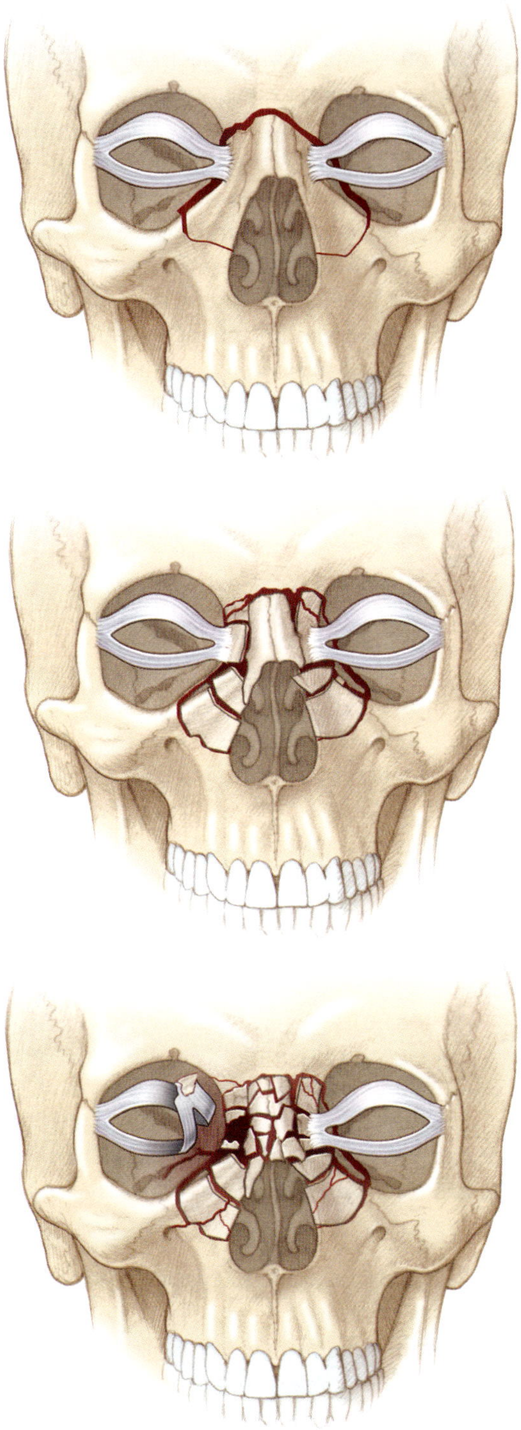


**Figure 6-4** Naso-orbital-ethmoidal fractures result in traumatic telecanthus with rounding of the medial canthus. Types I–III are described depending on the severity of the injury. *(Illustration by Christine Gralapp.)*

fracture and plate stabilization. Transnasal wiring of the medial canthus is used less frequently, as miniplate fixation often allows precise bony reduction.

*Indirect (blowout) fractures* are frequently extensions of blowout fractures of the orbital floor. Isolated blowout fractures of the medial orbital wall may also occur. Surgical intervention is indicated in the setting of muscle and associated tissue entrapment, enophthalmos, and large fracture size. Large, isolated medial wall fractures may result in cosmetically noticeable enophthalmos; however, the risk of enophthalmos is greatest when both the floor and the medial wall are fractured. If surgery is required, the medial orbital wall may be approached by continuing the exploration of the floor up along the medial wall via the eyelid or transconjunctival approach. An alternative approach is a medial orbitotomy through a Lynch (frontoethmoidal) incision in the skin or a transcaruncular approach. See Chapter 7 for discussion of some of the incisions mentioned in this chapter.

Shorr N, Baylis HI, Goldberg RA, Perry JD. Transcaruncular approach to the medial orbit and orbital apex. *Ophthalmology.* 2000;107(8):1459–1463.

## Orbital Floor Fractures

Direct fractures of the orbital floor can extend from fractures of the inferior orbital rim. Indications for repair of the orbital floor in these cases are the same as those for indirect (blowout) fractures. Indirect fractures of the orbital floor are not associated with fracture of the inferior orbital rim.

Past theory held that blowout fractures were caused by increased intraorbital pressure when the impact of a blunt object rapidly occluded the orbital aperture. According to this theory, the contents of the orbit are compressed posteriorly toward the apex of the orbit, and the orbital bones break at their weakest point, usually the posterior medial part of the floor in the maxillary bone. The orbital contents prolapse through the fracture into the maxillary sinus and may be entrapped. An alternative mechanism of action is demonstrated when an impacting object compresses the inferior rim, directly buckling the orbital floor. In this case, the degree of increased orbital pressure determines whether orbital tissues are pushed down through the fracture into the maxillary antrum.

The diagnosis of a blowout fracture of the orbital floor is suggested by the patient's history, physical examination, and radiographs. There is a history of the orbital entrance being struck by an object, usually one larger than the diameter of the orbital opening (eg, a ball, an automobile dashboard, or a fist). An orbital blowout fracture should be suspected in any patient who has received a periorbital blow forceful enough to cause ecchymosis. Physical examination typically reveals the following:

- *Eyelid signs.* Ecchymosis and edema of the eyelids may be present, but other external signs of injury can be absent *(white-eyed blowout).*
- *Diplopia with limitation of upgaze, downgaze, or both.* Limited vertical movement of the globe, vertical diplopia, and pain in the inferior orbit on attempted vertical movement of the globe are consistent with entrapment of the inferior rectus muscle or its adjacent septa in the fracture. Orbital edema and hemorrhage or damage to the extraocular muscles or their innervation can also limit movement of the globe. A significant limitation of both horizontal and vertical eye movements

may indicate nerve damage or generalized soft tissue injury. Limitations of globe movements caused by hemorrhage or edema generally improve during the first 1–2 weeks after injury. If entrapment is present, a *forced duction test (traction test)* shows restriction of passive movement of the eye. This test is performed with the instillation of anesthetic eyedrops followed by a cotton pledget of topical anesthetic in the inferior cul-de-sac for several minutes. Using either a cotton-tipped applicator or toothed forceps, the examiner engages the insertion of the inferior rectus muscle through the conjunctiva and attempts to rotate the globe gently up and down. Another characteristic finding of inferior rectus entrapment is an increase in intraocular pressure (IOP) in upgaze as compared to IOP in primary position.
- *Enophthalmos and ptosis of the globe.* These findings occur with large fractures in which the orbital soft tissues prolapse into the maxillary sinus. A medial wall fracture, if associated with the orbital floor fracture, may significantly contribute to enophthalmos because of prolapse of the orbital tissues into both the ethmoid and the maxillary sinuses. Enophthalmos may be masked by orbital edema immediately following the injury, but it becomes more apparent as the edema subsides.
- *Hypoesthesia in the distribution of the infraorbital nerve.*
- *Emphysema of the orbit and eyelids.* Any fracture that extends into a sinus may allow air to escape into the subcutaneous tissues. This occurs most commonly with medial wall fractures. Patients with fractures are advised to avoid nose blowing to prevent orbital emphysema.

In patients with orbital floor fractures, vision loss can result from globe trauma, injury to the optic nerve, or increased orbital pressure causing a *compartment syndrome* (discussed in the section Traumatic Vision Loss With Clear Media). An orbital hemorrhage should be suspected if loss of vision is associated with proptosis and increased IOP. (Orbital hemorrhage is discussed later in this chapter.) Injuries to the globe and ocular adnexa may also be present.

### *Management*

Computed tomography scans with coronal or sagittal views help guide treatment. They allow evaluation of fracture size and extraocular muscle relationships, providing information that can be used to help predict enophthalmos and muscle entrapment. Despite the publication of multiple studies suggesting neuroimaging criteria for extraocular muscle entrapment, restrictive strabismus related to blowout fracture remains a clinical diagnosis.

Most blowout or other orbital floor fractures do not require surgical intervention. When swelling and orbital hemorrhage are present, patients with orbital blowout fractures are usually observed for 5–10 days to allow time for this to subside. Oral steroids (1 mg/kg per day for the first 7 days) decrease edema and may help hasten the decision of whether surgery for diplopia is necessary.

An exception to initial observation occurs in pediatric patients, in whom the inferior rectus muscle may become tightly trapped beneath a trapdoor fracture (Fig 6-5). In these patients, vertical globe excursion is significantly limited, and CT reveals the inferior rectus muscle within the maxillary sinus. Eye movement may stimulate the oculocardiac

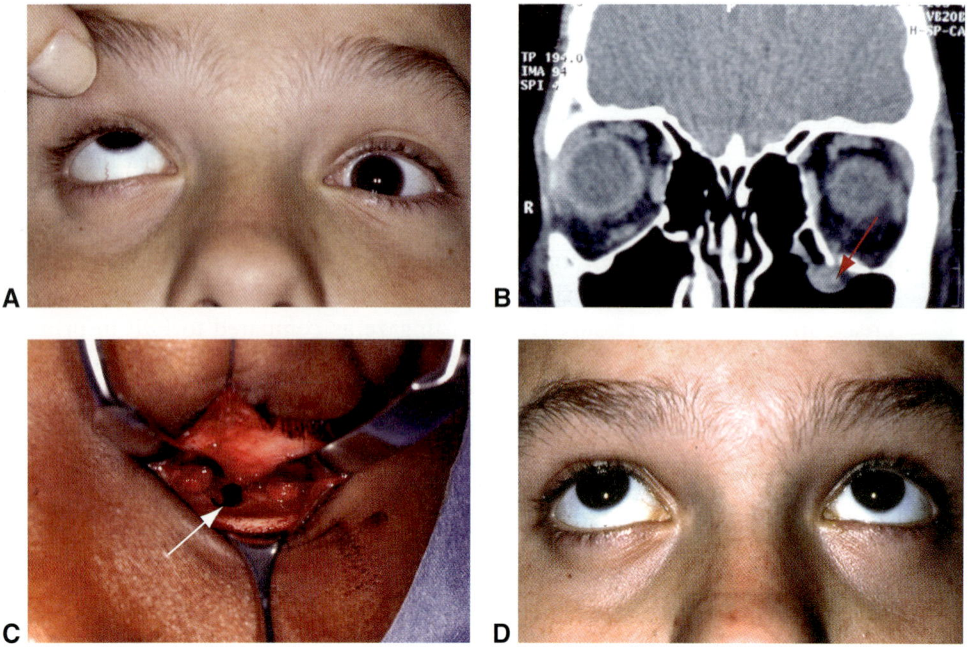


**Figure 6-5** **A,** Teenaged patient following blunt trauma to the eye and orbit. Attempted gaze up and left. The left eye is unable to elevate to midline. (Note: The pupillary dilation is pharmacologic). **B,** Coronal CT scan of the orbit showing a small orbital floor fracture and inferior rectus muscle prolapsing into the maxillary sinus *(arrow)*. **C,** Intraoperative view of a similar case showing an orbital floor defect *(arrow)* enlarged surgically to release and extract inferior rectus muscle. **D,** Two months postoperatively, the patient demonstrates resolution of upgaze limitation. *(Courtesy of John B. Holds, MD.)*

reflex, causing pain, nausea, and bradycardia. Urgent repair should be undertaken in these cases. Release of the entrapped muscle without delay may improve the final ocular motility result by limiting fibrosis.

Although the indications for surgery are controversial, the following general guidelines are helpful for the clinician in determining when surgery is advisable:

- *Diplopia with the following: limitation of upgaze and/or downgaze within 30° of the primary position; positive forced duction test after resolution of the edema; and radiologic confirmation of an orbital floor fracture.* These findings indicate functional entrapment of tissues affecting the inferior rectus muscle. Diplopia may improve significantly over the course of the first 2 weeks as orbital edema, hemorrhage, or both resolve and as some of the entrapped tissues stretch. However, if the findings are still present after 2 weeks and if the entrapped tissues are not freed, vertical diplopia is likely to persist. As mentioned previously, tight entrapment of the inferior rectus muscle with possible muscle ischemia is an indication for immediate repair.
- *Enophthalmos that exceeds 2 mm and is cosmetically unacceptable to the patient.* Enophthalmos is often masked by orbital edema immediately after the injury, and

then gradual fat atrophy due to trauma may delay recognition of the enophthalmos for weeks to months. Exophthalmometry measurements are taken at the initial evaluation and at subsequent visits to monitor for enophthalmos. If significant enophthalmos is present within the first 2 weeks in association with a large orbital floor fracture, even greater enophthalmos can be anticipated in the future.
- *Large fractures involving at least half of the orbital floor, particularly when associated with large medial wall fractures (determined by CT).* Orbital fractures of this size have a high incidence of subsequent significant enophthalmos and are usually repaired as part of initial management.

Burnstine MA. Clinical recommendations for repair of isolated orbital floor fractures: an evidence-based analysis. *Ophthalmology.* 2002;109(7):1207–1210.

Egbert JE, May K, Kersten RC, Kulwin DR. Pediatric orbital floor fracture: direct extraocular muscle involvement. *Ophthalmology.* 2000;107(10):1875–1879.

Harris GJ, Garcia GH, Logani SC, Murphy ML. Correlation of preoperative computed tomography and postoperative ocular motility in orbital blowout fractures. *Ophthal Plast Reconstr Surg.* 2000;16(3):179–187.

Jordan DR, Allen LH, White J, Harvey J, Pashby R, Esmaeli B. Intervention within days for some orbital floor fractures: the white-eyed blowout. *Ophthal Plast Reconstr Surg.* 1998; 14(6):379–390.

**Surgical management of orbital fractures** When surgery is indicated for blowout fractures of the orbital floor, it generally is preferable to proceed with the repair within 2 weeks of the initial trauma. Formation of scar tissue and contracture of the prolapsed tissue make later correction of entrapment and diplopia difficult. Larger fractures in which eventual enophthalmos is anticipated are also more easily repaired within the first 2 weeks of the trauma; however, satisfactory correction of enophthalmos is often obtainable even if surgery is delayed.

The surgical approach to blowout fractures of the orbital floor can be made through an infraciliary incision or a conjunctival (inferior fornix) incision combined with or without a lateral canthotomy and inferior cantholysis. The approaches through the lower eyelid have the following steps in common: elevation of the periorbita from the orbital floor, release of the prolapsed tissues from the fracture, and, usually, placement of an implant over the fracture to prevent recurrent adhesions and prolapse of the orbital tissues.

The development of miniplating and microplating systems and their various metallic orbital implants has significantly improved the management of large, unstable orbital floor fractures. Orbital implants can be alloplastic (porous polyethylene, nylon foil, polytetrafluoroethylene, silicone sheet, or titanium mesh) or autogenous (split cranial bone, iliac crest bone, or fascia). The harvesting of autogenous grafts requires an additional operative site, and bone grafts are rarely indicated.

Delayed treatment of blowout fractures to correct debilitating strabismus and diplopia or cosmetically unacceptable enophthalmos may include exploration of the orbital floor in an attempt to free the scarred tissues entrapped or prolapsed through the fracture and to replace them in the orbit. In late surgery for enophthalmos, placement of an implant to reposition the globe anteriorly or superiorly may be necessary. Other treatment options include strabismus surgery and procedures to camouflage the narrowed palpebral fissure and deep superior sulcus associated with enophthalmos.

Complications of blowout fracture surgery include decreased vision or blindness, persistent or new diplopia, undercorrection or overcorrection of enophthalmos, retraction of the lower eyelid, hypoesthesia of the infraorbital nerve, infection, early or late extrusion of the implant, lymphedema, and damage to the lacrimal drainage system.

## Intraorbital Foreign Bodies

If foreign bodies within the orbit are radiopaque, they can be localized by plain-film radiographs, CT, or magnetic resonance imaging (MRI). Some wooden foreign bodies may be missed on CT and are seen better on MRI. However, MRI should be avoided if there is a possibility that the foreign object is ferromagnetic. If an embedded foreign body causes an orbital infection that drains to the skin surface, it is sometimes possible to locate the object by surgically following the fistulous tract posteriorly. Orbital ultrasonography may be helpful for foreign bodies positioned more anteriorly. Treatment of orbital foreign bodies initially involves culturing the wound (or the foreign body if it is removed) and administering antibiotics. Foreign bodies should be removed if they are composed of vegetable matter or if they are easily accessible in the anterior orbit. In many cases, objects can be safely observed without surgery if they are inert and have smooth edges or are located in the posterior orbit. BBs are common intraorbital foreign bodies and are usually best left in place. MRI can be safely performed with a BB in the orbit.

Finkelstein M, Legmann A, Rubin PA. Projectile metallic foreign bodies in the orbit: a retrospective study of epidemiologic factors, management, and outcomes. *Ophthalmology.* 1997;104(1):96–103.

Ho VH, Wilson MW, Fleming JC, Haik BG. Retained intraorbital metallic foreign bodies. *Ophthal Plast Reconstr Surg.* 2004;20(3):232–236.

## Orbital Hemorrhage

Hemorrhage into the orbit can arise after trauma or surgery; it can also occur spontaneously in association with an underlying vascular tumor of the orbit or blood dyscrasias. Urgent lateral canthotomy and cantholysis, orbital decompression, or surgical drainage is seldom necessary unless visual function is compromised by compression of the optic nerve or by increased orbital pressure that impedes arterial perfusion. Occasionally, a hematic cyst may form following accidental trauma, usually beneath the periosteum.

## Traumatic Vision Loss With Clear Media

Many patients report decreased vision following periocular trauma. The decrease may be due to associated injuries of the cornea, lens, vitreous, or retina. In addition, swelling of the eyelids may cause difficulty in opening the eyes sufficiently to clear the visual axis.

However, a small percentage of patients have true vision loss without any evidence of globe injury. Vision loss in this setting suggests traumatic dysfunction of the optic nerve *(traumatic optic neuropathy)*. Such vision loss usually results from 1 of 3 mechanisms:

- direct injury to the optic nerve from a penetrating wound
- disruption of the blood supply to the optic nerve due to a compartment syndrome, in which posttraumatic orbital edema or hemorrhage causes orbital pressure to increase above arterial perfusion pressure
- indirect injury caused by force from a frontal blow transmitted to the optic nerve in the orbital apex and optic canal

All patients with decreased vision following periorbital trauma should be urgently examined for evidence of direct globe injury. Two key diagnostic questions should be answered when the patient has reduced vision with an apparently normal globe:

- Is an afferent pupillary defect present?
- Is there a "tight" orbit?

Detection of an afferent pupillary defect in the presence of an intact globe strongly suggests traumatic optic neuropathy. However, the examiner must remember that detection of an afferent defect may be difficult if the patient has received narcotics that cause pupillary constriction. The second key diagnostic indicator is intraorbital pressure. Periorbital trauma may cause significant retrobulbar hemorrhage or edema, which can lead to proptosis, ptosis, and limitation of extraocular motility. A portable applanation tonometer may be used in the emergency department to measure IOP, which is increased in the tight orbit in response to the underlying increased orbital pressure. Although fundus examination may reveal a central retinal artery occlusion, vision loss is more often caused by occlusion of the posterior ciliary arteries, which have a lower perfusion pressure than does the central retinal artery.

Patients with a tight orbit, increased IOP, and decreased vision with afferent pupillary defect should undergo emergent decompression of the orbit. This is most easily achieved by disinsertion of the eyelids from the lateral canthus (lateral canthotomy and cantholysis), allowing the orbital volume to expand anteriorly. Lateral canthotomy alone does not sufficiently decrease orbital pressure; inferior cantholysis and sometimes superior cantholysis are also required. Surgical relief of the increased orbital pressure is a priority. Although IOP is elevated in the setting of traumatic orbital hemorrhage, the elevation reflects the increased orbital pressure and is not indicative of glaucoma (although angle-closure glaucoma occurs rarely following retrobulbar hemorrhages).

If a tight orbit has been ruled out, a mechanism other than an ischemic compartment syndrome should be sought to explain the vision loss. The circumstances suggest indirect trauma to the optic nerve. Patients with this disorder usually have a history of blunt trauma to the frontal region or rapid deceleration of the cranium and often have experienced loss of consciousness associated with frontal head trauma. Thin-section CT scans of the orbital apex and anterior clinoid process show fractures through or adjacent to the optic canal in many cases.

The proper management of neurogenic vision loss after blunt head trauma is controversial. Observation alone, high-dose corticosteroids, and surgical decompression of the optic canal have been considered as treatment options for traumatic optic neuropathy. However, recent studies have shown that high-dose corticosteroid therapy may not provide any additional visual benefit over observation alone and could potentially be harmful in patients with traumatic optic neuropathy who have concomitant head trauma. Recent studies have also shown that decompression of the optic nerve provides no additional benefit over observation alone while subjecting patients to the risks associated with surgery. The optimal management of traumatic optic neuropathy remains unresolved. Future studies focusing on neuroprotection are needed.

Steinsapir KD, Goldberg RA. Traumatic optic neuropathy: an evolving understanding. *Am J Ophthalmol.* 2011;151(6):928–933.

Yu-Wai-Man P, Griffiths PG. Steroids for traumatic optic neuropathy. *Cochrane Database Syst Rev.* 2013;6:CD006032.

Yu-Wai-Man P, Griffiths PG. Surgery for traumatic optic neuropathy. *Cochrane Database Syst Rev.* 2005;4:CD005024.

CHAPTER 7

# Orbital Surgery

Orbital surgery requires the delicacy of a neurosurgeon, the strength of an orthopedic surgeon, and the 3-dimensional sense of a general surgeon. Few other locations of the body have so many surgical spaces and so many vital structures within such a small area. Surgical comfort and success are based on the surgeon's knowledge of the relationships among the orbital structures and ability to approach the orbit from different directions and angles to achieve the best access to the pathology.

## Surgical Spaces

There are 5 surgical spaces within the orbit (Fig 7-1):

- the *subperiosteal (subperiorbital) surgical space,* which is the potential space between the bone and the periorbita
- the *extraconal surgical space* (peripheral surgical space), which lies between the periorbita and the muscle cone with its fascia
- the *sub-Tenon (episcleral) surgical space,* which lies between the Tenon capsule and the globe

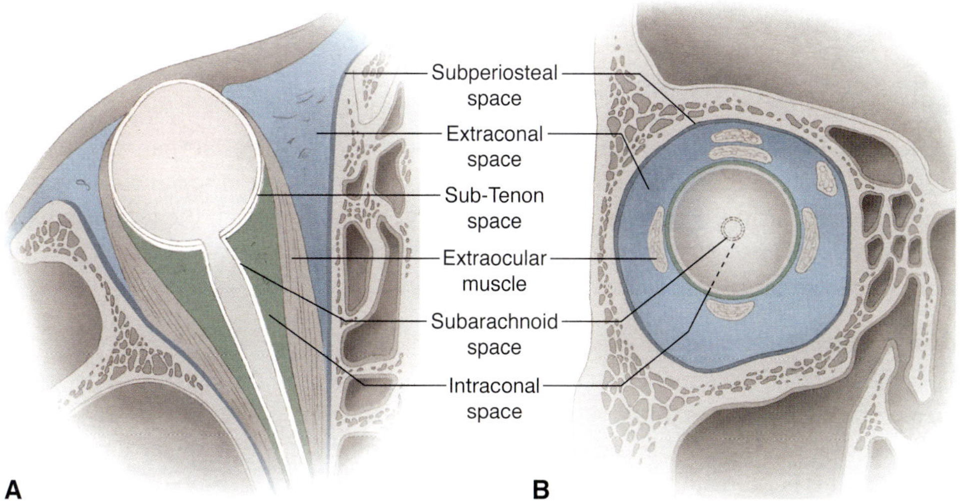


**Figure 7-1** Surgical spaces of the orbit. **A,** Axial view. **B,** Coronal view. *(Illustration by Cyndie C. H. Wooley.)*

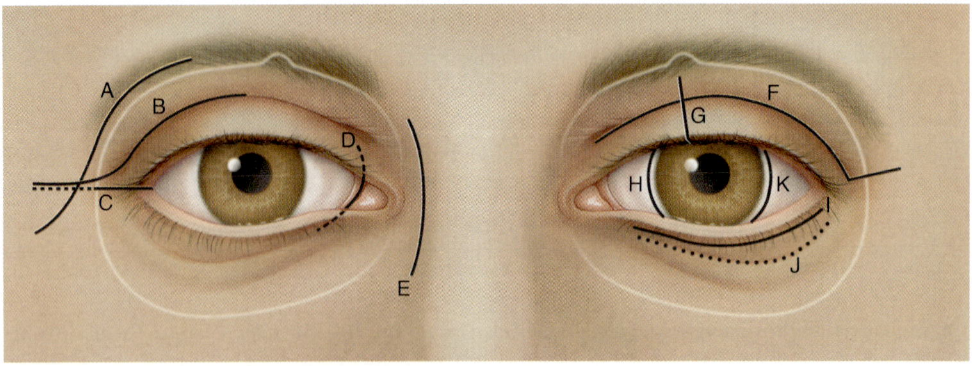


**Figure 7-2** Sites of surgical entry into the orbit. *A,* Classic Stallard-Wright lateral orbitotomy. *B,* Eyelid crease lateral orbitotomy. *C,* Lateral canthotomy/cantholysis orbitotomy. *D,* Transcaruncular medial orbitotomy. *E,* Frontoethmoidal (Lynch) medial orbitotomy. *F,* Upper eyelid crease anterior orbitotomy. *G,* Vertical eyelid split superomedial orbitotomy. *H,* Medial bulbar conjunctival orbitotomy. *I,* Subciliary inferior orbitotomy. *J,* Transconjunctival inferior orbitotomy. *K,* Lateral bulbar conjunctival orbitotomy. *(Illustration by Christine Gralapp after a drawing by Jennifer Clemens.)*

- the *intraconal surgical space* (central surgical space), which lies within the muscle cone
- the *subarachnoid surgical space,* which lies between the optic nerve and the nerve sheath

A single orbital lesion may involve more than 1 surgical space, and a combination of approaches may be necessary for pathologic processes affecting the orbit. The approaches to these spaces—superior, inferior, medial, and lateral—are discussed in the following sections. Incisions used to reach these surgical spaces are shown in Figure 7-2.

## Orbitotomy

### Superior Approach

More orbital lesions are found in the superoanterior part of the orbit than in any other location. Lesions in this area can usually be reached through a transcutaneous incision. With this approach, the surgeon must take care to avoid damaging the levator muscle, superior oblique muscle, trochlea, lacrimal gland, and sensory nerves and vessels entering or exiting the orbit along the superior orbital rim.

#### *Transcutaneous incisions*

For procedures in the superior subperiosteal space, an incision through the upper eyelid crease offers good access to the superior orbital rim and periosteum, with a well-hidden scar (Fig 7-3). Although this incision requires additional soft tissue dissection, the cosmetic result is better with an eyelid crease incision than with an incision directly over the superior orbital rim. After making an upper eyelid crease incision, the surgeon obtains access to the superior orbital rim by dissecting superiorly in the postorbicularis fascial plane anterior to the orbital septum. After the rim is exposed, an incision is made in the arcus

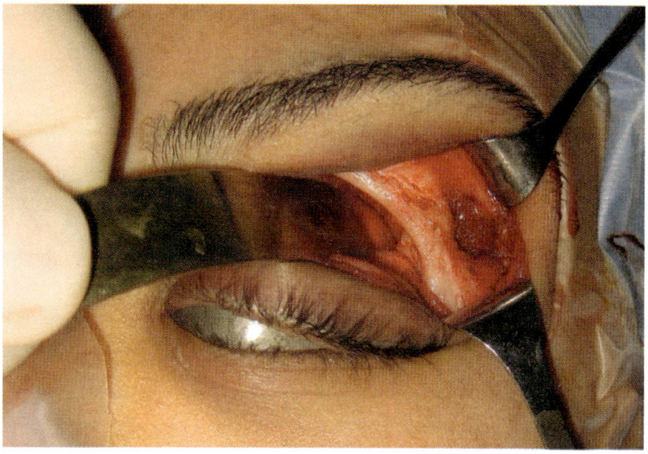

**Figure 7-3** The eyelid crease incision allows access to the superior and lateral orbit, as demonstrated in this surgical excision of a dumbbell dermoid in the lateral orbital wall and temporal fossa. *(Courtesy of Morris E. Hartstein, MD.)*

marginalis of the rim, and a periosteal elevator is then used to separate the periosteum from the frontal bone of the orbital roof. The periosteal dissection is facilitated by initially keeping the periorbita intact, which prevents orbital fat from obscuring the view during reflection of the periosteum.

Upper eyelid crease incisions may also be used for entry into the medial intraconal space, which requires exposure of the medial edge of the levator muscle and dissection through the intermuscular septum extending from the superior rectus to the medial rectus muscles. This approach may be used for exposure and biopsy of the optic nerve or for fenestration of the retrobulbar optic nerve sheath in cases of idiopathic intracranial hypertension.

The coronal approach to the superior orbit is most often used in conjunction with trauma or craniofacial surgery. This approach is also used for transcranial orbitotomies to expose extensive lesions of the superior and posterior orbit and sinuses that require bone removal for access. Although the coronal incision may be used to gain access for lateral orbitotomy, this incision requires extensive elevation of the temporalis muscle, which may result in postoperative temporalis atrophy. Alopecia may occur at the site of the coronal scalp incision.

Stewart WB, Levin PS, Toth BA. Orbital surgery. The technique of coronal scalp flap approach to the lateral orbitotomy. *Arch Ophthalmol.* 1988;106(12):1724–1726.

### *Transconjunctival incision*

Incisions in the superior conjunctiva can be used to reach the superonasal, sub-Tenon, intraconal, or extraconal surgical spaces; but dissection must be performed medial to the levator muscle to prevent postoperative ptosis.

### *Vertical eyelid splitting*

Vertical splitting of the upper eyelid at the junction of the medial and central thirds allows extended transconjunctival exposure for the removal of superomedial intraconal tumors.

The surgeon incises the eyelid and levator aponeurosis vertically to expose the superomedial intraconal space. Realignment of the tarsal plate and aponeurosis with vertical closure prevents postoperative ptosis and eyelid retraction.

Kersten RC, Kulwin DR. Vertical lid split orbitotomy revisited. *Ophthal Plast Reconstr Surg.* 1999;15(6):425–428.

## Inferior Approach

The inferior approach is suitable for masses that are visible or palpable in the inferior conjunctival fornix of the lower eyelid, as well as for deeper inferior extraconal orbital masses. The surgeon can also gain access to intraconal lesions by dissecting between the inferior rectus and lateral rectus muscles. The inferior oblique muscle inserts over the macula and may be identified and retracted while intraconal lesions are accessed. This route is commonly used to approach the orbital floor for fracture repair or decompression.

### *Transcutaneous incisions*

Visible scarring can be minimized by the use of an infraciliary blepharoplasty incision (2.5–4.0 mm below the margin) in the lower eyelid skin, followed by inferior dissection beneath the orbicularis oculi muscle to expose the inferior orbital septum and inferior orbital rim. An incision in the lower eyelid crease or directly over the inferior orbital rim can provide similar exposure, but it leaves a slightly more obvious scar. Once the skin–muscle flap is created, the surgeon can open the septum to expose the extraconal surgical space. Alternatively, for access to the inferior subperiosteal space the periosteum is incised and elevated at the arcus marginalis to expose the orbital floor. Fractures of the orbital floor are reached by the subperiosteal route.

### *Transconjunctival incisions*

The transconjunctival approach (Fig 7-4) has largely replaced the transcutaneous route for exposure of tumors in the inferior orbit and for management of fractures of the orbital floor and medial wall. To reach the extraconal surgical space and the orbital floor, the surgeon may make an incision through the inferior conjunctiva and lower eyelid retractors. The optical cavity can be enlarged by adding a lateral canthotomy and cantholysis. The transconjunctival incision is made either just below the inferior tarsal border or in the conjunctival fornix. When using cutting cautery, the surgeon should take care not to cause thermal damage to the conjunctiva and tarsus. Opening the reflected periosteum and then retracting the muscles and intraconal fat provide access to not only the orbital floor but also the intraconal space.

Working on the globe surface and using an incision of the bulbar conjunctiva and Tenon capsule allows entry to the sub-Tenon surgical space. This technique is used to reach the extraocular muscles. If the inferior rectus is retracted, the intraconal surgical space can be accessed through this incision.

## Medial Approach

When dissecting in the medial orbit, the surgeon should be careful to avoid damaging the medial canthal tendon, lacrimal canaliculi and sac, trochlea, superior oblique tendon

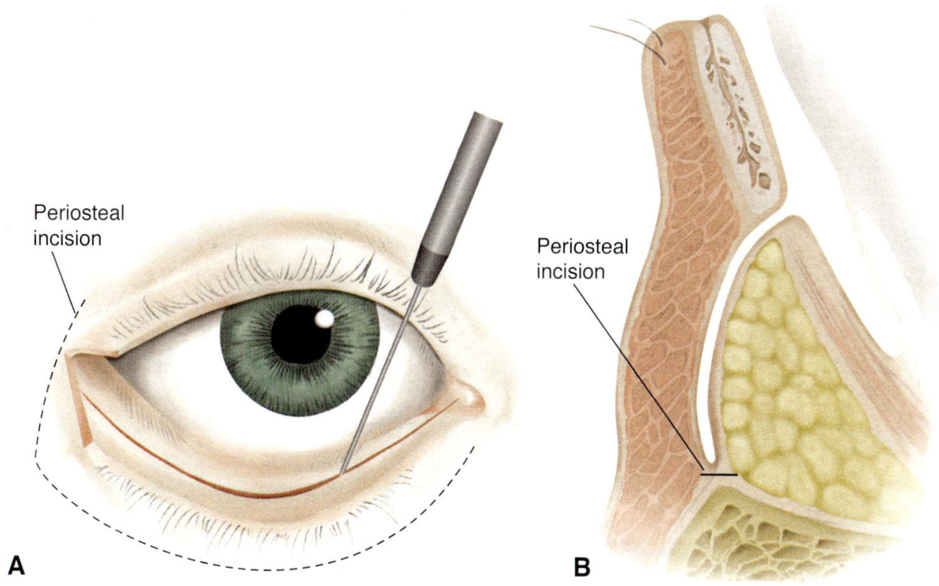


**Figure 7-4** Inferior transconjunctival approach to the orbital floor. **A,** Canthotomy, cantholysis, and conjunctival incision. **B,** Plane of dissection anterior to orbital septum. *(Illustration by Cyndie C. H. Wooley.)*

and muscle, inferior oblique muscle, and the sensory nerves and vessels along the medial aspect of the superior orbital rim.

#### *Transcutaneous incision*

Tumors within or near the lacrimal sac, the frontal or ethmoid sinuses, or the medial rectus muscle can be approached through a skin incision (*Lynch,* or *frontoethmoidal, incision*) placed vertically just medial to the insertion of the medial canthal tendon (approximately 9–10 mm medial to the medial canthal angle). This route is generally used to enter the subperiosteal space. The medial canthal tendon can be reflected with the periosteum and, therefore, does not need to be incised.

Superomedial intraconal lesions can be approached through a medial upper eyelid crease incision. The superior oblique tendon must be identified, and dissection is then carried out medial to the medial horn of the levator muscle, providing access to the intraconal space.

Pelton RW, Patel BC. Superomedial lid crease approach to the medial intraconal space: a new technique for access to the optic nerve and central space. *Ophthal Plast Reconstr Surg.* 2001; 17(4):241–253.

#### *Transconjunctival incision*

An incision in the bulbar conjunctiva allows entry into the extraconal or sub-Tenon surgical space. If the medial rectus muscle is detached, the surgeon can then enter the intraconal surgical space to expose the region of the anterior optic nerve for examination, biopsy, or sheath fenestration (Fig 7-5). If the posterior optic nerve or muscle cone needs

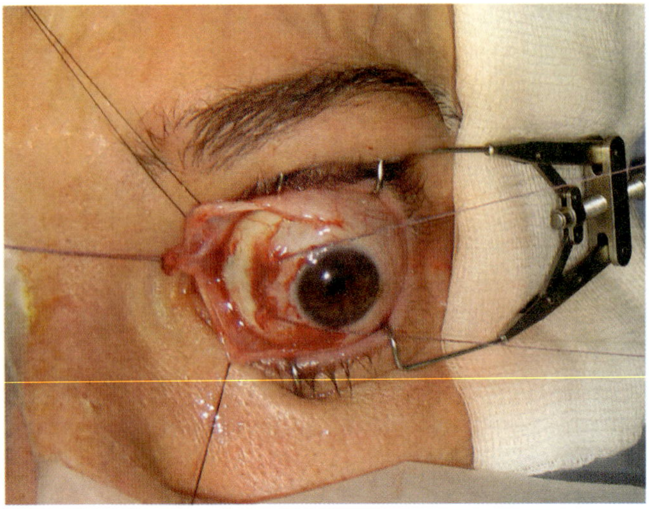

**Figure 7-5** Medial transconjunctival approach for optic nerve sheath fenestration. The medial rectus muscle has been disinserted. There is a traction suture at the muscle insertion site to rotate the globe, and the muscle is imbricated with a suture. *(Courtesy of Morris E. Hartstein, MD.)*

to be seen well, a combined lateral/medial orbitotomy can be performed. A lateral orbitotomy with removal of the lateral orbital wall allows the globe to be displaced temporally, thus maximizing medial access to the deeper orbit.

#### *Transcaruncular incision*

An incision through the posterior third of the caruncle allows excellent exposure of the medial periosteum. Blunt dissection carried medially, just posterior to the lacrimal sac, allows access to the subperiosteal space along the medial wall. Incision and elevation of the medial periorbita allow exposure of the medial orbital wall. This incision has the advantage of providing better cosmetic results than the traditional Lynch, or frontoethmoidal, incision, but the surgeon must be careful to protect the lacrimal canaliculi and to remain posterior to the lacrimal apparatus. The combination of the transcaruncular route with an inferior transconjunctival incision allows extensive exposure of the inferior and medial orbit. This approach provides access for repair of medial wall fractures, for medial orbital bone decompression, and for drainage of medial subperiosteal abscesses.

Goldberg RA, Mancini R, Demer JL. The transcaruncular approach: surgical anatomy and technique. *Arch Facial Plast Surg.* 2007;9(6):443–447.

### Lateral Approach

A lateral orbitotomy approach is used when a lesion is located within the lateral intraconal space, behind the equator of the globe, or in the lacrimal gland fossa. As the orbits are relatively shallower in children than in adults, extensive exposure of the orbits without the need for bone removal may be possible in children. The traditional S-shaped Stallard-Wright skin incision (see Fig 7-2), extending from beneath the eyebrow laterally and curving down along the zygomatic arch, allowed good exposure of the lateral rim but left a noticeable scar. It has largely been replaced by approaches through either an upper eyelid crease incision or an extended lateral canthotomy incision. Both of these approaches allow exposure of the lateral orbital rim and anterior portion of the zygomatic arch after reflection of the temporalis muscle and the periosteum of the orbit. Dissecting through the periorbita and then intermuscular septum either above or below the lateral rectus muscle and posterior to the equator of the globe provides access to the intraconal retrobulbar space. The retrobulbar optic nerve may be reached this way and fenestrated in cases of idiopathic intracranial hypertension.

If a lesion cannot be adequately exposed through a soft tissue lateral incision, an oscillating saw is used to remove the bone of the lateral rim to expose the underlying periorbita, which is then opened. An operating microscope is often useful during intraorbital surgery, especially if dissection proceeds inside the muscle cone. Good exposure of the intraconal surgical space can be achieved with retraction of the lateral rectus muscle. Tumors can occasionally be prolapsed into the incision by application of gentle pressure over the eyelids. A cryosurgical probe or Allis forceps can be used to provide firm traction on encapsulated tumors. In cavernous hemangiomas, a suture through the lesion allows not only traction but also slow decompression of the tumor to facilitate its removal.

Complete hemostasis should be accomplished before closure. To help prevent postoperative intraorbital hemorrhage, an external drain may be placed through the skin to reach the deep orbital tissues. The lateral orbital rim is usually replaced and may be sutured back into place through predrilled tunnels in the rim. Alternatively, the surgeon may use rigid fixation with plating systems. The overlying tissues are then returned to their normal positions and sutured. The use of steel wire is avoided because it can cause artifacts on follow-up computed tomography scans. The surgeon closes the periosteum loosely to allow postoperative hemorrhage to decompress.

Kersten RC, Kulwin DR. Optic nerve sheath fenestration through a lateral canthotomy incision. *Arch Ophthalmol.* 1993;111(6):870–874.

## Orbital Decompression

Orbital decompression is a surgical procedure used to improve the volume-to-space discrepancy that occurs primarily in thyroid eye disease (TED). The goal of orbital decompression is to allow the enlarged muscles and orbital fat to expand into the additional space that has been created by the surgery (Fig 7-6). This expansion relieves pressure on the optic nerve and its blood supply and reduces proptosis.

Decompression historically involved removal of the medial orbital wall and much of the orbital floor to allow orbital tissues to expand into the ethmoid and maxillary sinuses. The approach was made through the maxillary sinus (Caldwell-Luc) or transcutaneous anterior orbitotomy incision. However, when used in patients with inflammatory eye disease featuring enlarged, restricted inferior rectus muscles, this type of decompression with removal of the medial orbital strut may result in or exacerbate globe ptosis and upper eyelid retraction and disrupt globe excursion due to prolapse of the muscles into the ethmoid

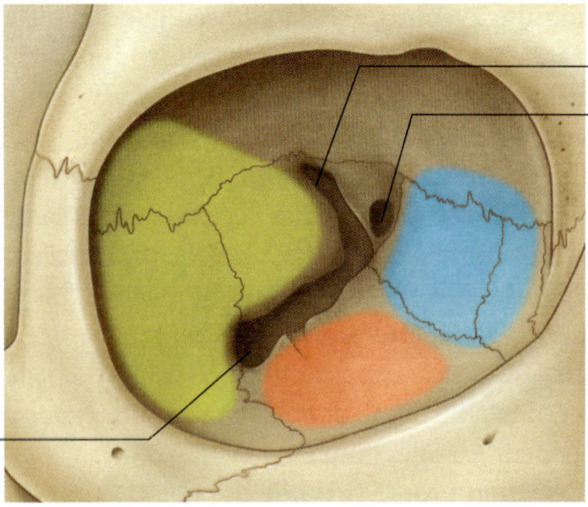


**Figure 7-6** Potential sites for orbital decompression include the medial wall *(blue),* lateral wall *(yellow),* and floor of the orbit *(orange). (Courtesy of Bobby S. Korn, MD, PhD.)*

or maxillary sinuses and displacement of the orbital contents. The approach currently used by many orbital surgeons is a transconjunctival incision combined with a lateral canthotomy/cantholysis to evert the lower eyelid for exposure of the inferior and lateral orbital rims (Fig 7-7). Extension of this incision superonasally with a transcaruncular approach allows excellent access to the medial orbital wall for bone removal and decompression. (A transnasal endoscopic approach to the medial orbit via the ethmoid sinus may also be useful for the medial wall.) To allow further decompression into the infratemporal fossa, the surgeon may remove the lateral orbital rim and reposition it anteriorly at the time of closure. Anterior displacement of the lateral canthus may also aid in the reduction of eyelid retraction. Burring down the orbital surface of the lateral wall and the sphenoid wing results in additional decompression. This type of procedure maximizes volume expansion and "balances" the decompression (Fig 7-8).

Removal of retrobulbar fat at the time of decompression further reduces proptosis and has also been shown to be beneficial in compressive optic neuropathy. Decompression through the orbital roof into the anterior cranial fossa is rarely advisable.

**Figure 7-7** Surgical approach to the orbit combining lateral canthotomy/cantholysis, inferior transconjunctival incision, and medial Lynch (frontoethmoidal) incision. Lateral orbital rim bone removed. *(Courtesy of Jill Foster, MD.)*

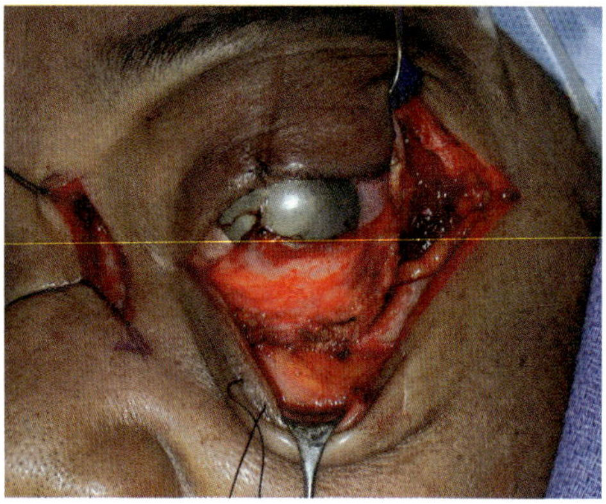

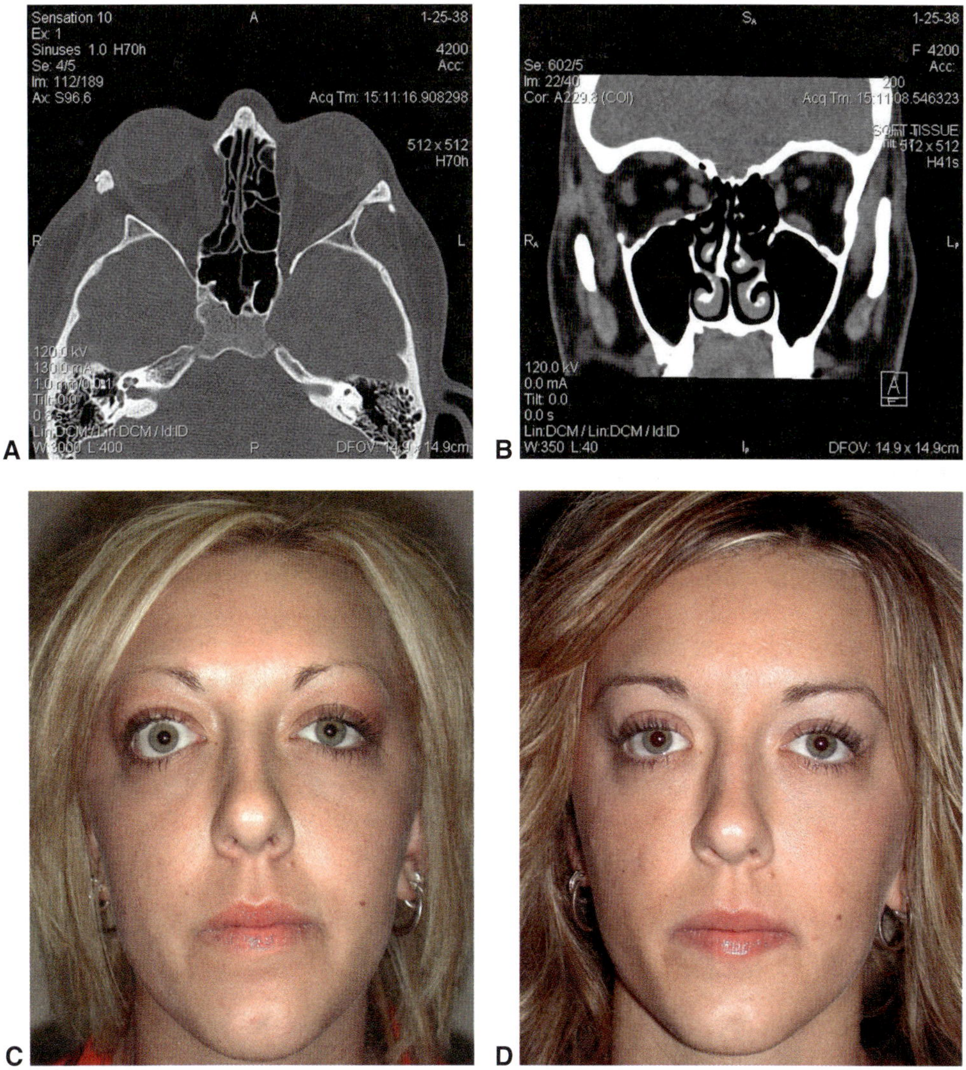


**Figure 7-8** "Balanced" orbital decompression. **A,** Axial view computed tomography (CT) scan showing surgical removal of areas of the lateral and medial walls on the right side. **B,** Coronal CT of same patient with views of medial, lateral, and inferior medial bone removal. **C,** Clinical photograph of this patient before surgery. **D,** Clinical photo of same patient following surgery. *(Courtesy of Jill Foster, MD.)*

Kacker A, Kazim M, Murphy M, Trokel S, Close LG. "Balanced" orbital decompression for severe Graves' orbitopathy: technique with treatment algorithm. *Otolaryngol Head Neck Surg.* 2003;128(2):228–235.

Perry JD, Kadakia A, Foster JA. Transcaruncular orbital decompression for dysthyroid optic neuropathy. *Ophthal Plast Reconstr Surg.* 2003;19(5):353–358.

White WA, White WL, Shapiro PE. Combined endoscopic medial and inferior orbital decompression with transcutaneous lateral orbital decompression in Graves' orbitopathy. *Ophthalmology.* 2003;110(9):1827–1832.

## Postoperative Care for Orbital Surgery

Measures used to reduce postoperative edema are elevation of the head, iced compresses on the eyelids, administration of systemic steroids, and optional placement of a drain (if used, the drain is removed in 24–48 hours). Visual acuity is checked in the first 12 hours after surgery. Systemic antibiotics may be given. Ice packs minimize swelling and still allow frequent observation of the operative site and vision monitoring.

## Special Surgical Techniques in the Orbit

Fine-needle aspiration biopsy (FNAB) may have value in selected cases of lymphoid lesions, secondary tumors invading the orbit from the sinuses, suspected metastatic tumors, and blind eyes with optic nerve tumors. The technique is not very effective for obtaining tissue from fibrous lesions because of the difficulty in successfully aspirating cells. Although FNAB has not been considered a good technique for biopsy in lymphoproliferative disorders, it may assist in the diagnosis of selected cases when used with flow cytometry with monoclonal antibodies or polymerase chain reaction analysis. FNAB is performed with a 4-cm 22- or 23-gauge needle attached to a syringe in a pistol-grip syringe holder. If necessary, the needle can be guided into the tumor by ultrasonography or computed tomography. Cells (and occasionally a small block of tissue) are aspirated from the lesion. A skilled cytologist is required to study the specimen. See BCSC Section 4, *Ophthalmic Pathology and Intraocular Tumors,* for further discussion of FNAB.

Masses or traumatic injuries may involve the skull base, including posterior and superior aspects of the orbit. Advanced surgical techniques provide access to these areas via a frontal craniotomy or frontotemporal-orbitozygomatic approach. Such operations often require the combined efforts of the orbital surgeon, neurosurgeon, and otorhinolaryngologist. The neurosurgeon provides orbital access for the oculofacial surgeon by removing the frontal bar and the orbital roof, giving unparalleled access to superior apical lesions. These techniques allow removal of tumors such as meningiomas, fibrous dysplasia, hemangiomas, hemangiopericytomas, schwannomas, and gliomas that might not otherwise be resectable. In addition, the frontotemporal-orbitozygomatic approach provides access to the intracranial optic canal for decompression.

McDermott MW, Durity FA, Rootman J, Woodhurst WB. Combined frontotemporal-orbitozygomatic approach for tumors of the sphenoid wing and orbit. *Neurosurgery.* 1990;26(1):107–116.

## Complications of Orbital Surgery

The surgeon can reduce complications from orbital surgery by performing a complete preoperative evaluation with orbital imaging when indicated, choosing the appropriate surgical approach, obtaining adequate exposure, carefully manipulating the tissues, employing proper instrumentation and illumination, maintaining good hemostasis, and using a team approach when appropriate.

Decreased or lost vision is a serious complication of surgery that may be caused by excessive traction on the globe and optic nerve, contusion of the optic nerve, postoperative infection, or hemorrhage, which leads to increased orbital pressure and consequent ischemic injury to the optic nerve. A patient who has severe orbital pain postoperatively should be evaluated immediately for possible orbital hemorrhage. If this pain is associated with decreased vision, proptosis, ecchymosis, increased intraocular pressure, and an afferent pupillary defect, the surgeon should consider opening the wound to minimize the effects of the compartment syndrome (see Chapter 6), evacuating any hematoma, and controlling active bleeding.

Hypoesthesia in the distribution of the infraorbital nerve may follow manipulation of the orbital floor after fracture repair or orbital floor decompression. Other complications of decompression, such as downward displacement of the globe and postoperative exacerbation of upper eyelid retraction, were discussed previously. Motility disorders may be caused or exacerbated by orbital surgery. The active, or inflammatory, phase of TED may increase the risks of postoperative restrictive myopathy and enlarged muscle displacement in orbital decompression. In tumor resection in the superior orbit, the superior division of the third cranial nerve is especially susceptible to intraoperative injury. The ciliary ganglion is at risk in lateral approaches to the intraconal space. Other complications of orbital surgery include ptosis, neuroparalytic keratopathy, pupillary changes, vitreous hemorrhage, detached retina, hypoesthesia of the forehead, keratitis sicca, cerebrospinal fluid leak, and infection.

Purgason PA, Hornblass A. Complications of surgery for orbital tumors. *Ophthal Plast Reconstr Surg.* 1992;8(2):88–93.

CHAPTER 8

# The Anophthalmic Socket

It is occasionally necessary to remove an eye or the contents of an orbit to enhance patient comfort and cosmesis, to protect the vision in the fellow eye, or to safeguard life. The indications for anophthalmic surgery are diverse, and the procedure of choice varies. *Enucleation* involves removal of the entire globe while preserving other orbital tissues. *Evisceration* is the removal of the intraocular contents (lens, uvea, retina, and vitreous), leaving the sclera, extraocular muscles, and optic nerve intact. *Exenteration* refers to the removal of some or all of the orbital tissues, including the globe. The cosmetic goals in anophthalmic surgery are to minimize any condition that draws attention to the anophthalmia. Surgical efforts to produce orbital and eyelid symmetry and to promote good prosthetic position and motility enhance cosmesis.

Congenital anophthalmia (absence of the globe) and microphthalmia (globe diminished in size) and their management are discussed in Chapter 3. Management of infants with these disorders differs from that of anophthalmic adults because of the opportunity for orbital and tissue expansion in infants. However, the principles of socket surgery described in this chapter also apply to these children.

With loss of an eye, the patient can become depressed or have a degraded self-image. The ophthalmologist can assist the patient both before and after surgery by providing reassurance and psychological support. Discussions of the procedure, the rehabilitation process, and expected functional changes can help the patient with adjustment. With very few exceptions, the monocular patient may resume the full range of home, vocational, and recreational activities. When resuming full activity, patients should take a cautious approach to allow adjustment to the loss of some depth perception and visual field. This loss may result in occupational limitations. One of the most important roles for the ophthalmologist is to help safeguard the remaining eye through regular follow-up examinations and the prescription of polycarbonate safety glasses for full-time wear.

Brady FB. *A Singular View: The Art of Seeing With One Eye.* 6th ed. Vienna, VA: Michael O. Hughes; 2004.

Coday MP, Warner MA, Jahrling KV, Rubin PA. Acquired monocular vision: functional consequences from the patient's perspective. *Ophthal Plast Reconstr Surg.* 2002;18(1): 56–63.

# Enucleation and Evisceration

## Enucleation

In enucleation, the extraocular muscles are released from the sclera, and then the sclera and the entire globes are removed. Enucleation allows for complete histologic examination of the eye and optic nerve. It reduces the concern that surgery might contribute to the risk of sympathetic ophthalmia (discussed below) in the fellow eye. Enucleation is the procedure of choice if the nature of the intraocular pathology is unknown or if ocular tumor is suspected in an eye with no view of the posterior pole.

Enucleation is indicated for primary intraocular malignancies not amenable to alternative modes of therapy (eg, external-beam irradiation, episcleral plaque brachytherapy). Retinoblastoma and choroidal melanoma are the ocular tumors that most commonly require enucleation. When enucleation is performed for an intraocular tumor, the surgeon must take care to avoid penetrating the globe during surgery and to handle the globe gently to minimize the risk of disseminating tumor cells. In cases of suspected retinoblastoma, the surgeon should obtain a long segment of optic nerve with the enucleation specimen to increase the chance of complete resection of the tumor. Blind eyes with opaque media should be suspected of harboring an occult neoplasm unless another cause of ocular disease can be surmised. Although blind or phthisical eyes are not at increased risk for malignancy, a tumor can occasionally be the cause of globe degeneration. Ultrasonography is useful in evaluating these eyes and planning proper management.

In severely traumatized eyes, early enucleation may be considered if the risk of sympathetic ophthalmia and harm to the remaining eye is judged to be greater than the likelihood of recovering useful vision in the traumatized eye. Sympathetic ophthalmia is thought to be a delayed hypersensitivity immune response to the uveal antigens. Enucleation with complete removal of the uveal pigment may be beneficial in preventing the subsequent immune response. The incidence rate of sympathetic ophthalmia is estimated to be 0.03 cases per 100,000 per year. The condition has been reported to occur from 9 days to 50 years after corneoscleral perforation. The infrequency of sympathetic ophthalmia, coupled with improved medical therapy for uveitis, has made early enucleation strictly for prophylaxis a debatable practice. (See BCSC Section 9, *Intraocular Inflammation and Uveitis,* for additional detailed information.)

Painful eyes without useful vision can be managed with enucleation or evisceration. Patients with end-stage neovascular glaucoma, chronic uveitis, or previously traumatized blind eyes can obtain dramatic relief from discomfort and improved cosmesis with either procedure. Enucleation can be performed satisfactorily under local or general anesthesia; however, most patients prefer general anesthesia or sedation when an eye is removed. For debilitated patients unable to undergo surgery and rehabilitation, retrobulbar injection of ethanol may provide adequate pain relief. Serious complications of retrobulbar injections of ethanol include chronic orbital inflammation, fibrosis, and pain.

For nonpainful, disfigured eyes, it is generally advisable to consider a trial of a cosmetic scleral shell prior to removal of the eye. If tolerated, scleral shells can provide excellent cosmesis and motility.

Galor A, Davis JL, Flynn HW Jr, et al. Sympathetic ophthalmia: incidence of ocular complications and vision loss in the sympathizing eye. *Am J Ophthalmol.* 2009;148(5): 704–710.e2.

Yousuf SJ, Jones LS, Kidwell ED Jr. Enucleation and evisceration: 20 years of experience. *Orbit.* 2012;31(4):211–215.

### *Goals for the surgical anophthalmic socket*

After enucleation or evisceration is performed, the following components are necessary in order for an anophthalmic socket to be functionally acceptable and to promote cosmesis:

- an implant of sufficient volume centered within the orbit (implants and prostheses are discussed later in the chapter)
- a socket lined with conjunctiva or mucous membrane with fornices deep enough to hold a prosthesis
- eyelids with normal appearance and adequate tone to support a prosthesis
- good transmission of motility from the implant to the overlying prosthesis
- a comfortable ocular prosthesis that looks similar to the normal eye

### *Enucleation in childhood*

Enucleation in early childhood, as well as congenital anophthalmia or microphthalmia, may lead to underdevelopment of the involved bony orbit with secondary facial and eyelid asymmetry. Orbital soft-tissue volume is a critical determinant of orbital bone growth. Thus, for an anophthalmic socket in a young child, the surgeon aims to select an implant that maximally replaces the lost orbital volume but exerts minimal tension on the wound. Sometimes an implant no larger than 10–16 mm is used.

Autogenous dermis-fat grafts can be used successfully as primary anophthalmic implants in young children. These grafts have been shown to grow along with the expanding orbit. The opposite effect has been observed in adults, in whom a loss of volume generally occurs when dermis-fat grafts are used as primary anophthalmic implants.

Heher KL, Katowitz JA, Low JE. Unilateral dermis-fat graft implantation in the pediatric orbit. *Ophthal Plast Reconstr Surg.* 1998;14(2):81–88.

## Evisceration

Evisceration involves the removal of the contents of the globe, leaving the sclera, extraocular muscles, and optic nerve intact. Evisceration should be considered *only* if the presence of an intraocular malignancy has been ruled out.

The goals for the anophthalmic socket after evisceration were discussed in the subsection "Goals for the surgical anophthalmic socket."

### *Advantages of evisceration*

- *Less disruption of orbital anatomy.* With less dissection within the orbit, there is a lower chance of injury to the extraocular muscles and nerves and of fat atrophy. The relationships between the muscles, globe, eyelids, and fornices remain undisturbed.
- *Better motility of the prosthesis.* The extraocular muscles remain attached to the sclera.

- *Treatment of endophthalmitis.* Evisceration is preferred by some surgeons in cases of endophthalmitis because extirpation and drainage of the ocular contents can occur without invasion of the orbit. The chance of contamination of the orbit with possible subsequent orbital cellulitis or intracranial extension is therefore theoretically reduced.
- *A technically simpler procedure.* Performing this less invasive procedure may be important when general anesthesia is contraindicated or when bleeding disorders increase the risk of orbital dissection. Because evisceration requires less manipulation of the orbital contents, less anesthetic sedation may be necessary.
- *Lower rate of migration or extrusion of the implant, and reoperation.*

#### *Disadvantages of evisceration*

- *Not every patient is a candidate.* Evisceration should never be performed if a malignant ocular tumor is suspected. Severe phthisis bulbi limits the size of the orbital implant that can be placed unless posterior sclerotomies are performed.
- *Theoretical increased risk of sympathetic ophthalmia.* Initial report of 4 cases more than 25 years ago has not been subsequently confirmed by additional case reports.
- *Evisceration affords a less complete specimen for pathologic examinations.*

Levine MR, Pou CR, Lash RH. Evisceration: is sympathetic ophthalmia a concern in the new millennium? The 1998 Wendell Hughes Lecture. *Ophthal Plast Reconstr Surg.* 1999;15(1):4–8.

Lucarelli MJ, Kaltreider SA. Advances in evisceration and enucleation. *Focal Points: Clinical Modules for Ophthalmologists.* San Francisco: American Academy of Ophthalmology; 2004, module 6.

Massry GG, Holds JB. Evisceration with scleral modification. *Ophthal Plast Reconstr Surg.* 2001;17(1):42–47.

### Intraoperative Complications of Enucleation and Evisceration

#### *Removal of the wrong eye*

This is one of the most feared complications in ophthalmology. Taking a “time-out” to reexamine the patient’s medical record, the operative permit, and the patient with ophthalmoscopy in the operating room immediately before enucleation or evisceration is of critical importance. Marking the skin near the eye to be enucleated or eviscerated after having the patient and family point to the involved eye gives further assurance.

AAO Wrong-Site Task Force, Hoskins Center for Quality Eye Care. Patient Safety Statements. *Recommendations of American Academy of Ophthalmology Wrong-Site Task Force.* San Francisco: American Academy of Ophthalmology; 2008. Available at: http://one.aao.org/patient-safety-statement/recommendations-of-american-academy-ophthalmology-. Accessed July 8, 2014.

#### *Ptosis and extraocular muscle damage*

Avoiding excessive dissection, especially near the orbital roof and apex, reduces the chance of damaging the extraocular muscles, the levator muscle, and/or their innervation.

## Orbital Implants

The implant's function is to replace lost orbital volume, maintain the structure of the orbit, and impart motility to the overlying ocular prosthesis. Modern implants are usually either spheres or implants with anterior surface projections to which the extraocular muscles can be attached. Spherical implants may be grouped according to the materials from which they are manufactured: *inert materials,* such as glass, silicone, or methylmethacrylate; and *biointegrated materials,* such as hydroxyapatite or porous polyethylene (Fig 8-1). The latter are designed to be incorporated by soft-tissue ingrowth from the socket.

Inert spherical implants provide comfort, have low extrusion rates, and are considered an appropriate cost-effective choice in patients not requiring implant integration. Disadvantages of nonporous implants include the possibilities of decreased motility and implant migration. Spheres of inert materials may be wrapped in sclera, vicryl mesh, or autogenous materials (eg, fascia, dermis, or muscle) to provide a substrate for attachment of the extraocular muscles. Inert implants transfer motility to the prosthesis only through passive movement of the socket. Buried motility implants with anterior surface projections push the overlying prosthesis with direct force and can improve prosthetic motility. The anterior surface projections, however, may pinch the conjunctiva between the implant and the prosthesis, leading to a painful socket or implant erosion.

Hydroxyapatite and porous polyethylene implants allow for drilling and placement of a peg to integrate the prosthesis directly with the moving implant (see Fig 8-1B). Pegging is usually carried out 6–12 months after enucleation. Although pegged porous implants offer excellent motility, they also have a higher rate of postoperative complications, including inflammation and exposure. It should be noted that most porous implants are never pegged and are able to achieve adequate motility.

Locations for implants after evisceration are behind or within the sclera. After enucleation, they are placed either within the Tenon capsule or behind the posterior Tenon capsule, in the muscle cone. Spheres may be covered with materials such as sclera (homologous or cadaveric), autogenous fascia, or vicryl mesh, which serve as further barriers to migration and extrusion. Secure closure of Tenon capsule over the anterior surface of an

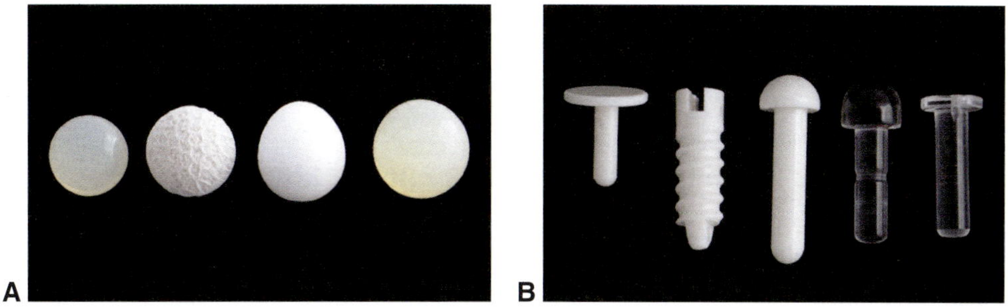

**Figure 8-1** **A,** Examples of various orbital implants *(from left to right)*: silicone, 18 mm; hydroxyapatite, 20 mm; porous polyethylene, 20 mm; silicone, 22 mm. **B,** Various pegs and rescue screws for integrated orbital implants. *(Courtesy of Christine C. Nelson, MD.)*

anophthalmic implant is an important barrier to later extrusion. A dermis-fat graft may be placed instead of an implant or to increase the surface area of the conjunctiva. As the conjunctiva reepithelializes over the dermis, it adds to the socket mucosa.

Extraocular muscles should not be crossed over the front surface of a spherical implant or purse-stringed anteriorly because the implant migrates when the muscles slip off the anterior surface. Muscles sutured into the normal anatomical locations, either directly to the implant or to added material (sclera, autogenous fascia, vicryl mesh) surrounding the implant, allow superior motility and prevent migration.

Following enucleation or evisceration surgery, an acrylic or silicone conformer is placed in the conjunctival fornices to maintain the conjunctival space that will eventually accommodate the prosthesis.

Fahim D, Frueh BR, Musch DC, Nelson CC. Complications of pegged and non-pegged hydroxyapatite orbital implants. *Ophthal Plast Reconstr Surg.* 2007;23(3):206–210.

Kaltreider SA, Lucarelli MJ. A simple algorithm for selection of implant size for enucleation and evisceration: a prospective study. *Ophthal Plast Reconstr Surg.* 2002;18(5):336–341.

Smit TJ, Koornneef L, Zonneveld FW, Groet E, Otto AJ. Primary and secondary implants in the anophthalmic orbit: preoperative and postoperative computed tomographic appearance. *Ophthalmology.* 1991;98(1):106–110.

### Prostheses

An ocular prosthesis is fitted within 4–8 weeks after enucleation or evisceration. The ideal prosthesis is custom fitted to the exact dimensions of the conjunctival fornices after postoperative edema has subsided. Premade or stock eyes are less satisfactory cosmetically, and they limit prosthetic motility. In addition, they may trap secretions between the prosthesis and the socket. Typically, the patient might remove the prosthesis once a month for cleaning.

The American Society of Ocularists is an international nonprofit professional and educational organization founded by technicians specializing in the fabrication and fitting of custom ocular prosthetics. Its website includes information for both patients and physicians (www.ocularist.org).

Custer PL, Kennedy RH, Woog JJ, Kaltreider SA, Meyer DR. Orbital implants in enucleation surgery: a report by the American Academy of Ophthalmology. *Ophthalmology.* 2003; 110(10):2054–2061.

Custer PL, Trinkaus KM, Fornoff J. Comparative motility of hydroxyapatite and alloplastic enucleation implants. *Ophthalmology.* 1999;106(3):513–516.

## Anophthalmic Socket Complications and Treatment

### Deep Superior Sulcus

Deep superior sulcus deformity is caused by decreased orbital volume (Fig 8-2). The surgeon can correct this deformity by increasing the orbital volume through placement of a subperiosteal secondary implant on the orbital floor. This implant pushes the initial implant and superior orbital fat upward to fill out the superior sulcus. Dermis-fat grafts may

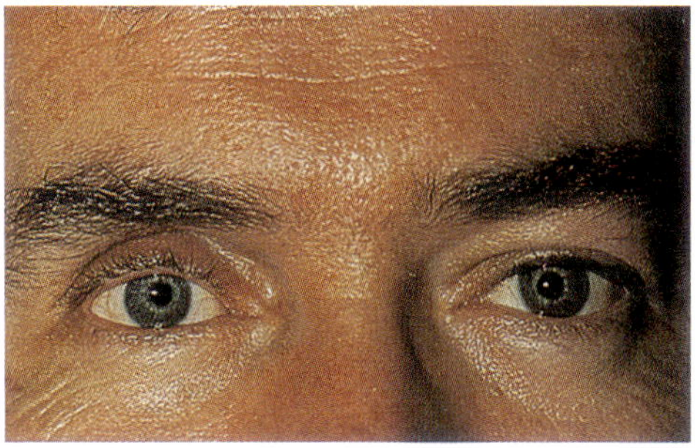

**Figure 8-2** Superior sulcus deformity following enucleation of the right eye.

be implanted in the upper eyelid to fill out the sulcus, but eyelid contour and function may be damaged and the graft may undergo resorption. Superior sulcus deformity can also be corrected with replacement of the original implant with a larger secondary implant or dermis-fat graft. Alternatively, modification of the ocular prosthesis may be used to correct a deep superior sulcus.

A related problem occurs when the superior conjunctival fornix is too deep. This leads to retention of mucus and debris, which build up, causing chronic discharge and infection. This condition is called "giant fornix syndrome" and is treated with a superior conjunctival resection.

Jones DF, Lyle CE, Fleming JC. Superior conjunctivoplasty-mullerectomy for correction of chronic discharge and concurrent ptosis in the anophthalmic socket with enlarged superior fornix. *Ophthal Plast Reconstr Surg.* 2010;26(3):172–175.

## Contracture of Fornices

Preventing contracted fornices includes preserving as much conjunctiva as possible and limiting dissection in the fornices. Placing extraocular muscles in their normal anatomical positions also minimizes shortening of the fornices. It is recommended that the patient wear a conformer in the immediate postoperative period to maintain soft-tissue anatomy and minimize conjunctival shortening. Conformers and prostheses should not be removed for periods greater than 24 hours. The prosthesis can be removed and cleaned, especially in the presence of infection, but should be replaced promptly after irrigation of the socket.

## Exposure and Extrusion of the Implant

Implants may extrude if placed too far forward, if closure of anterior Tenon capsule is not meticulous, or if the irregular surface of the implant mechanically erodes through the conjunctiva (Fig 8-3). Postoperative infection, poor wound healing, poorly fitting prostheses or conformers, and pressure points between the implant and prosthesis may also contribute to extrusion of the implant. Exposed implants are subject to infection. Although small defects over porous implants may, in rare instances, close spontaneously, most exposures should be covered with scleral patch grafts or autogenous tissue grafts to promote conjunctival healing.

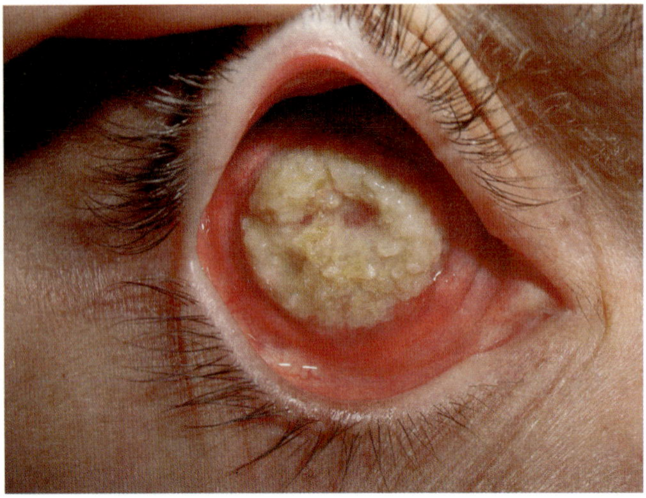

**Figure 8-3** Large exposure of the porous polyethylene orbital implant in a patient who had undergone evisceration for trauma. *(Courtesy of Martín Devoto, MD.)*

A dermis-fat graft may be used when a limited amount of conjunctiva remains in the socket. This graft increases the net amount of conjunctiva available as the conjunctiva reepithelializes over the front surface of the dermis. Unpredictable fat resorption is a serious drawback to the dermis-fat graft technique in adults. However, as stated earlier, dermis-fat grafts in children appear to grow along with the surrounding orbit and may help stimulate orbital development if enucleation is required during infancy or childhood.

## Contracted Sockets

Causes of contracted sockets include

- radiation treatment (usually as treatment of the tumor that necessitated removal of the eye)
- extrusion of an enucleation implant
- severe initial injury (alkali burns or extensive lacerations)
- poor surgical techniques (excessive sacrifice or destruction of conjunctiva and Tenon capsule; traumatic dissection within the socket causing excessive scar tissue formation)
- multiple socket operations
- removal of the conformer or prosthesis for prolonged periods

Sockets are considered to be contracted when the fornices are too small to retain a prosthesis (Fig 8-4). Socket reconstruction procedures involve incision or excision of the scarred tissues and placement of a graft to enlarge the fornices. Full-thickness mucous membrane grafting is preferred because it allows the grafted tissue to match conjunctiva histologically. Amniotic membrane may also be used. Buccal mucosal grafts may be taken from the cheeks (avoid the duct from the parotid gland), the lower lip, or the upper lip or from the hard palate for rigid tissue. Goblet cells and mucus production are preserved.

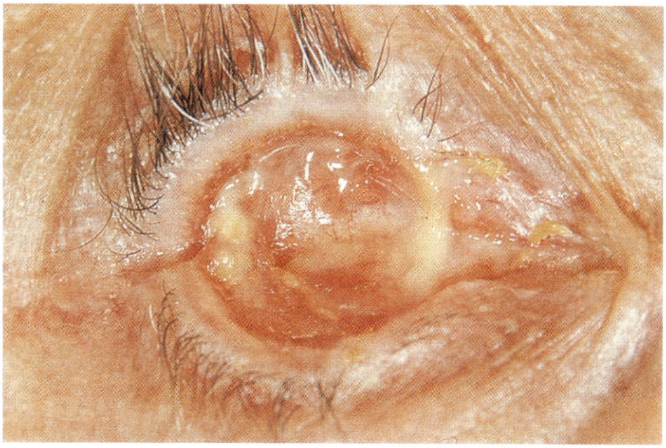

**Figure 8-4** Socket contraction of right anophthalmic orbit. Note obliteration of conjunctival fornices. The patient is unable to wear an ocular prosthesis.

Contracture of the fornices alone (more common with the inferior fornix) is usually associated with milder degrees of socket contracture. In these cases, the buccal mucosal graft is placed in the defect, and a silicone sheet is attached by sutures to the superior or inferior orbital rim, depending on which fornix is involved. In 2 weeks, the sheet may be removed and a prosthesis placed.

Neuhaus RW, Hawes MJ. Inadequate inferior cul-de-sac in the anophthalmic socket. *Ophthalmology.* 1992;99(1):153–157.

## Anophthalmic Ectropion

Lower eyelid ectropion may result from the loosening of lower eyelid support under the weight of a prosthesis. Frequent removal of the prosthesis or use of a larger prosthesis accelerates the development of lid laxity. Tightening the lateral or medial canthal tendon may correct the ectropion. Surgeons may combine ectropion repair with deepening of the inferior fornix by recessing the inferior retractor muscle and grafting mucous membrane tissue.

## Anophthalmic Ptosis

Ptosis of the anophthalmic socket results from superotemporal migration of sphere implants, cicatricial tissue in the upper fornix, or damage to the levator muscle or nerve. Small amounts of ptosis may be managed by modification of the prosthesis. Greater amounts of ptosis require tightening of the levator aponeurosis. This procedure is best done under local anesthesia with intraoperative adjustment of eyelid height and contour because mechanical forces may cause the surgeon to underestimate true levator function. Ptosis surgery usually improves a deep sulcus by bringing the preaponeurotic fat forward. Mild ptosis may be corrected with Müller muscle–conjunctival resection. Frontalis suspension is usually a less useful procedure because there is no visual drive to stimulate contracture of the frontalis muscle to elevate the eyelid.

### Lash Margin Entropion

Lash margin entropion, trichiasis, and ptosis of the eyelashes are common in patients with an anophthalmic socket. Contracture of fornices or cicatricial tissue near the lash margin contributes to these abnormalities. Horizontal tarsal incisions and rotation of the lash margin may correct the problem. In more severe cases, splitting of the eyelid margins at the gray line with mucous membrane grafting to the eyelid margin may correct the entropic lash margin.

### Cosmetic Optics

Spectacles with particular frame styles and tinted lenses can be used to help camouflage residual defects in reconstructed sockets in addition to protecting the contralateral eye. Plus (convex) lenses or minus (concave) lenses may be placed in the glasses in front of the prosthesis to alter the apparent size of the prosthesis. Prisms in the glasses may be used to change the apparent vertical position of the prosthesis.

Smit TJ, Koornneef L, Zonneveld FW, Groet E, Otto AJ. Computed tomography in the assessment of the postenucleation socket syndrome. *Ophthalmology.* 1990;97(10): 1347–1351.

## Exenteration

Exenteration involves the removal of some or all of the soft tissues of the orbit, including the globe.

### Considerations for Exenteration

Exenteration should be considered in the following circumstances:

- *Destructive tumors extending into the orbit from the sinuses, face, eyelids, conjunctiva, or intracranial space* (Fig 8-5). However, exenteration is not indicated for all such tumors: some are responsive to radiation, and some have extended too far to be completely removed by surgical excision.
- *Intraocular melanomas or retinoblastomas that have extended outside the globe (if evidence of distant metastases is excluded).* When local control of the tumor would benefit the nursing care of the patient, exenteration is indicated.
- *Malignant epithelial tumors of the lacrimal gland.* Although the procedure is somewhat controversial, these tumors may require extended exenteration with radical bone removal of the roof, lateral wall, and floor.
- *Fungal infection.* Subtotal or total exenteration (discussed in the next section) may be necessary for the management of orbital mucormycosis, which occurs most commonly in patients who are diabetic or immunosuppressed. In some cases, it may be possible to control and treat the infection through more limited debridement of involved orbital tissues.
- *Sarcomas and other primary orbital malignancies that do not respond to nonsurgical therapy.* Some tumors such as rhabdomyosarcomas that were previously treated by exenteration are now initially treated by radiation and chemotherapy.

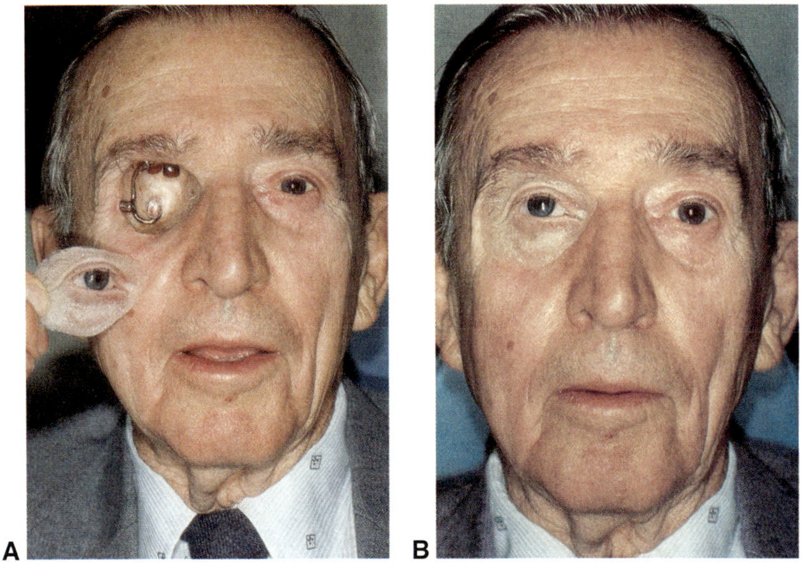


**Figure 8-5** Orbital exenteration and osseointegrated prosthesis. **A,** Exenterated socket for sebaceous cell carcinoma. **B,** Prosthesis in place; fixation is achieved with magnets attached to the bone-anchored framework. *(Courtesy of Jeffrey A. Nerad, MD.)*

## Types of Exenteration

Exenterations vary in the amount of tissue that is removed. Following are the types of exenteration:

- *Subtotal.* The eye and adjacent intraorbital tissues are removed such that the lesion is locally excised (leaving part of the periorbita and eyelids). This technique is used for some locally invasive tumors, for debulking of disseminated tumors, or for partial treatment in selected patients.
- *Total.* All intraorbital soft tissues, including periorbita, are removed, with or without the skin of the eyelids.
- *Extended.* All intraorbital soft tissues are removed, together with adjacent structures (usually bony walls and sinuses).

The technique selected depends on the pathologic process. The goal is to remove all lesions along with appropriate margins of adjacent tissue while retaining as much healthy tissue as possible. Following removal of the orbital contents, the bony socket may be allowed to spontaneously granulate and epithelialize or may be covered by a split-thickness skin graft, which may be placed onto bare bone or over a temporalis muscle or temporoparietal fascial flap. Rehabilitation after exenteration may include a prosthesis attached to either the eyeglasses frame, the periorbital area (with adhesive), or an osseointegrated implant (with magnets). The exenteration prosthesis restores the tissues that have been removed, including eyelids and an eye, but it does not blink or move.

Levin PS, Dutton JJ. A 20-year series of orbital exenteration. *Am J Ophthalmol.* 1991;112(5):496–501.

Yeatts RP, Marion JR, Weaver RG, Orkubi GA. Removal of the eye with socket ablation: a limited subtotal exenteration. *Arch Ophthalmol.* 1991;109(9):1306–1309.

# PART II

# Periocular Soft Tissues

CHAPTER 9

# Facial and Eyelid Anatomy

## Face

The surgeon who undertakes surgical manipulation of the face should understand its anatomy. The structural planes of the face include skin; subcutaneous tissue; the *superficial musculoaponeurotic system (SMAS)* and mimetic muscles; the deep facial fascia; and the plane containing the facial nerve, parotid duct, and buccal fat pad.

The superficial facial fascia, an extension of the superficial cervical fascia in the neck, invests the facial mimetic muscles (platysma, zygomaticus major, zygomaticus minor, and orbicularis oculi), making up the SMAS (Figs 9-1A, B). The SMAS distributes facial muscle contractions, facilitating facial expression. These muscle actions are transmitted to the skin by ligamentous attachments located between the SMAS and the dermis. The SMAS is also connected to the underlying bone by a network of fibrous septa and ligaments. Thus, facial support is transmitted from the deep fixed structures of the face to the overlying dermis. Two major components of this system are the osteocutaneous ligaments (orbitomalar, zygomatic, and mandibular) and the fascial cutaneous ligaments formed by a condensation of superficial and deep facial fasciae (parotidocutaneous and masseteric). As these ligaments become attenuated in conjunction with facial dermal elastosis, facial aging becomes apparent. Dissection and repositioning of the SMAS have important implications for facial cosmetic surgery.

As the SMAS continues superiorly over the zygomatic arch, it becomes continuous with the *temporoparietal fascia* (also called the *superficial temporal fascia*); more superiorly, the SMAS becomes continuous with the galea aponeurotica. Beneath the loose areolar tissue and the temporoparietal fascia, the deep temporal fascia of the temporal muscle splits and envelops the temporal fat pad, creating deep and superficial layers of the deep temporal fascia (Fig 9-1C).

The mimetic muscles (Fig 9-2) can be grouped into those of the upper face and those of the lower face. In the upper face, the frontalis, corrugator supercilii, and procerus muscles animate the forehead and glabella. The orbicularis oculi depresses the eyebrows and closes the eyelids. The frontalis elevates the eyebrows, and contraction of the muscle causes transverse forehead rhytids.

In the lower face, mimetic muscles can be further categorized as superficial or deep. The *superficial mimetic muscles,* which receive their neurovascular supply on the posterior surfaces, include the platysma, zygomaticus major, zygomaticus minor, and risorius. The *deep mimetic muscles* receive their neurovascular supply anteriorly and include the buccinator, mentalis, and levator anguli oris. Other facial muscles include the orbicularis oris,

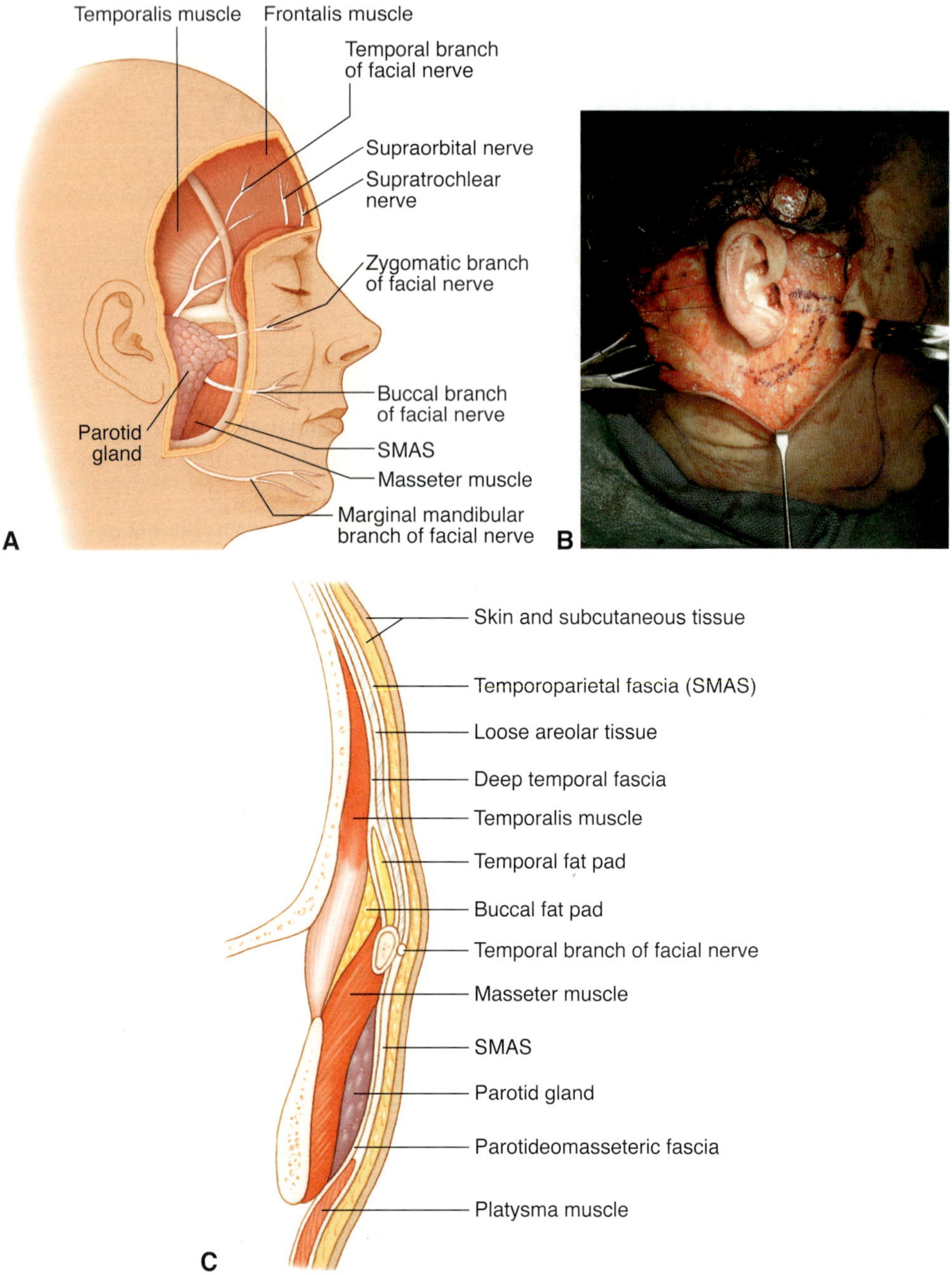


**Figure 9-1** **A,** Superficial musculoaponeurotic system (SMAS). Note that the facial nerve branches inferior to the zygomatic arch are deep to the SMAS. **B,** The SMAS exposed during a face-lift procedure. The horizontal surgical markings indicate the border of the zygomatic arch, and the oblique lines mark the area of planned excision of the SMAS during the procedure. **C,** Coronal section of the face. The temporal branch of the facial nerve is found within the superficial portion of the temporoparietal fascia (extension of the SMAS). *(Illustrations by Christine Gralapp. Clinical photo courtesy of Jill Foster, MD.)*

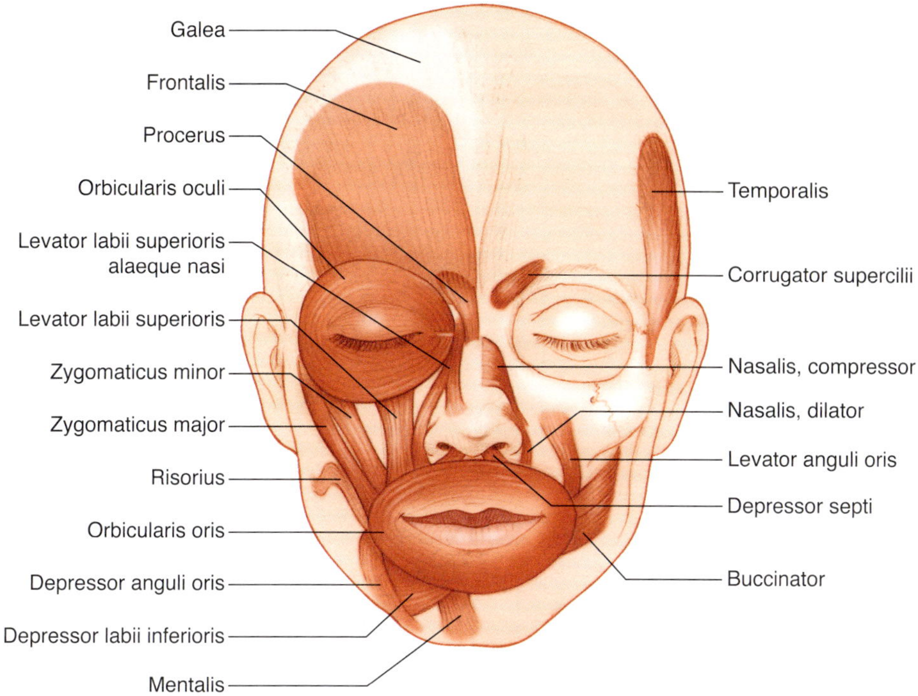


**Figure 9-2** Facial mimetic muscles. *(Illustration by Christine Gralapp.)*

the levator labii superioris, the levator labii superioris alaeque nasi, the depressor anguli oris and the depressor labii inferioris, the masseter, and the temporalis.

In the neck, the superficial cervical fascia and platysma are continuous with the SMAS, and the deep cervical fascia is found on the superficial surface of the strap muscles, superior to the hyoid bone. The deep cervical fascia overlies the myelohyoid muscle and extends superiorly over the body of the mandible. The parotideomasseteric fascia is a continuation of the deep cervical fascia of the neck. The facial nerve lies deep to this thin layer in the lower face. In the temporal region, above the zygomatic arch, the parotideomasseteric fascia is continuous with the deep temporal fascia, and the temporal (frontal) branch of the facial nerve lies superficial to this fascial layer. The transition of the temporal branch of the facial nerve from deep to superficial occurs as the temporal branch crosses over the zygomatic arch. Care is taken when biopsy of the superficial temporal artery is performed, because of the proximity of the temporal branch of the facial nerve, which, like the artery, is in the temporoparietal fascial plane.

The facial nerve, cranial nerve VII (CN VII), innervates the mimetic muscles and divides into 5 major branches within or deep to the parotid gland (Fig 9-3): temporal (frontal), zygomatic, buccal, marginal mandibular, and cervical. Landmarks identifying the depth of the nerve have special significance. There are 2 surgical planes that help surgeons avoid CN VII when operating: dissection deep to the SMAS and deep to CN VII (on top of the deep temporal fascia) in the upper face and temporal region; and dissection

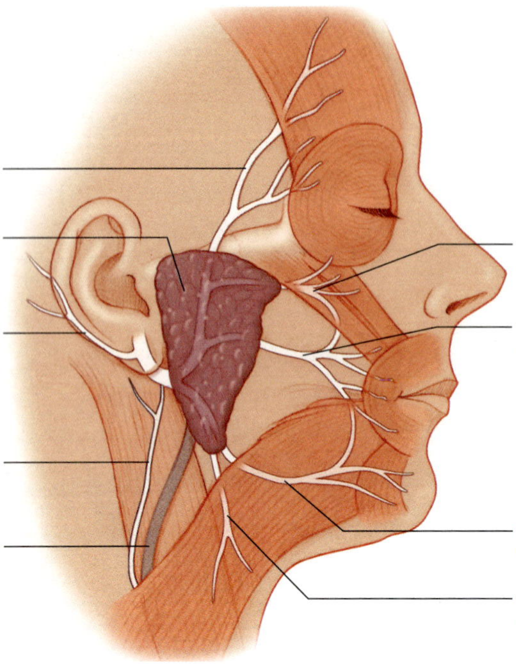


**Figure 9-3** The 5 major branches of the facial nerve. Note that the branches progress from deep beneath the parotid gland to more superficial layers as they cross the zygomatic arch or reach the anterior edge of the SMAS. CN = cranial nerve. *(Illustration by Christine Gralapp.)*

superficial to the SMAS and the branches of CN VII in the lower face. Both of these planes avoid the branches of the facial nerve.

In the temporal area, the temporal branch of CN VII (see Fig 9-3) crosses the zygomatic arch and courses superomedially in the deep layers of the temporoparietal fascia. The temporoparietal fascia bridges the SMAS of the lower face to the galea aponeurosis of the upper face. Deep to the temporoparietal fascia is the previously mentioned *deep temporal fascia*, a dense, immobile fascia that overlies the temporalis muscle (see Fig 9-1C). Dissection along this fascia allows mobilization of the temporal forehead while avoiding the overlying temporal branch of the facial nerve. This is an important anatomical principle in brow-lifting and forehead-lifting procedures.

In the lower face, the facial nerve branches, sensory nerves, vascular networks, and parotid gland and duct are deep to the SMAS (see Figs 9-1A, 9-3) Dissection just superficial to the SMAS, parotid gland, and parotideomasseteric fascia in the lower face avoids injury to these structures. The face receives its sensory innervation from the 3 branches of CN V: $V_1$, ophthalmic; $V_2$, maxillary; and $V_3$, mandibular (Fig 9-4). Damage to these nerves causes facial numbness and paresthesia. Fortunately, overlapping of the distal branches makes permanent sensation loss unusual unless injury occurs at the proximal neurovascular bundles or with extensive distal disruption, as can be seen with a coronal incision.

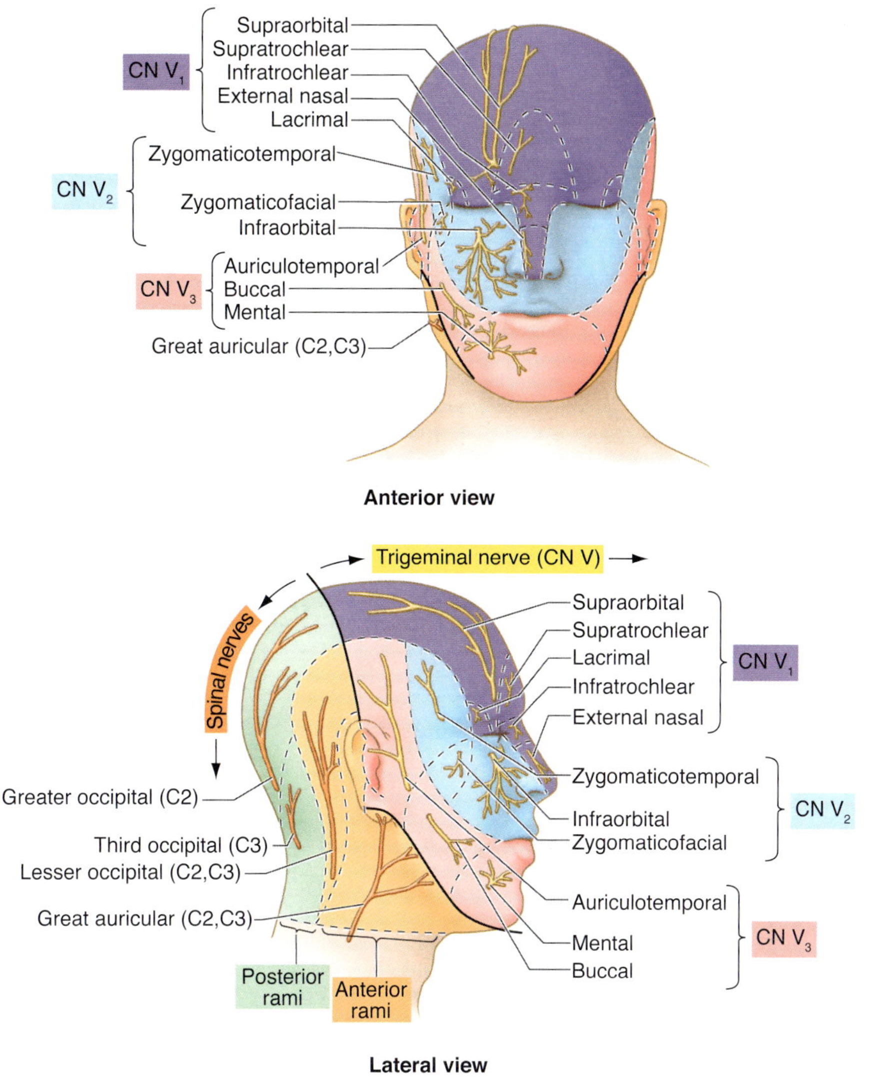


**Figure 9-4** The face receives its sensory innervation from the 3 branches of CN V: $V_1$, ophthalmic; $V_2$, maxillary; and $V_3$, mandibular. *(Modified with permission from Moore KL, Dalley AF, Agur AMR.* Clinically Oriented Anatomy. *7th ed. Baltimore: Lippincott Williams & Wilkins; 2013:851.)*

# Eyelids

For discussion purposes, the eyelids can be conveniently divided into the following 7 structural layers:

- skin and subcutaneous connective tissue
- muscles of protraction
- orbital septum

- orbital fat
- muscles of retraction
- tarsus
- conjunctiva

Figure 9-5 details the anatomy of the eyelids. See also BCSC Section 2, *Fundamentals and Principles of Ophthalmology,* for additional discussion and numerous illustrations.

## Skin and Subcutaneous Tissue

Eyelid skin is the thinnest of the body and is unique in having no subcutaneous fat layer. Because the thin skin of the eyelids is subjected to constant movement with each blink, the laxity that often occurs with age is not surprising. In both the upper and the lower eyelids,

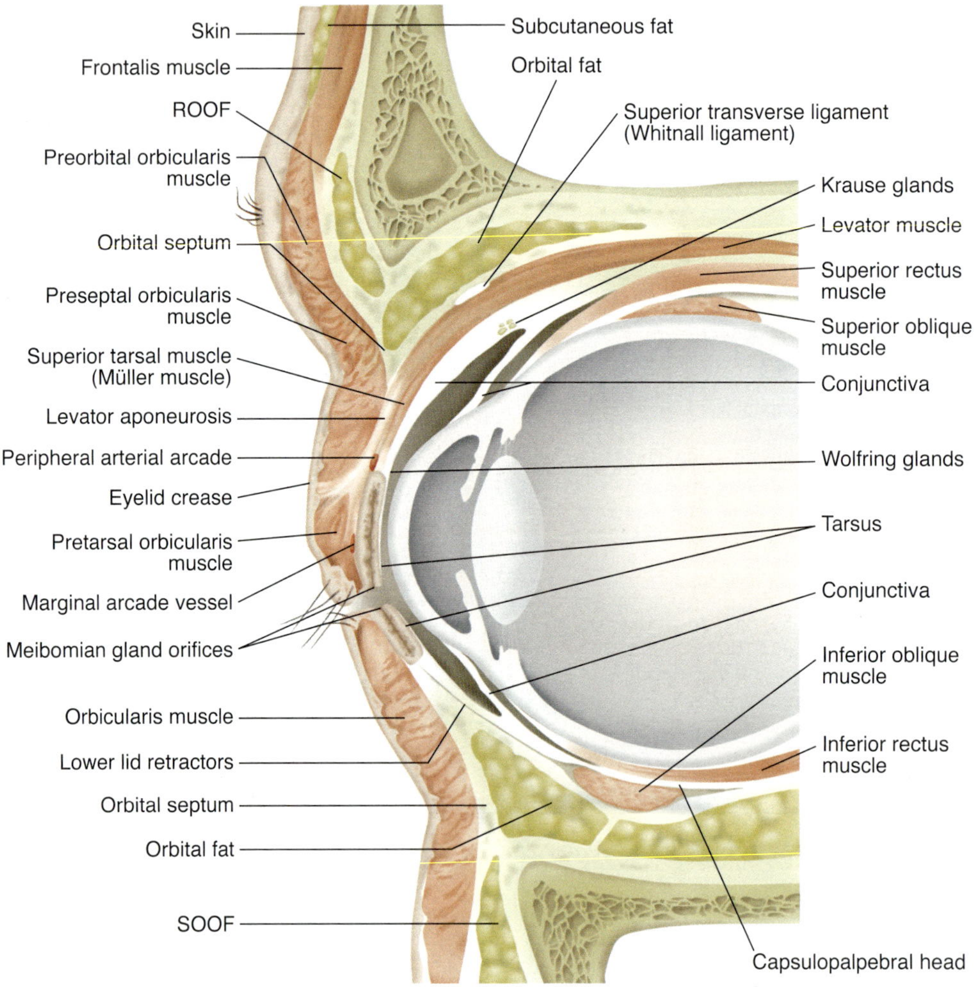


**Figure 9-5** Upper and lower eyelid anatomy. ROOF = retro-orbicularis oculi fat; SOOF = sub-orbicularis oculi fat. *(Modified from Stewart WB.* Surgery of the Eyelid, Orbit, and Lacrimal System. *Ophthalmology Monograph 8, vol 2. San Francisco: American Academy of Ophthalmology; 1994:23, 85. Illustration by Cyndie C. H. Wooley.)*

the pretarsal tissues are normally firmly attached to the underlying tissues, whereas the preseptal tissues are more loosely attached, creating potential spaces for fluid accumulation. The contours of the eyelid skin are defined by the *eyelid crease* and the *eyelid fold.* The upper eyelid crease approximates the attachments of the levator aponeurosis to the pretarsal orbicularis bundles and skin. In the Caucasian eyelid, this site is near or at the level of the superior border of the tarsus. The upper eyelid fold consists of the loose preseptal skin and subcutaneous tissues above the confluence of the levator aponeurosis and the septum.

Racial variation can be noted in the location of the eyelid crease and eyelid fold. The Asian eyelid normally has a relatively low upper eyelid crease because, in contrast to the supratarsal fusion, the orbital septum in the Asian eyelid fuses with the levator aponeurosis between the eyelid margin and the superior border of the tarsus (Fig 9-6). This also allows preaponeurotic fat to occupy a position more inferior and anterior in the eyelid. Although the lower eyelid crease is less well defined than the upper eyelid crease, these racial differences are apparent in the lower eyelid as well.

## Protractors

The orbicularis oculi muscle is the main protractor of the eyelid. Contraction of this muscle, which is innervated by CN VII, narrows the palpebral fissure. Specific portions of this muscle also constitute the lacrimal pump.

The orbicularis oculi muscle is divided into *pretarsal, preseptal,* and *orbital* parts (Fig 9-7). The palpebral (pretarsal and preseptal) parts are integral to involuntary eyelid movements (blinking), whereas the orbital portion is primarily involved in forced eyelid closure. The pretarsal orbicularis muscle arises from deep origins at the posterior

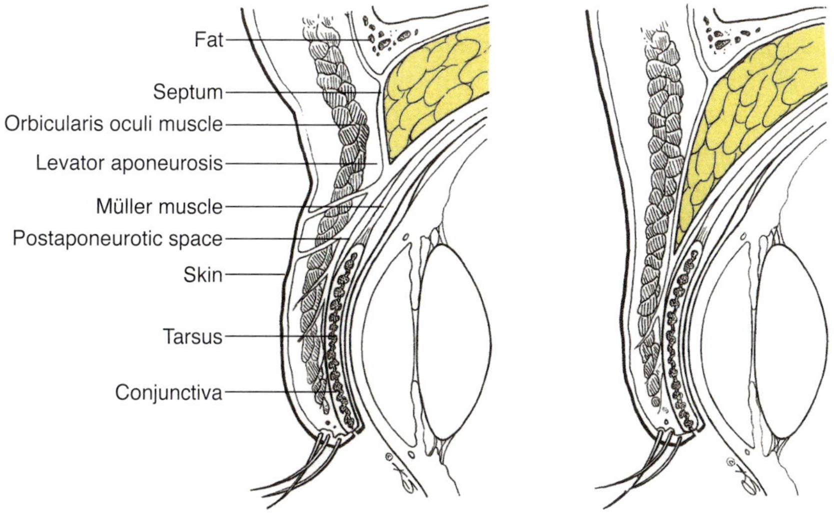


**Figure 9-6** Racial variations in eyelid anatomy. Variant I *(left)*: the orbital septum fuses with the levator aponeurosis above the tarsus. Variant II (Asian, *right*): the orbital septum fuses with the levator aponeurosis between the eyelid margin and the superior border of the tarsus, and there are fewer aponeurotic attachments to the skin. *(Reproduced with permission from Katowitz JA, ed.* Pediatric Oculoplastic Surgery. *Philadelphia: Springer-Verlag; 2002.)*

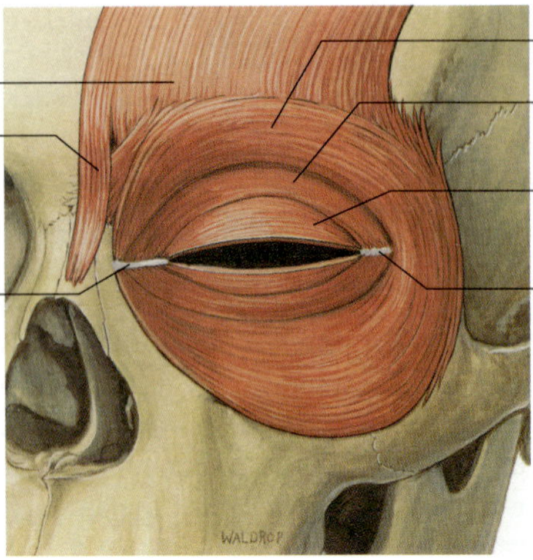


**Figure 9-7** Segments of the orbicularis oculi muscle. *(Reproduced with permission from Dutton JJ.* Atlas of Clinical and Surgical Orbital Anatomy. *Philadelphia: Saunders; 1994:132.)*

lacrimal crest and superficial origins at the anterior limb of the medial canthal tendon (Fig 9-8). Near the common canaliculus, the deep heads of the pretarsal orbicularis fuse to form a prominent bundle of fibers known as the *Horner muscle,* which runs just behind the posterior arm of the canthal tendon. The Horner muscle continues posteriorly to the posterior lacrimal crest, just behind the posterior arm of the medial canthal tendon. The upper and lower eyelid segments of the pretarsal orbicularis fuse in the lateral canthal area to become the lateral canthal tendon.

The preseptal orbicularis arises from the upper and lower borders of the medial canthal tendon. The inferior preseptal muscle arises as a single head from the common tendon. In the upper eyelid, the preseptal muscle has an anterior head from the common tendon and a posterior head from both the superior and posterior arms of the tendon. Laterally, the preseptal muscles form the lateral palpebral raphe.

The orbital portions of the orbicularis muscle arise from the anterior limb of the medial canthal tendon, the orbital process of the frontal bone, and the frontal process of the

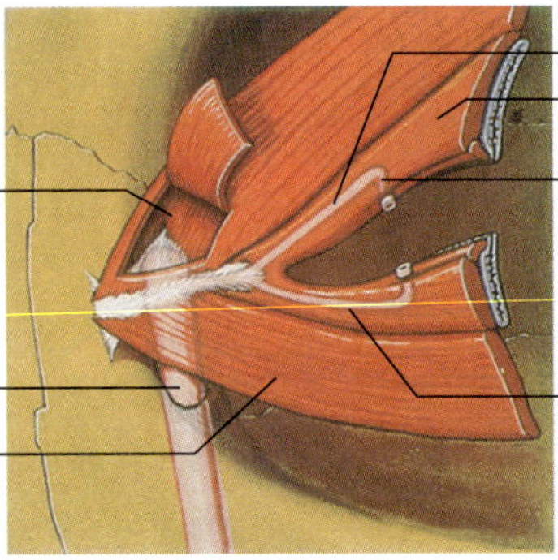


**Figure 9-8** Medial attachments of the orbicularis oculi muscle. *(Reproduced with permission from Dutton JJ.* Atlas of Clinical and Surgical Orbital Anatomy. *Philadelphia: Saunders; 1994:146.)*

maxillary bone in front of the anterior lacrimal crest. Its fibers form a continuous ellipse and insert just below the point of origin. At the eyelid margin, a specialized bundle of striated muscle fibers, the *muscle of Riolan,* lies more posterior than the main portion of the orbicularis and creates the gray line (see Fig 9-11). The muscle of Riolan may play a role in meibomian glandular discharge, blinking, and the position of the eyelashes.

Dutton JJ. *Atlas of Clinical and Surgical Orbital Anatomy.* Philadelphia: Saunders; 1994.

Muzaffar AR, Mendelson BC, Adams WP Jr. Surgical anatomy of the ligamentous attachments of the lower lid and lateral canthus. *Plast Reconstr Surg.* 2002;110(3):873–884; discussion 897–911.

Wulc AE, Dryden RM, Khatchaturian T. Where is the gray line? *Arch Ophthalmol.* 1987; 105(8):1092–1098.

## Orbital Septum

The orbital septum, a thin, multilayered sheet of fibrous tissue, arises from the periosteum over the superior and inferior orbital rims at the arcus marginalis. In the upper eyelid, the orbital septum fuses with the levator aponeurosis 2–5 mm above the superior tarsal border in non-Asian persons (see Fig 9-6). In the lower eyelid, the orbital septum fuses with the capsulopalpebral fascia at or just below the inferior tarsal border. The fused capsulopalpebral orbital septum complex, along with a small contribution from the inferior tarsal smooth muscle, inserts on the posterior and anterior tarsal surfaces as well as the tapered inferior border of the tarsus. As a result of aging, the septum in both the upper and the lower eyelids may become quite attenuated. Thinning of the septum and laxity of the orbicularis muscle contribute to anterior herniation of the orbital fat in the aging eyelid.

Meyer DR, Linberg JV, Wobig JL, McCormick SA. Anatomy of the orbital septum and associated eyelid connective tissues. Implications for ptosis surgery. *Ophthal Plast Reconstr Surg.* 1991;7(2):104–113.

## Orbital Fat

Orbital fat lies posterior to the orbital septum and anterior to the levator aponeurosis (upper eyelid) or the capsulopalpebral fascia (lower eyelid). In the upper eyelid, there are 2 fat pockets: nasal and central. In the lower eyelid, there are 3 fat pockets: nasal, central, and temporal. These pockets are surrounded by thin fibrous capsules that are forward continuations of the anterior orbitoseptal system. The central orbital fat pad is an important landmark in both elective eyelid surgery and lid laceration repair because it lies directly behind the orbital septum and in front of the levator aponeurosis.

## Retractors

The retractors of the upper eyelid are the levator palpebrae superioris muscle with its aponeurosis and the superior tarsal muscle *(Müller muscle).* In the lower eyelid, the retractors are the capsulopalpebral fascia and the inferior tarsal muscle.

### *Upper eyelid retractors*

The levator muscle originates in the apex of the orbit, arising from the periorbita of the lesser wing of the sphenoid, just above the annulus of Zinn. The muscular portion of the levator is approximately 40 mm long; the aponeurosis is 14–20 mm in length. The superior transverse ligament *(Whitnall ligament)* is a sleeve of elastic fibers around the levator muscle. It is located in the area where the levator muscle transitions into the levator aponeurosis (Fig 9-9).

The Whitnall ligament functions primarily as a suspensory support for the upper eyelid and the superior orbital tissues. The ligament also acts as a fulcrum for the levator, transferring its vector force from an anterior–posterior to a superior–inferior direction. Its analogue in the lower eyelid is the *Lockwood ligament.* Medially, the Whitnall ligament attaches to connective tissue around the trochlea and superior oblique tendon. Laterally, it forms septa through the stroma of the lacrimal gland, then arches upward to attach to the inner aspect of the lateral orbital wall approximately 10 mm above the lateral orbital tubercle, with a small group of fibers extending inferiorly to insert onto the lateral retinaculum. The Whitnall ligament has sometimes been confused with the horns of the levator aponeurosis. However, the horns of the levator aponeurosis lie more inferior and toward the canthi. The lateral horn inserts onto the lateral orbital tubercle; the medial horn inserts onto the posterior lacrimal crest. The lateral horn of the levator aponeurosis is strong, and it divides the lacrimal gland into orbital and palpebral lobes, attaching firmly to the orbital tubercle. The medial horn of the aponeurosis is more delicate and forms loose connective attachments to the posterior aspect of the medial canthal tendon and to the posterior lacrimal crest.

As the levator aponeurosis continues toward the tarsus, it divides into an anterior and posterior portion a variable distance above the superior tarsal border. The anterior portion is composed of fine strands of aponeurosis that insert into the septa between the pretarsal orbicularis muscle bundles and skin. These fine attachments are responsible for the close apposition of the pretarsal skin and orbicularis muscle to the underlying tarsus. The upper eyelid crease is formed by the most superior of these attachments and by contraction of the underlying levator complex. The upper eyelid fold is created by the overhanging skin, fat, and orbicularis muscle superior to the crease.

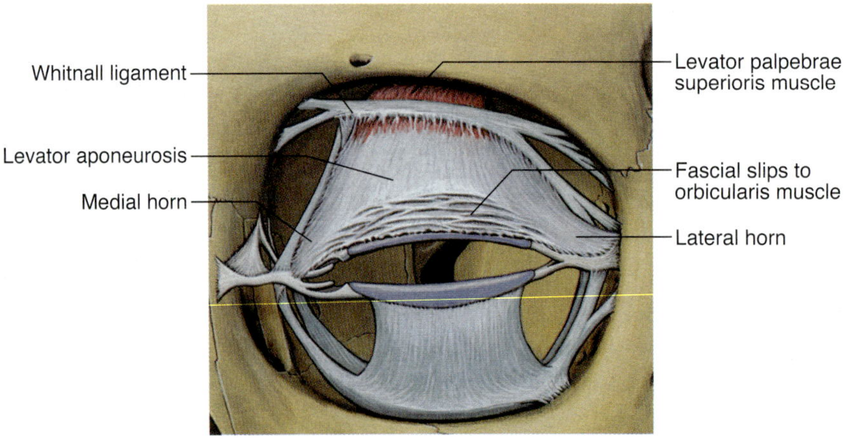


**Figure 9-9** The suspensory and fibrous anatomy of the eyelid. *(Reproduced with permission from Dutton JJ.* Atlas of Clinical and Surgical Orbital Anatomy. *Philadelphia: Saunders; 1994:129.)*

The levator muscle is innervated by the superior division of CN III, which also supplies the superior rectus muscle. A superior division palsy, resulting in ptosis and decreased upgaze, implies an intraorbital disruption of CN III.

The posterior portion of the levator aponeurosis inserts firmly onto the anterior surface of the lower half of the tarsus. It is most firmly attached approximately 3 mm above the eyelid margin and is only very loosely attached to the superior 2–3 mm of the tarsus. Disinsertion, dehiscence, or rarefaction of the aponeurosis following ocular surgery or due to intraocular inflammation, eyelid trauma, or senescence may give rise to ptosis.

The Müller muscle originates in the undersurface of the levator palpebrae superioris muscle approximately at the level of the Whitnall ligament, 12–14 mm above the upper tarsal margin. The levator muscle divides into an anterior branch, which becomes the aponeurosis, and a posterior branch, which becomes the Müller muscle. This sympathetically innervated smooth muscle extends inferiorly to insert along the upper border of the superior tarsus. The muscle provides approximately 2 mm of elevation of the upper eyelid; if it is interrupted (as in Horner syndrome), mild ptosis results. The Müller muscle is firmly attached to the adjacent conjunctiva posteriorly, especially just above the superior tarsal border. The peripheral arterial arcade is found between the levator aponeurosis and the Müller muscle, just above the superior tarsal border. This vascular arcade serves as a useful surgical landmark to identify the Müller muscle.

Codère F, Tucker NA, Renaldi B. The anatomy of Whitnall ligament. *Ophthalmology.* 1995; 102(12):2016–2019.

Kakizaki H, Prabhakaran V, Pradeep T, Malhotra R, Selva D. Peripheral branching of levator superioris muscle and Müller muscle origin. *Am J Ophthalmol.* 2009;148(5):800–803.e1.

Ng SK, Chan W, Marcet MM, Kakizaki H, Selva D. Levator palpebrae superioris: an anatomical update. *Orbit.* 2013;32(1):76–84.

Stasior GO, Lemke BN, Wallow IH, Dortzbach RK. Levator aponeurosis elastic fiber network. *Ophthal Plast Reconstr Surg.* 1993;9(1):1–10.

#### *Lower eyelid retractors*

The capsulopalpebral fascia in the lower eyelid is analogous to the levator aponeurosis in the upper eyelid. The fascia originates as the capsulopalpebral head from attachments to the terminal muscle fibers of the inferior rectus muscle. The capsulopalpebral head divides as it encircles the inferior oblique muscle and fuses with the sheath of the inferior oblique muscle. Anterior to the inferior oblique muscle, the 2 portions of the capsulopalpebral head join to form the Lockwood suspensory ligament. The capsulopalpebral fascia extends anteriorly from this point, sending strands to the inferior conjunctival fornix. The capsulopalpebral fascia wraps around the inferior tarsal border, just after it fuses with the orbital septum.

The inferior tarsal muscle in the lower eyelid is analogous to the Müller muscle. The poorly developed inferior tarsal muscle runs posterior to the capsulopalpebral fascia. The smooth muscle fibers are most abundant in the area of the inferior fornix.

### Tarsus

The tarsi are firm, dense plates of connective tissue that serve as the structural support of the eyelids (Fig 9-10). The upper eyelid tarsal plates measure 10–12 mm vertically in the

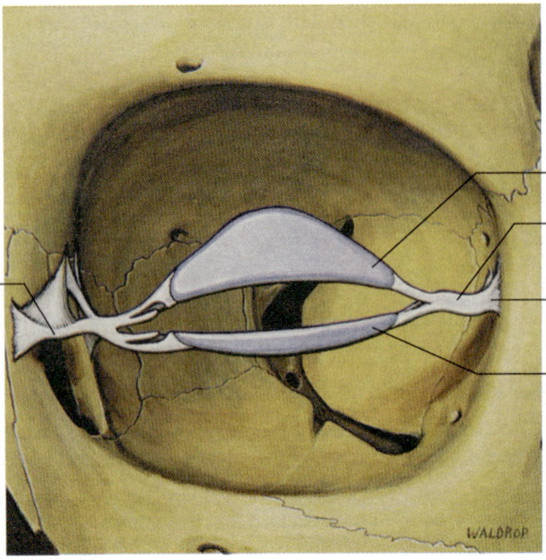


**Figure 9-10** Tarsal plates and suspensory tendons of the eyelid. *(Reproduced with permission from Dutton JJ.* Atlas of Clinical and Surgical Orbital Anatomy. *Philadelphia: Saunders; 1994.)*

center of the eyelid; the maximum lower eyelid tarsal plate measurement is 4 mm. The tarsal plates have rigid attachments to the periosteum through the canthal tendons medially and laterally. The tarsal plates may become horizontally displaced with age as a result of stretching of the medial and lateral supporting tendons. Both tarsal plates are usually 1 mm thick and taper at the medial and lateral ends as they approach the canthal tendons. Located within the tarsus, the meibomian glands are modified holocrine sebaceous glands.

## Conjunctiva

The conjunctiva is composed of nonkeratinizing squamous epithelium. It forms the posterior layer of the eyelids and contains the mucin-secreting goblet cells and the accessory lacrimal *glands of Wolfring* and *Krause.* The accessory lacrimal glands are found in the subconjunctival tissue mainly in the upper and lower eyelids. The glands of Wolfring are found primarily along the nonmarginal tarsal borders, and the glands of Krause are found in the fornices.

## Additional Anatomical Considerations

### *Connective tissue*

**Suborbicularis fat pads** Deep to the orbicularis muscle overlying the maxillary and zygomatic periosteum is a plane of nonseptate fat called the *suborbicularis oculi fat (SOOF).* This fat is analogous to the superiorly located *retro-orbicularis oculi fat (ROOF),* which is situated deep to the eyebrow and extends into the eyelid, where it merges with postorbicularis fascia in the upper eyelid (see Fig 9-5).

The SOOF plays an important role in the aging process of gradual gravitational descent of the midfacial soft tissues. Repositioning of the SOOF is performed to support involutional and cicatricial retraction of the lower eyelid. In aesthetic procedures, elevation of the SOOF restores more youthful contours in the lower eyelid and midfacial soft tissues.

Similarly, the *ROOF* undergoes gravitational descent, compounding a redundant upper eyelid skin fold. The displaced ROOF can be confused with a coexisting redundant upper eyelid fold and prominent prolapsed preaponeurotic fat pad in the upper eyelid. In some patients, it is necessary to modify the descended ROOF during blepharoplasty to achieve an adequate functional and aesthetic result.

Lucarelli MJ, Khwarg SI, Lemke BN, Kozel JS, Dortzbach RK. The anatomy of midfacial ptosis. *Ophthal Plast Reconstr Surg.* 2000;16(1):7–22.

Mendelson BC, Muzaffar AR, Adams WP Jr. Surgical anatomy of the midcheek and malar mounds. *Plast Reconstr Surg.* 2002;110(3):885–896; discussion 897–911.

**Canthal tendons** The configuration of the palpebral fissure is maintained by the medial and lateral canthal tendons in conjunction with the attached tarsal plates. The 2 origins of the medial canthal tendon from the anterior and posterior lacrimal crests fuse just temporal to the lacrimal sac and then again split into an upper limb and a lower limb that attach to the upper and lower tarsal plates. The attachment of the tendon to the periosteum overlying the anterior lacrimal crest is diffuse and strong; the attachment to the posterior lacrimal crest is more delicate but important in maintaining apposition of the eyelids to the globe, allowing the puncta to lie in the tear lake.

The lateral canthal tendon attaches at the lateral orbital tubercle on the inner aspect of the orbital rim. It splits into superior and inferior branches that attach to the respective tarsal plates. Cutting, stretching, or disinsertion of either of the canthal tendons usually causes cosmetic or functional problems such as telecanthus and horizontal eyelid laxity. Horizontal eyelid instability is frequently the result of lateral canthal lengthening. The lateral canthal tendon usually inserts 2 mm higher than does the medial canthal tendon, giving the normal horizontal palpebral fissure an upward slope medial to lateral. Insertion of the lateral canthal tendon inferior to the medial canthal tendon causes the horizontal palpebral fissure to be slanted downward.

### *Eyelid margin*

The eyelid margin is the confluence of the mucosal surface of the conjunctiva, the edge of the orbicularis, and the cutaneous epithelium. Along the margin are eyelashes and glands, which provide protection for the ocular surface. The mucocutaneous junction of the eyelid margin is often erroneously referred to as the *gray line.* The gray line is an isolated section of pretarsal orbicularis muscle (Riolan) just anterior to the tarsus. The mucocutaneous junction is located posterior to the meibomian gland orifices on the eyelid margin (Fig 9-11). The horizontal palpebral fissure is approximately 30 mm long. The main portion of the margin, called the *ciliary margin,* has a rather well-defined anterior and posterior edge. Medial to the punctum and in the lateral quarter of the eyelid, the eyelid margin is thinner.

### *Eyelashes*

There are approximately 100 eyelashes, or cilia, on the upper eyelid and 50 on the lower eyelid. The lashes usually originate in the anterior aspect of the eyelid margin just anterior to the tarsal plate and form 2 or 3 irregular rows. A few cilia may be found in the caruncle.

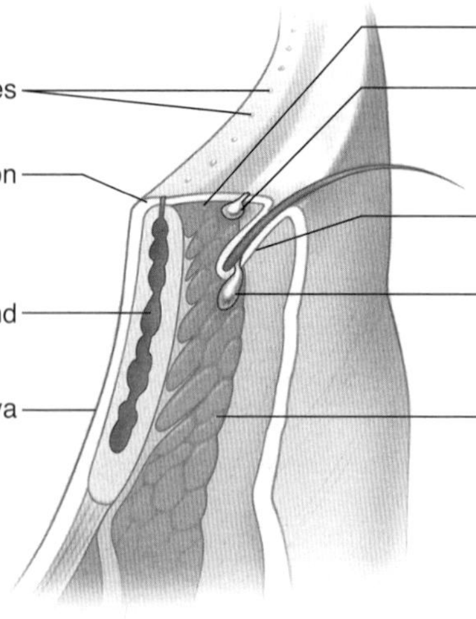


**Figure 9-11** Eyelid margin anatomy. *(Illustration by Christine Gralapp.)*

### *Meibomian glands*

The meibomian glands originate in the tarsus and number approximately 25 in the upper eyelid and 20 in the lower eyelid. During the second month of gestation, both the eyelashes and the meibomian glands differentiate from a common pilosebaceous unit. This dual potentiality explains why, following trauma or chronic irritation, a lash follicle may develop from a meibomian gland *(acquired distichiasis).* Similarly, an extra row of lashes arising from the meibomian orifices may be present from birth *(congenital distichiasis).* The meibomian glands are sebaceous glands that contribute to the lipid layer of the tear film via modified holocrine secretion.

### *Vascular and lymphatic supply*

The extensive vascularity of the eyelids promotes healing and helps defend against infection. The arterial supply of the eyelids comes from 2 main sources: (1) the internal carotid artery by way of the ophthalmic artery and its branches (supraorbital and lacrimal) and (2) the external carotid artery by way of the arteries of the face (angular and temporal). Collateral circulation between these 2 systems is extensive, anastomosing throughout the upper and lower eyelids and forming the marginal and peripheral arcades.

The *marginal arterial arcade* should not be confused with the peripheral arterial arcade. In the upper eyelid, the marginal arcade lies 2 mm superior to the margin, near the follicles of the cilia and anterior to the tarsal plate. The *peripheral arcade* lies superior to the tarsus, between the levator aponeurosis and the Müller muscle (see Fig 9-5). The lower eyelid often has only 1 arterial arcade, located at the inferior tarsal border.

Eyelid venous drainage may be divided into a *preseptal* system, in which the preseptal tissues drain into the angular vein medially and into the superficial temporal vein laterally, and a *postseptal* system, in which drainage flows into the orbital veins and the deeper branches of the anterior facial vein and pterygoid plexus. Lymphatic vessels serving the medial portion of the eyelids drain into the submandibular lymph nodes. Lymph channels serving the lateral portions of the eyelids drain first into the superficial preauricular nodes and then into the deeper cervical nodes.

CHAPTER 10

# Classification and Management of Eyelid Disorders

The eyelids can be affected by various congenital, acquired, infectious, inflammatory, neoplastic, and traumatic conditions. These disorders and their management are discussed in this chapter. In addition, the eyelids are subject to various positional abnormalities and involutional changes, which are discussed in Chapter 11.

## Congenital Anomalies

Congenital anomalies of the eyelid may be isolated or associated with other eyelid, facial, or systemic anomalies. Careful evaluation of patients in cases of hereditary syndromes is helpful before proceeding with treatment. Most congenital anomalies of the eyelids occur during the second month of gestation because of failure of fusion or an arrest of development. Most of the defects described in this section are rare. (See also BCSC Section 6, *Pediatric Ophthalmology and Strabismus.*)

### Blepharophimosis–Ptosis–Epicanthus Inversus Syndrome

Blepharophimosis–ptosis–epicanthus inversus syndrome (BPES), also called *blepharophimosis syndrome,* is an autosomal dominantly inherited blepharophimosis, usually presenting with telecanthus, epicanthus inversus (fold of skin extending from the lower to upper eyelid), and severe ptosis. The syndrome is caused by mutations in the *FOXL2* gene, located on chromosome 3. There are 2 types of BPES; both types I and II involve abnormalities of the eyelids. Type I also includes an early loss of ovarian function in women. Additional findings may include lateral lower eyelid ectropion secondary to vertical eyelid deficiency, a poorly developed nasal bridge, hypoplasia of the superior orbital rims, ear deformities, and hypertelorism (Fig 10-1).

Surgical modification may require multiple surgeries. Visually disruptive ptosis should be addressed promptly. Whether performed simultaneously with the ptosis repair or separately, medial canthal repositioning places traction on the upper eyelid and may exacerbate the ptosis. Repair of the ptosis usually requires frontalis suspension for adequate lift. Multiple Z-plasties or Y–V-plasties, sometimes combined with transnasal wiring of the medial canthal tendons, are used to modify the telecanthus and epicanthus. Additional procedures may be necessary to correct ectropion or orbital rim hypoplasia.

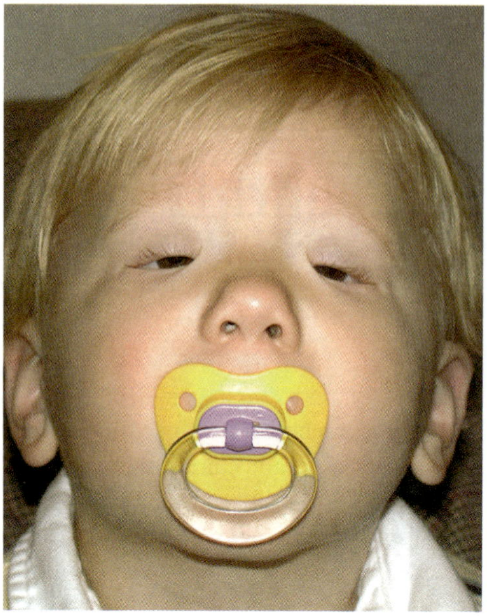

**Figure 10-1** Young child with blepharophimosis–ptosis–epicanthus inversus syndrome (blepharophimosis syndrome). *(Courtesy of Jill Foster, MD.)*

Allen CE, Rubin PA. Blepharophimosis-ptosis-epicanthus inversus syndrome (BPES): clinical manifestation and treatment. *Int Ophthalmol Clin.* 2008;48(2):15–23.

Anderson RL, Nowinski TS. The five-flap technique for blepharophimosis. *Arch Ophthalmol.* 1989;107(3):448–452.

## Congenital Ptosis of the Upper Eyelid

Congenital ptosis of the upper eyelid is discussed in Chapter 11.

## Congenital Ectropion

Congenital ectropion rarely occurs as an isolated finding. It is more often associated with BPES (blepharophimosis syndrome), Down syndrome, or ichthyosis. Congenital ectropion is caused by a vertical insufficiency of the anterior lamella of the eyelid and may give rise to chronic epiphora and exposure keratitis. Mild congenital ectropion usually requires no treatment. If it is severe and symptomatic, congenital ectropion is treated like a cicatricial ectropion, with horizontal tightening of the lateral canthal tendon and vertical lengthening of the anterior lamella with full-thickness skin grafting.

Complete eversion of the upper eyelids occasionally occurs in newborns (Fig 10-2). Possible causes include inclusion conjunctivitis, anterior lamellar inflammation or shortage, and Down syndrome. Topical lubrication and short-term patching of both eyes may be curative. Full-thickness sutures or a temporary tarsorrhaphy is used when necessary, followed by definitive repair.

## Euryblepharon

Euryblepharon is associated with both vertical shortening and horizontal lengthening of the involved eyelids (Figs 10-3, 10-4). The lateral portion of the eyelids is typically more

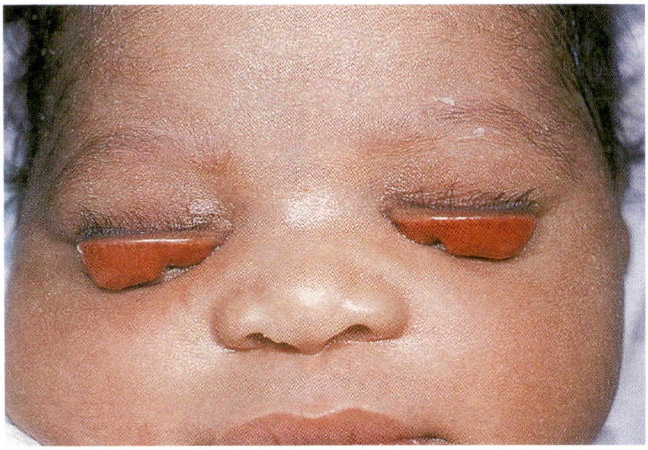

**Figure 10-2** Congenital eyelid eversion. *(Courtesy of Thaddeus S. Nowinski, MD.)*

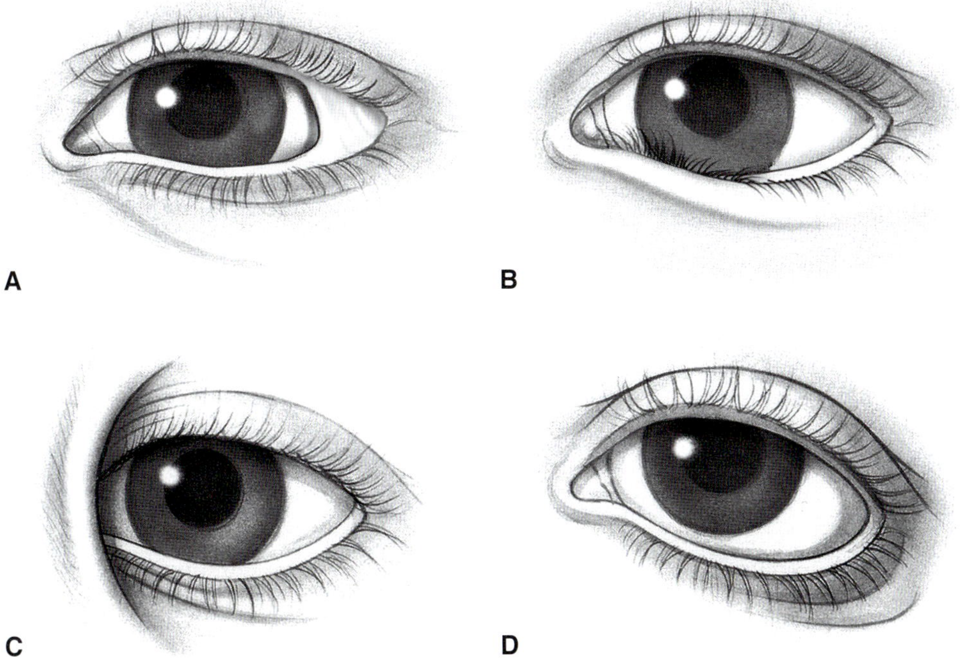

**Figure 10-3** Congenital eyelid deformities. **A,** Ankyloblepharon. **B,** Epiblepharon. **C,** Epicanthus. **D,** Euryblepharon. *(Illustration by Christine Gralapp.)*

involved than the medial aspect, and the condition may be associated with BPES (blepharophimosis syndrome). The palpebral fissure often has a downward slant because of the inferiorly displaced lateral canthal tendon. Impaired blinking, poor closure, and lagophthalmos may result in exposure keratitis. If the condition is symptomatic, reconstruction may include lateral canthal repositioning along with suspension of the suborbicularis

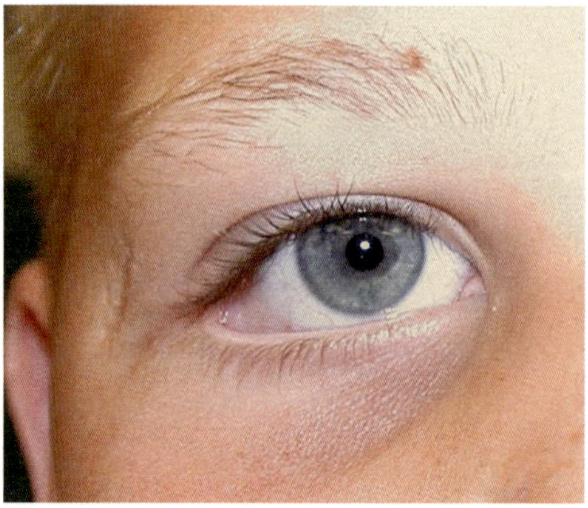

**Figure 10-4** Patient with euryblepharon. *(Courtesy of Jill Foster, MD.)*

oculi fat to the lateral orbital rim so that the lower eyelid is supported. If excess horizontal length is still apparent, a lateral tarsal strip or eyelid margin resection may be added. Skin grafts may occasionally be necessary.

## Ankyloblepharon

Ankyloblepharon is partial (ankyloblepharon filiforme adnatum) or complete fusion of the eyelids by webs of skin (see Fig 10-3A). These webs can usually be opened with scissors after being clamped for a few seconds with a hemostat.

## Epicanthus

Epicanthus is a medial canthal fold that may result from immature midfacial bones or a fold of skin and subcutaneous tissue (Fig 10-5; see also Fig 10-3C). The condition is usually bilateral. An affected child may appear esotropic because of decreased scleral exposure nasally *(pseudostrabismus).* Traditionally, 4 types of epicanthus have been described: (1) *epicanthus tarsalis,* in which the fold is most prominent in the upper eyelid; (2) *epicanthus inversus,* in which the fold is most prominent in the lower eyelid; (3) *epicanthus palpebralis,* in which the fold involves the upper and lower eyelids equally; and (4) *epicanthus supraciliaris,* in which the fold arises from the eyebrow region and runs to the lacrimal sac. Epicanthus tarsalis can be a normal variation of the Asian eyelid, whereas epicanthus inversus is frequently associated with BPES (blepharophimosis syndrome).

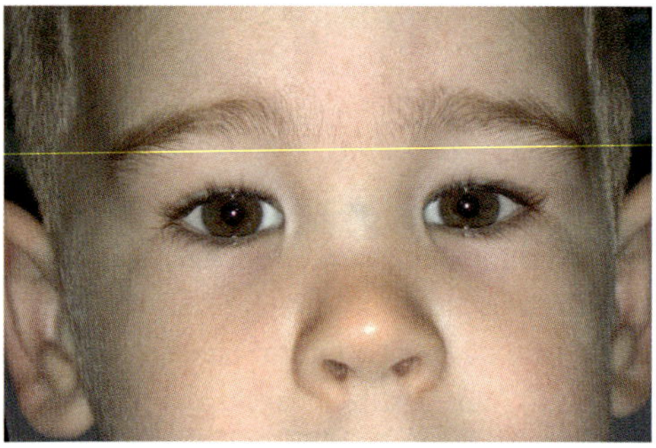

**Figure 10-5** Child with epicanthal folds. *(Courtesy of Jill Foster, MD.)*

Most forms of epicanthus become less apparent with normal growth of the facial bones. If no associated eyelid anomalies are present, observation is recommended until the face achieves maturity. Epicanthus inversus, however, rarely resolves with facial growth. Most cases of isolated epicanthus requiring treatment respond well to linear revisions such as Z-plasty or Y–V-plasty. Epicanthus tarsalis in the Asian patient may be eliminated by a Y–V-plasty with or without construction of an upper eyelid crease.

## Epiblepharon

In epiblepharon, the lower eyelid pretarsal muscle and skin ride above the lower eyelid margin to form a horizontal fold of tissue that causes the cilia to assume a vertical position (Fig 10-6; see also Fig 10-3B). The eyelid margin, therefore, is in normal position with respect to the globe. Epiblepharon is most common in Asian children.

The cilia often do not touch the cornea except in downgaze, and this rarely causes corneal staining. Epiblepharon may not require surgical treatment, because it tends to diminish with the maturation of the facial bones. However, epiblepharon occasionally results in acute or chronic corneal epithelial irritation; in that case, the excess skin and muscle fold are excised just inferior to the eyelid margin.

## Congenital Entropion

In contrast to epiblepharon, eyelid margin inversion is present in congenital entropion (Fig 10-7). Developmental factors that lead to this rare condition include lower eyelid retractor dysgenesis, structural defects in the tarsal plate, and relative shortening of the posterior lamella. Unlike epiblepharon, congenital entropion is unlikely to improve spontaneously and may require surgical correction. Congenital entropion may be repaired through removal of a small amount of the skin and orbicularis along the subciliary portion of the eyelid, in conjunction with advancement of the lower eyelid retractors to the tarsus.

*Tarsal kink* is an unusual form of congenital entropion in which the tarsal plate of the upper eyelid is folded, resulting in entropion. It may be repaired by removal of the kink in combination with a margin rotation. In some cases, skin grafting for the anterior lamella may be necessary.

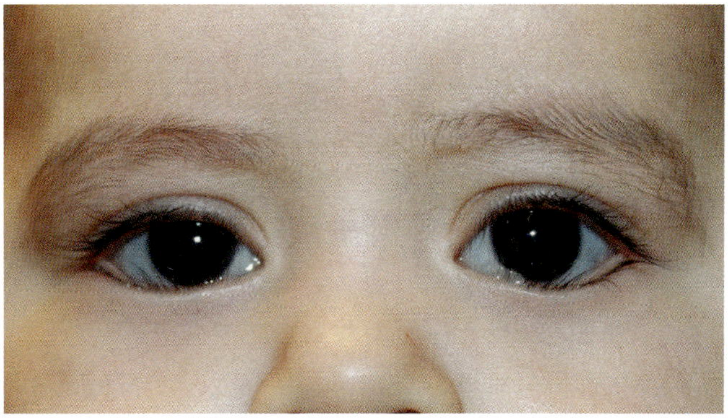

**Figure 10-6** Epiblepharon. *(Courtesy of Jill Foster, MD.)*

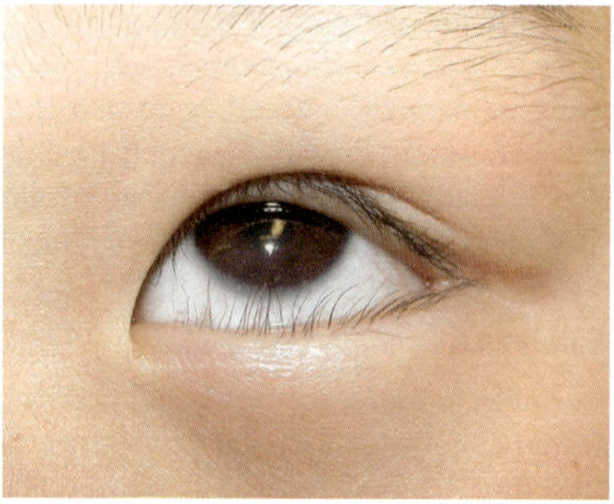

**Figure 10-7** Congenital entropion. *(Courtesy of Jill Foster, MD.)*

Dailey RA, Harrison AR, Hildebrand PL, Wobig JL. Levator aponeurosis disinsertion in congenital entropion of the upper eyelid. *Ophthal Plast Reconstr Surg.* 1999;15(5):360–362.

## Congenital Distichiasis

Distichiasis is a rare, sometimes hereditary condition in which an extra row of eyelashes is present in place of the orifices of the meibomian glands. Congenital distichiasis occurs when embryonic pilosebaceous units improperly differentiate into hair follicles (Fig 10-8). Treatment is indicated if the patient is symptomatic or if keratopathy develops. Lubricants and soft contact lenses may be sufficient, but electrolysis, cryoepilation, and eyelid splitting with removal of the follicles are alternatives.

Vaughn GL, Dortzbach RK, Sires BS, Lemke BN. Eyelid splitting with excision or microhyfrecation for distichiasis. *Arch Ophthalmol.* 1997;115(2):282–284.

## Congenital Coloboma

A *coloboma* is an embryologic cleft that is usually an isolated anomaly when it occurs in the medial upper eyelid. A true coloboma includes a defect in the eyelid margin (Fig 10-9). When found in the lower eyelid, however, the coloboma is frequently associated with other congenital conditions such as facial clefts (eg, Goldenhar syndrome) and lacrimal deformities.

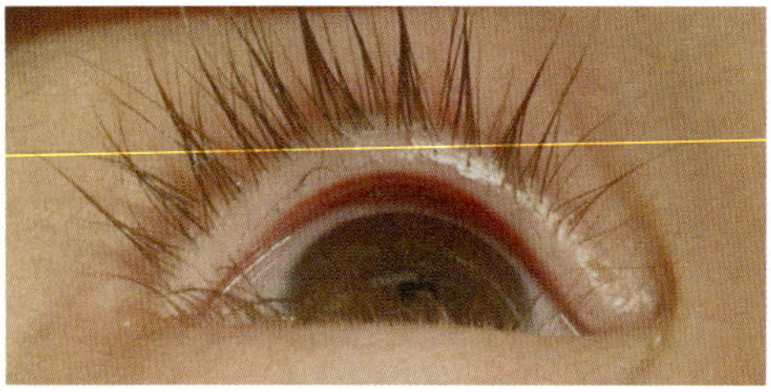

**Figure 10-8** Congenital distichiasis. *(Courtesy of Jill Foster, MD.)*

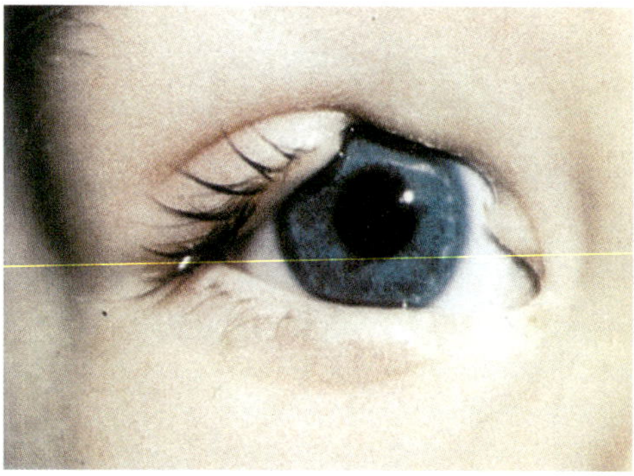

**Figure 10-9** True coloboma of upper eyelid.

Full-thickness defects affecting up to one-third of the eyelid can usually be repaired by creating raw vertical margins and sliding flaps along the eyelid crease. A lateral cantholysis may provide additional horizontal relaxation. Almost all large defects can be repaired with use of a variation of the lateral canthal semicircular flap (see the section Eyelid Defects Involving the Eyelid Margin, later in this chapter). Because of the risk of amblyopia, eyelid-sharing procedures that occlude the visual axis are avoided unless there is no other reconstructive alternative.

## Cryptophthalmos

Cryptophthalmos is a rare condition that presents with partial or complete absence of the eyebrow, palpebral fissure, eyelashes, and conjunctiva (Fig 10-10). The partially developed adnexa are fused to the anterior segment of the globe. Cryptophthalmos may be unilateral or bilateral. Histologically, the levator, orbicularis oculi muscle, tarsus, conjunctiva, and meibomian glands are attenuated or absent; thus, attempts at reconstruction are difficult. Severe ocular defects are present in the underlying eye.

## Congenital Eyelid Lesions: Infantile (Capillary) Hemangioma

Although infantile (capillary) hemangiomas sometimes occur as congenital eyelid lesions, most are not apparent at birth. Rather, they usually appear over the first weeks or months of life. Hemangiomas may also involve the orbit (see the section Vascular Tumors, Malformations, and Fistulas in Chapter 5). They are associated with a high incidence of amblyopia; therefore, treatment is recommended for patients who present with occlusion of the visual axis, anisometropia, strabismus, or lesions causing significant disfigurement. In the typical natural course of infantile hemangioma, the lesion becomes apparent shortly after birth, increases in size until the patient is 1 year old, and then decreases over the next 3–7 years.

In cases in which vision is threatened by the hemangioma, lesions limited to the eyelid may be treated with topical timolol gel or intralesional steroids; more widespread involvement is addressed with systemic propranolol or oral corticosteroids (see Chapter 5). Topical timolol gel appears to have the fewest adverse effects. For patients who cannot take β-blockers or do not respond to timolol, intralesional steroids are considered. Intralesional steroids may act by rendering the tumor's vascular bed more sensitive to the body's circulating catecholamines. Intralesional steroid injection is relatively safe, simple, and

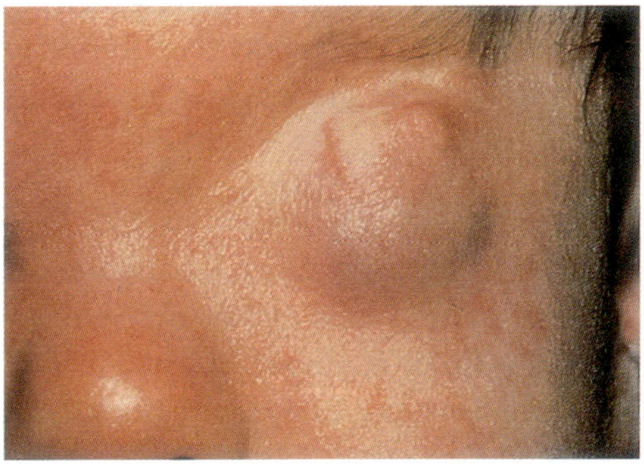

**Figure 10-10** Cryptophthalmos.

repeatable. However, rare cases of eyelid necrosis, embolic retinal vascular occlusion, and systemic adrenal suppression may occur following even a single injection. Treatment with systemic steroids eliminates the risks attributed to the injection delivery, but the dosage and risk of systemic adverse effects are increased.

Other treatment options may be considered for vision-compromising lesions that persist despite intervention. Topical treatment with clobetasol propionate has also been reported to successfully shrink eyelid hemangiomas. However, topical treatment does not eliminate the risks of systemic steroid exposure. Interferon-α is usually reserved for life-threatening or sight-threatening lesions unresponsive to other forms of treatment because of the risk of serious adverse effects. Surgical excision may be used for rare well-circumscribed lesions. Meticulous control of hemostasis is advised. Use of the carbon-dioxide laser as an incisional device is helpful for controlling bleeding when lesions must be removed. Topical skin lasers may be used on the superficial (1–2 mm) layers of the skin to diminish the redness of a lesion. However, cutaneous lasers do not penetrate deeply enough to shrink a visually disabling lesion.

Chambers CB, Katowitz WR, Katowitz JA, Binenbaum G. A controlled study of topical 0.25% timolol maleate gel for the treatment of cutaneous infantile capillary hemangiomas. *Ophthal Plast Reconstr Surg.* 2012;28(2):103–106.

Missoi TG, Lueder GT, Gilbertson K, Bayliss SJ. Oral propranolol for treatment of periocular infantile hemangiomas. *Arch Ophthalmol.* 2011;129(7):899–903.

Price CJ, Lattouf C, Baum B, et al. Propranolol vs corticosteroids for infantile hemangiomas: a multicenter retrospective analysis. *Arch Dermatol.* 2011;147(12):1371–1376.

## Acquired Eyelid Disorders

### Chalazion

Chalazion is a focal inflammation of the eyelids that results from an obstruction of the meibomian glands (an internal posterior hordeolum). This common disorder is often associated with rosacea and chronic blepharitis and may occasionally be confused with a malignant neoplasm.

The *meibomian glands* are oil-producing sebaceous glands located in the tarsal plate. The oil is an essential component of the tear film. If the gland orifices on the eyelid margin become plugged, the contents of the glands *(sebum)* are released into the tarsus and the surrounding eyelid soft tissue, eliciting an acute inflammatory response accompanied by pain and erythema. The exact role of bacterial agents (most commonly *Staphylococcus aureus*) in the production of chalazia is not clear. Histologically, these lesions are characterized by chronic lipogranulomatous inflammation.

#### Treatment

In the acute inflammatory phase, treatment consists of warm compresses and appropriate eyelid hygiene. Topical antibiotic or anti-inflammatory ocular medications may provide comfort. Acute secondary infection may be treated with an antibiotic directed at skin flora. Oral doxycycline or tetracycline may be appropriate when a case requires long-term suppression of meibomian gland inflammation or ocular rosacea.

Occasionally, chalazia become chronic, requiring surgical management. In most cases, the greatest inflammatory response is on the posterior eyelid margin, and an incision through tarsus and conjunctiva is appropriate for drainage. Sharp dissection and excision of all necrotic material, including the cyst wall, are indicated. This procedure results in a posterior marsupialization of the chalazion (Fig 10-11). The clinician should exercise caution in removing inflammatory tissue at the eyelid margin or adjacent to the punctum. In rare cases, the greatest inflammatory response is anterior; in such cases, a skin incision is used. Given the risk of masquerade conditions, including sebaceous cell carcinoma, pathologic examination is appropriate for atypical or recurrent chalazia.

Though sometimes employed as a less invasive option, local injection of corticosteroids in chalazia can cause depigmentation of the overlying skin and is not as effective as surgical treatment. The combination of excision and steroid injection yields a 95% resolution rate.

## Hordeolum

An acute infection (usually staphylococcal) can involve the sebaceous secretions in the glands of Zeis *(external hordeolum,* or *stye)* or the meibomian glands *(internal hordeolum).* In the case of external hordeola, the infection often appears to center around an eyelash follicle, and the eyelash can be plucked to promote drainage. The condition often resolves spontaneously. If needed, diligent application of hot compresses and topical

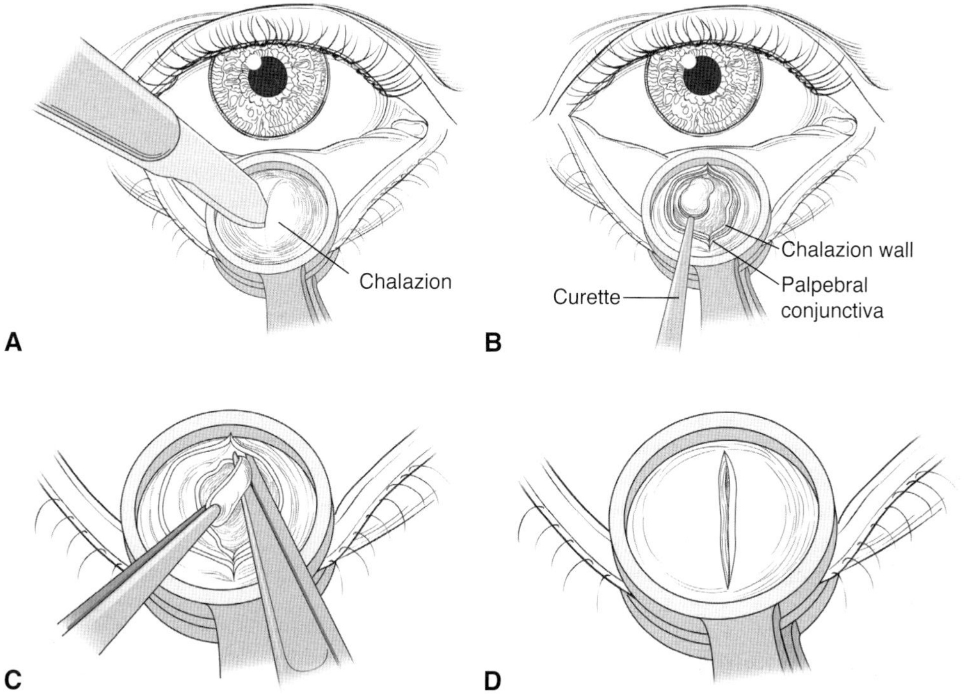


**Figure 10-11** Excision of chalazion. **A,** After a clamp is placed around the chalazion, a blade is used to make a vertical incision into the tarsus. **B,** The cyst contents are removed. **C,** The lining walls are excised with scissors. **D,** The defect is allowed to heal by secondary intention. *(Original illustration by Jeanne C. Koelling; revision by Mark Miller.)*

antibiotic ointment usually cures the infection. In rare cases, hordeola may progress to true superficial cellulitis, or even abscesses, of the eyelid. In such cases, systemic antibiotic therapy and possible surgical incision and drainage may be required.

## Eyelid Edema

Swelling of the eyelids may be caused by local conditions, such as insect bites or allergy, or by systemic conditions, such as cardiovascular disease, renal disease, collagen vascular diseases, or thyroid eye disease. Cerebrospinal fluid leakage into the orbit or eyelids following trauma may mimic eyelid edema. Lymphedema may be present if the lymphatic drainage system from the eyelid is interrupted.

## Floppy Eyelid Syndrome

Floppy eyelid syndrome is characterized by ocular irritation and mild mucus discharge that is frequently worse on awakening. Patients have a chronic papillary conjunctivitis. The superior tarsal plate is soft, rubbery, flaccid, and easily everted (Fig 10-12). During examination, if the clinician pulls the upper eyelid up toward the forehead, the upper eyelid everts spontaneously, especially laterally. Associations have been reported with obesity, keratoconus, eyelid rubbing, hyperglycemia, and sleep apnea. Histologic examination has revealed a marked decrease in the number of elastin fibers in the tarsal plate. Often, patients have a history of sleeping prone; this position can cause mechanical upper eyelid eversion, allowing the superior palpebral conjunctiva to rub against the pillow or bedding. Initial conservative treatment using viscous lubrication and a patch or eyelid shield at night is helpful. Frequently, surgical correction by horizontal tightening of the eyelid is indicated. Sleep studies are recommended to rule out sleep apnea.

*Eyelid imbrication syndrome* occurs when a lax upper eyelid with a normal tarsal plate overrides the lower eyelid margin during closure; this results in chronic conjunctivitis. Management consists of topical lubrication in mild cases. In more severe cases, horizontal tightening of the upper eyelid is indicated.

Ezra DG, Beaconsfield M, Sira M, et al. Long-term outcomes of surgical approaches to the treatment of floppy eyelid syndrome. *Ophthalmology.* 2010;117(4):839–846.

Karesh JW, Nirankari VS, Hameroff SB. Eyelid imbrications. An unrecognized cause of chronic ocular irritation. *Ophthalmology.* 1993;100(6):883–889.

Valenzuela AA, Sullivan TA. Medial upper eyelid shortening to correct medial eyelid laxity in floppy eyelid syndrome: a new surgical approach. *Ophthal Plast Reconstr Surg.* 2005;21(4): 259–263.

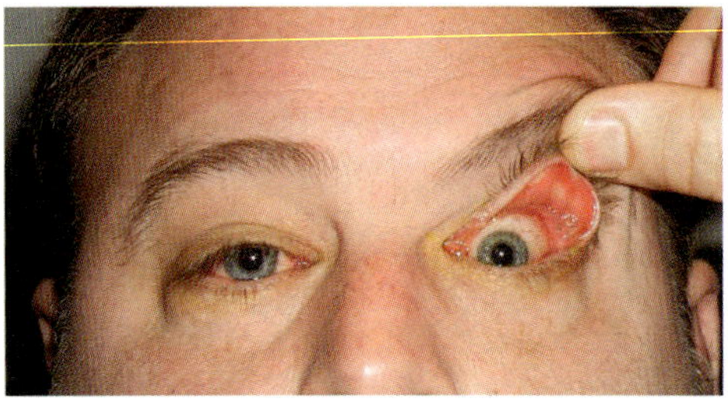

**Figure 10-12** Easy eversion of loose eyelid, characteristic of floppy eyelid syndrome. *(Courtesy of Morris E. Hartstein, MD.)*

### Trichotillomania

Trichotillomania is an impulse-control disorder most commonly seen in preteen or teenaged girls. It is characterized by the repeated desire to pull out hairs, frequently eyebrows or eyelashes. Diagnosis may be elusive, as affected patients usually deny the cause. Characteristically, multiple hairs are broken off and regrow at different lengths, a finding that guides the diagnosis.

## Eyelid Neoplasms

Numerous benign and malignant cutaneous neoplasms can develop in the periocular skin; they may arise from the epidermis, dermis, or eyelid adnexal structures. Most lesions, whether benign or malignant, develop from the epidermis, the rapidly growing superficial layer of the skin. Although many of these lesions may occur elsewhere on the body, their appearance and behavior in the eyelids may be unique owing to the particular characteristics of eyelid skin and the specialized adnexal elements. The malignant lesions that most frequently affect the eyelids are basal cell carcinoma, squamous cell carcinoma, sebaceous cell carcinoma, and melanoma. Histologic examination of suspected cutaneous malignancies is recommended.

### Clinical Evaluation of Eyelid Tumors

The history and physical examination of eyelid lesions offer important clues regarding the likelihood of malignancy. Predisposing factors in the development of skin cancer include

- a history of prior skin cancer
- excessive sun exposure, especially blistering sunburn
- previous radiation therapy
- a history of smoking
- Celtic or Scandinavian ancestry, with fair skin, red hair, and blue eyes
- immunosuppression

Signs suggesting malignancy are

- slow, painless growth of a lesion
- ulceration, drainage, bleeding, and crusting
- pigmentary changes
- destruction of normal eyelid margin architecture (especially meibomian orifices) and loss of cilia
- heaped-up, pearly, translucent margins with central ulceration
- fine telangiectasias
- loss of fine cutaneous wrinkles or vellus hair

Palpable induration extending well beyond visibly apparent margins suggests tumor infiltration into the dermis and subcutaneous tissue.

Lesions near the puncta should be evaluated for punctal or canalicular involvement. Probing and irrigation may be required to exclude lacrimal system involvement or to prepare for surgical resection.

Large lesions should be palpated for evidence of fixation to deeper tissues or bone. In addition, regional lymph nodes should be palpated for evidence of metastases in cases of suspected squamous cell carcinoma, sebaceous carcinoma, melanoma, or Merkel cell carcinoma. Lymphatic tumor spread may produce rubbery swelling along the line of the jaw or in front of the ear. Restriction of ocular motility and proptosis suggest orbital extension. The function of cranial nerves V and VII is assessed to enable detection of any deficiencies that may indicate perineural tumor spread. Perineural invasion is a characteristic of squamous cell carcinoma. Systemic evidence of liver, pulmonary, bone, or neurological involvement should be sought in cases of sebaceous adenocarcinoma or melanoma of the eyelid. It is important to obtain photographs and measurements prior to treatment of the lesion. For more extensive coverage and additional clinical and pathology photographs, see BCSC Section 4, *Ophthalmic Pathology and Intraocular Tumors.*

Cook BE Jr, Bartley GB. Epidemiologic characteristics and clinical course of patients with malignant eyelid tumors in an incidence cohort in Olmsted County, Minnesota. *Ophthalmology.* 1999;106(4):746–750.

de la Garza AG, Kersten RC, Carter KD. Evaluation and treatment of benign eyelid lesions. *Focal Points: Clinical Modules for Ophthalmologists.* San Francisco: American Academy of Ophthalmology; 2010, module 5.

## Benign Eyelid Lesions

### *Epithelial hyperplasias*

The terminology used to describe various benign epithelial proliferations continues to evolve. It is helpful to group the various benign epithelial proliferations under the clinical heading of *papillomas.* (This designation does not necessarily imply any association with the papillomavirus.) Clinical and histologic characterizations of the various benign epithelial proliferations overlap considerably. Included within this group are seborrheic keratosis, pseudoepitheliomatous hyperplasia, verruca vulgaris, acrochordon (also called skin tag, fibroepithelial polyp, squamous papilloma) (Fig 10-13), basosquamous acanthoma,

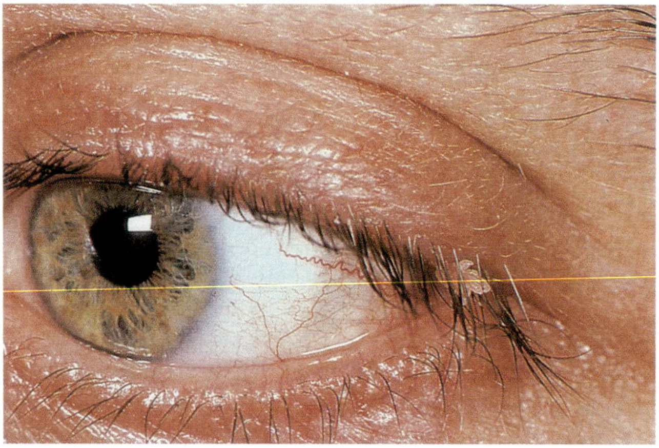

**Figure 10-13** Acrochordon (also called *skin tag* or *squamous papilloma*).

squamous acanthoma, and many others. All of these benign epithelial proliferations can be managed with shave excision at the dermal–epidermal junction.

*Seborrheic keratosis* is an example of acquired benign eyelid papilloma (Fig 10-14). It tends to affect middle-aged and elderly patients. Its clinical appearance varies; it may be sessile or pedunculated and have varying degrees of pigmentation and hyperkeratosis. On facial skin, seborrheic keratosis typically appears as a smooth, greasy, stuck-on lesion. On the thinner eyelid skin, this lesion can be more lobulated, papillary, or pedunculated with visible excrescences on its surface. The lesions can be managed by shave excision.

*Pseudoepitheliomatous hyperplasia* is not a discrete lesion but rather a pattern of reactive changes in the epidermis that may develop over areas of inflammation or neoplasia.

*Verruca vulgaris,* caused by epidermal infection with the human papillomavirus (type 6 or 11), rarely occurs in thin eyelid skin (Fig 10-15). Cryotherapy may eradicate the lesion and minimize the risk of viral spread.

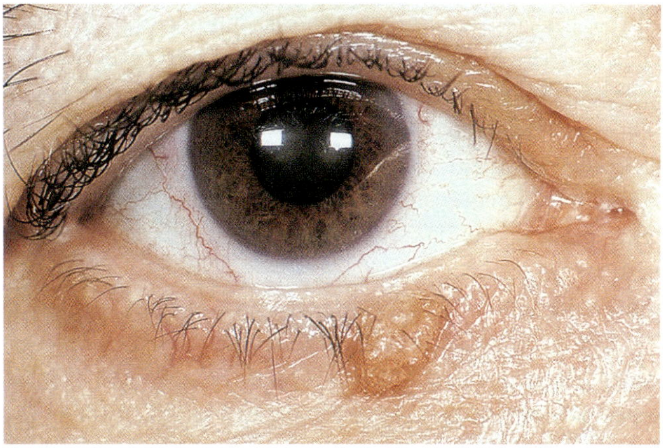

**Figure 10-14** Seborrheic keratosis.

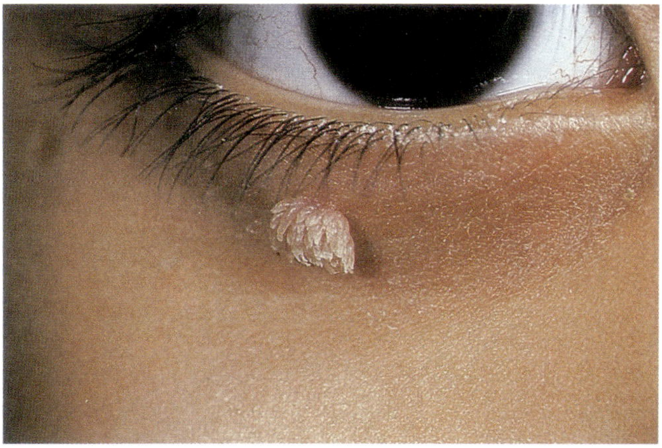

**Figure 10-15** Verruca vulgaris (wart).

*Cutaneous horn* is a descriptive, nondiagnostic term referring to *exuberant hyperkeratosis.* This lesion may be associated with various benign or malignant histologic processes, including seborrheic keratosis, verruca vulgaris, and squamous or basal cell carcinoma. Biopsy of the base of the cutaneous horn is recommended.

### Benign epithelial lesions

Cysts of the epidermis are the second most common type of benign periocular cutaneous lesions, accounting for approximately 18% of excised benign lesions. Most of these are *epidermal inclusion cysts,* which arise from the infundibulum of the hair follicle, either spontaneously or following traumatic implantation of epidermal tissue into the dermis (Fig 10-16). The lesions are slow-growing, elevated, round, and smooth. They often have a central pore, indicating the remaining pilar duct. Although these cysts are often called *sebaceous cysts,* they are actually filled with keratin. Rupture of the cyst wall may cause an inflammatory foreign-body reaction. The cysts may also become secondarily infected. Recommended treatment for small cysts is marsupialization, which involves excising around the periphery of the cyst but leaving the base of the cyst wall to serve as the new surface epithelium. Larger or deeper cysts may require complete excision, in which case the cyst wall should be removed intact to reduce the possibility of recurrence.

Multiple tiny epidermal inclusion cysts are called *milia.* They are particularly common in newborn infants. Generally, milia resolve spontaneously, but they may be marsupialized with a sharp blade or needle. Multiple confluent milia may be treated with topical retinoic acid cream.

A less common epidermal cyst is the *pilar,* or *trichilemmal, cyst.* Such cysts are clinically indistinguishable from epidermal inclusion cysts, but they tend to occur in areas containing large and numerous hair follicles. Approximately 90% of pilar cysts occur on the scalp; in the periocular region, they are generally found in the eyebrows. The cysts are filled with desquamated epithelium, and calcification occurs in approximately 25% of cases.

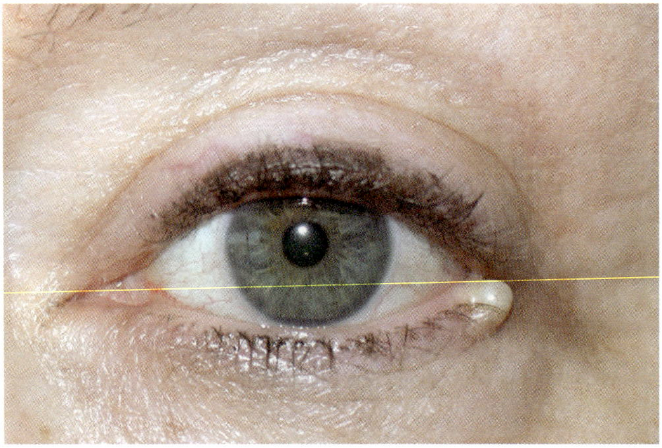

**Figure 10-16** Epidermal inclusion cyst. *(Courtesy of Jill Foster, MD.)*

*Molluscum contagiosum* is a viral infection of the epidermis that often involves the eyelid in children (Fig 10-17). Occasionally, multiple exuberant lesions appear in adult patients with acquired immunodeficiency syndrome (AIDS). The lesions are characteristically waxy and nodular, with a central umbilication. They may produce an associated follicular conjunctivitis. Treatment is observation, oral cimetadine, excision, controlled cryotherapy, or curettage.

*Xanthelasmas* are yellowish plaques that occur commonly in the medial canthal areas of the upper and lower eyelids (Fig 10-18). They represent lipid-laden macrophages in the superficial dermis and subdermal tissues. Xanthelasmas are sometimes associated with hypercholesterolemia or congenital disorders of lipid metabolism, so patients whose lipid levels are unknown may benefit from having them checked by their primary care physician. When excising these lesions, the surgeon must be careful to avoid causing cicatricial ectropion or eyelid retraction. Xanthelasmas may recur. Other treatment options include serial excision, laser ablation, and topical trichloroacetic acid. Deep extension into the orbicularis oculi muscle can occur.

## Benign Adnexal Lesions

The term *adnexa* refers to skin appendages that are located within the dermis but communicate through the epidermis to the surface. They include oil glands, sweat glands, and

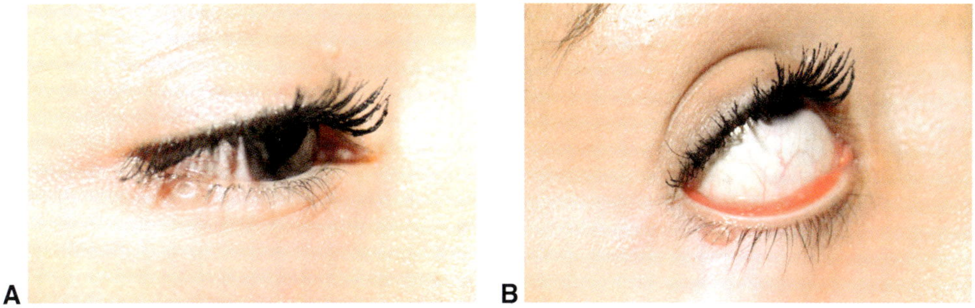

**Figure 10-17** Molluscum. **A,** Umbilicated eyelid lesion. **B,** Molluscum lesions can cause conjunctivitis, which typically resolves with removal of the lesion. *(Courtesy of Vikram Durairaj, MD.)*

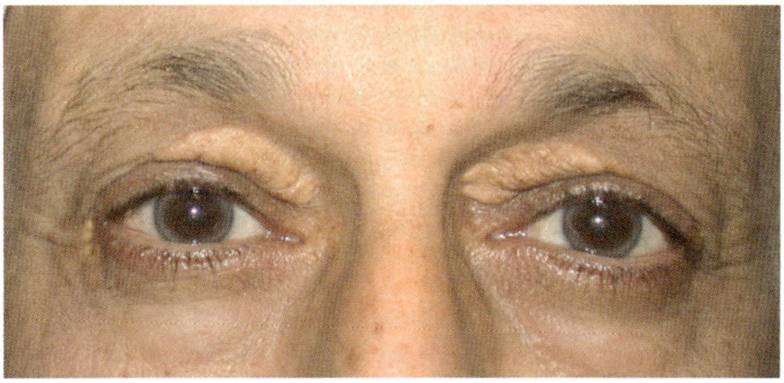

**Figure 10-18** Xanthelasma. *(Courtesy of Jill Foster, MD.)*

hair follicles. The eyelids contain both the specialized eyelashes and the normal vellus hairs found on skin throughout the body. Periocular adnexal oil glands include

- the *meibomian glands* within the tarsal plate
- the *glands of Zeis* associated with eyelash follicles
- normal *sebaceous glands* that are present as part of the pilosebaceous units in the skin hair

Sweat glands in the periocular region include the *eccrine sweat glands,* which have a general distribution throughout the body and are responsible for thermal regulation, and the eccrine glands with apocrine secretion (the *glands of Moll*), which are associated with the eyelid margin.

### *Lesions of oil gland origin*

**Chalazion and hordeolum** These common eyelid lesions are discussed earlier in this chapter in the section Acquired Eyelid Disorders.

**Sebaceous hyperplasia** Sebaceous gland hyperplasia presents as multiple small yellow papules that may have central umbilication. They tend to occur on the forehead and cheeks and are common in patients older than 40 years. These lesions may sometimes be mistaken for basal cell carcinoma because of their tendency to have central umbilication and fine telangiectasias. Patients with multiple acquired sebaceous gland adenomas, adenomatoid sebaceous hyperplasia, or basal cell carcinomas with sebaceous differentiation have an increased incidence of visceral malignancy *(Muir-Torre syndrome)* and should be evaluated accordingly.

**Sebaceous adenoma** This rare tumor appears as a yellowish papule on the face, scalp, or trunk and may mimic a basal cell carcinoma or seborrheic keratosis.

### *Tumors of eccrine sweat gland origin*

**Eccrine hidrocystoma** Eccrine hidrocystomas are common cystic lesions 1–3 mm in diameter that occur in groups and tend to cluster around the lower eyelids and canthi and the face. They are considered to be ductal retention cysts, and they often enlarge in conditions such as heat and increased humidity, which stimulate perspiration. Treatment consists of surgical excision.

**Syringoma** Benign eccrine sweat gland tumors found commonly in young females, syringomas present as multiple small, waxy, elevated nodules 1–2 mm in diameter on the lower eyelids (Fig 10-19). Syringomas can also be found in the axilla and sternal region. They become more apparent during puberty. Because the eccrine glands are located within the dermis, these lesions are too deep to allow shave excision. Removal requires complete surgical excision, which is often best accomplished in a staged fashion.

**Pleomorphic adenoma** This rare benign tumor occurs most commonly in the head and neck region and may involve the eyelids. Histologically, the tumor is identical to the pleomorphic adenoma of the salivary and lacrimal glands (discussed in Chapter 5). Treatment is complete surgical excision at the time of the primary exploration.

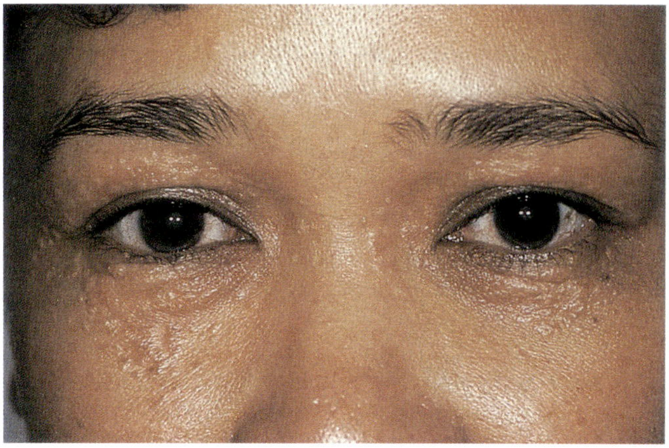

**Figure 10-19** Syringomas. *(Courtesy of Robert C. Kersten, MD.)*

***Tumors of apocrine sweat gland origin***

**Apocrine hidrocystoma** A very common solitary smooth cyst arising from the glands of Moll along the eyelid margin, apocrine hidrocystoma is considered to be an adenoma of the secretory cells of Moll rather than a retention cyst (Fig 10-20). These lesions typically are translucent or bluish, and they transilluminate. They may be multiple and often extend deep beneath the surface, especially in the canthal regions. Treatment for superficial cysts is marsupialization. Deep cysts require complete excision of the cyst wall.

**Cylindroma** Cylindromas are rare tumors that may be solitary or multiple and may be dominantly inherited. Lesions are dome-shaped, smooth, flesh-colored nodules of varying size that tend to affect the scalp and face. They may occur so profusely in the scalp that the scalp is entirely covered with lesions, in which case they are called *turban tumors.* Treatment is surgical excision, but it may prove difficult if there are multiple lesions over a large surface area.

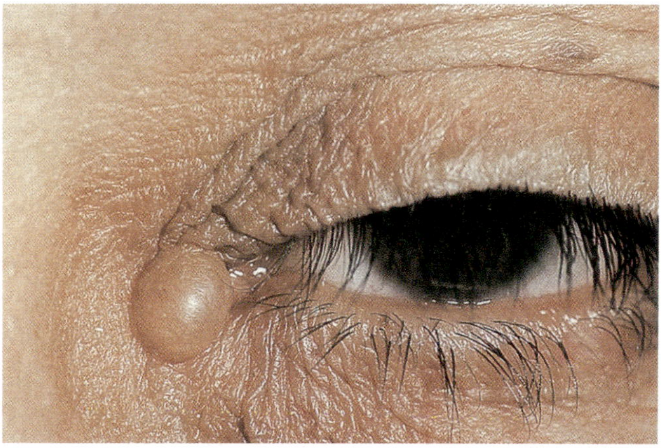

**Figure 10-20** Apocrine hidrocystoma. *(Courtesy of Robert C. Kersten, MD.)*

#### ***Tumors of hair follicle origin***

Several rare benign lesions may arise from the eyelashes, eyebrows, or vellus hairs in the periocular region.

**Trichoepithelioma** These lesions are small, flesh-colored papules with occasional telangiectasias that occur on the eyelids (Fig 10-21) or forehead. Histologically, trichoepitheliomas appear as basaloid islands and keratin cysts with immature hair follicle structures. If keratin is abundant, these lesions may clinically resemble an epidermal inclusion cyst. The individual histologic picture may be difficult to differentiate from that of basal cell carcinoma. Simple excision is curative.

**Trichofolliculoma** A trichofolliculoma is a single, sometimes umbilicated lesion found mainly in adults. Histologically, it represents a squamous cystic structure containing keratin and hair shaft components.

**Trichilemmoma** Another type of solitary lesion that occurs predominantly in adults, trichilemmomas resemble verrucae. Histologically, they show glycogen-rich cells oriented around hair follicles.

**Pilomatricoma** This lesion (sometimes spelled *pilomatrixoma*) most often affects young adults and usually occurs in the eyebrow and central upper eyelid as a reddish purple subcutaneous mass attached to the overlying skin (Fig 10-22). Pilomatricomas may become quite large. The tumor is composed of islands of epithelial cells surrounded by basophilic cells with shadow cells. Excision is curative.

### Benign Melanocytic Lesions

Melanocytic lesions of the skin arise from 3 sources: (1) nevus cells, (2) dermal melanocytes, and (3) epidermal melanocytes. Virtually any benign or malignant lesion may be pigmented, and lesions of melanocytic origin do not necessarily have visible pigmentation.

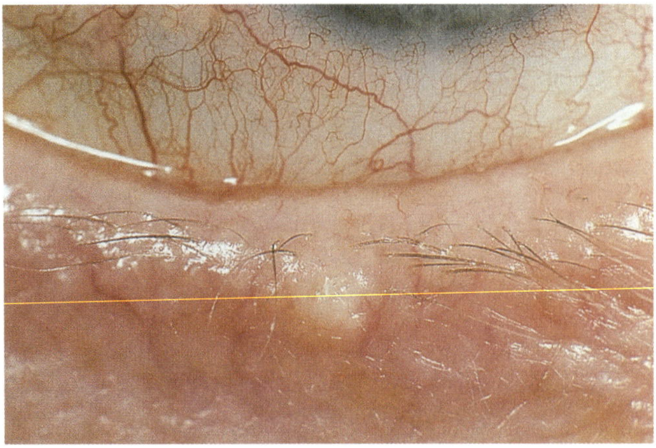

**Figure 10-21** Trichoepithelioma. *(Courtesy of Jeffrey A. Nerad, MD.)*

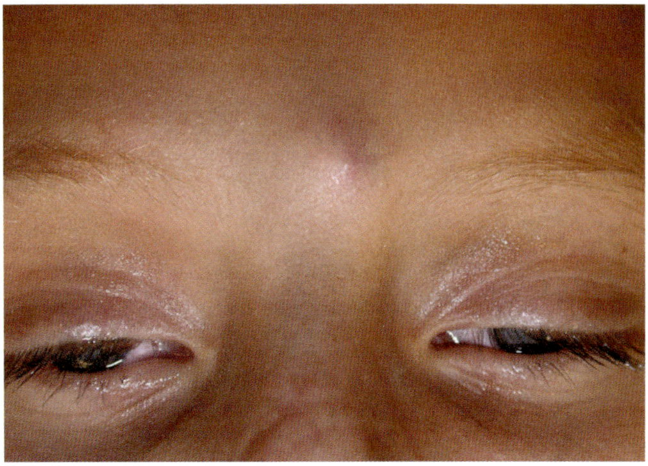

**Figure 10-22** Pilomatricoma of glabella. *(Courtesy of Jill Foster, MD.)*

For example, seborrheic keratoses are frequently pigmented, and basal cell carcinomas are occasionally pigmented, especially if they arise in persons with darker skin. In contrast, dermal nevi typically have no pigmentation in white individuals. Melanocytes are normally found distributed at the dermal–epidermal junction throughout the skin. Melanocytes are similar to nevus cells, but nevus cells are arranged in clusters and have ultrastructural differences. Both nevus cells and melanocytes give rise to several benign lesions. In addition to the individual lesions described next, diffuse eyelid skin hyperpigmentation called *melasma,* or *chloasma,* can occur in women who are pregnant or using oral contraceptives; in families with an autosomal dominant trait; and in patients with chronic atopic eczema, rosacea, and other inflammatory dermatoses.

### Nevi

Nevi are the third most common benign lesions encountered in the periocular region (after papillomas and epidermal inclusion cysts). They arise from *nevus cells,* which are incompletely differentiated melanocytes in the epidermis and dermis and in the junction zone between these 2 layers. Nevi are not apparent clinically at birth but begin to appear during childhood and often develop increased pigmentation during puberty.

All nevi tend to undergo evolution during life through 3 stages: (1) *junctional* (located in the basal layer of the epidermis at the dermal–epidermal junction), (2) *compound* (extending from the junctional zone up into the epidermis and down into the dermis), and (3) *dermal* (caused by involution of the epidermal component and persistence of the dermal component). In children, nevi arise initially as junctional nevi, which are typically flat, pigmented macules. Beyond the second decade, most nevi become compound, at which stage they appear as elevated, pigmented papules. Later in life, the pigmentation is lost, and the compound nevus remains as a minimally pigmented or amelanotic lesion. By age 70 years, virtually all nevi have become dermal nevi and have lost pigmentation.

Nevi are frequently found on the eyelid margin, characteristically molded to the ocular surface (Fig 10-23). Asymptomatic benign nevi require no treatment, but malignant

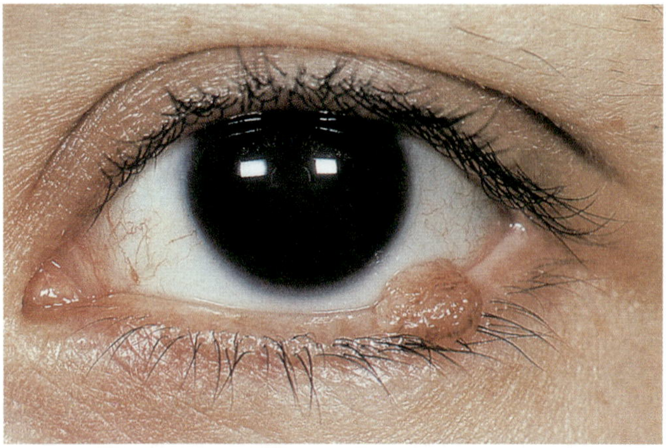

**Figure 10-23** Eyelid margin nevus.

transformation of a junctional or compound nevus can occur in rare cases. Nevi may become symptomatic if they rub on the ocular surface or enlarge and obstruct vision. They are managed with shave excision or wedge resection.

### Freckle

An *ephelis,* or *freckle,* is a small, flat, brown spot on the skin, the malar areas, eyelids, or the conjunctiva. Ephelides arise from hyperpigmentation of the basal layer of the epidermis. The number of epidermal melanocytes is not increased, but they extrude more than the usual amount of pigment into the epidermal basal cell layer. Ephelides are common in fair-skinned persons, and the hue of the ephelis darkens with sunlight exposure. No treatment is necessary other than sun protection.

### Lentigo simplex

*Simple lentigines* are flat, pigmented spots that are larger in diameter than ephelides. Occurring throughout life, lentigo simplex is not related to sun exposure. Lentigo simplex differs from a freckle in that the number of epidermal melanocytes is increased, and melanin is found in adjacent basal keratinocytes. Individual lesions are evenly pigmented and measure a few millimeters in diameter. Eyelid lentigines may be associated with Peutz-Jeghers syndrome (autosomal dominant polyposis of the intestinal tract). No treatment is necessary for lentigo simplex. Melanin-bleaching preparations may achieve cosmetic improvement.

### Solar lentigo

Multiple solar lentigines may occur in older persons, in which case they are called *senile lentigo.* Chronic sun exposure produces pigmented macules with an increased number of melanocytes. Solar lentigines are uniformly hyperpigmented and somewhat larger than simple lentigines. The dorsum of the hands and the forehead are the most frequently affected areas. No treatment is necessary, but sun protection is recommended. Melanin-bleaching preparations, intense pulsed light treatment, or cryotherapy may help fade the pigmentation of solar lentigines.

### *Blue nevi*

Blue nevi are dark blue-gray to blue-black, slightly elevated lesions that may be congenital or may develop during childhood. They arise from a localized proliferation of dermal melanocytes. The dark, dome-shaped lesions beneath the epidermis are usually 10 mm or less in diameter. Although the malignant potential is extremely low, these lesions are generally excised.

### *Dermal melanocytosis*

Also known as *nevus of Ota,* this diffuse, congenital blue nevus of the periocular skin most often affects persons of African, Hispanic, or Asian descent, especially females. Dermal melanocytes proliferate in the region of the first and second dermatomes of cranial nerve V. The eyelid skin is diffusely brown, gray, or blue, and pigmentation may extend to the adjacent forehead. Approximately 5% of cases are bilateral. When patchy slate-gray pigmentation also appears on the episclera and uvea, as occurs in two-thirds of affected patients, the condition is known as *oculodermal melanocytosis* (Fig 10-24). Although malignant transformation may occur, especially in white patients, no prophylactic treatment is recommended. Approximately 0.25% of patients with oculodermal melanocytosis develop a uveal melanoma. An additional concern is that 10% of patients with oculodermal melanocytosis also have glaucoma and pigmentation of the trabecular meshwork; thus, these patients should be monitored for glaucoma.

## Premalignant Epidermal Lesions: Actinic Keratosis

Actinic keratosis is the most common precancerous skin lesion. It usually affects fair-skinned, elderly persons with a history of chronic sun exposure (Fig 10-25). These lesions are typically round, scaly, keratotic plaques that on palpation have the texture of sandpaper. They often develop on the face, head, neck, forearms, and dorsum of the hands. These lesions are in a state of continual flux, increasing in size and darkening in response

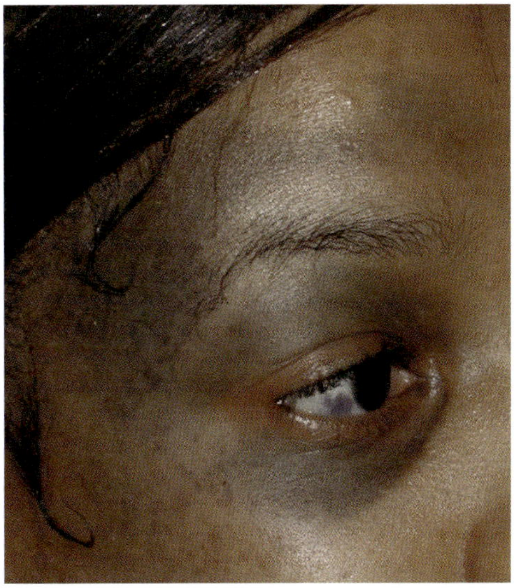

**Figure 10-24** Oculodermal melanocytosis. *(Courtesy of Jill Foster, MD.)*

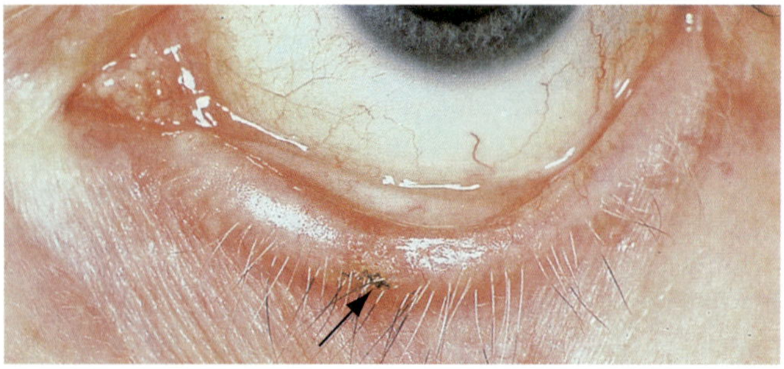

**Figure 10-25** Actinic keratosis *(arrow)*.

to sunlight exposure and remitting with reduced sun exposure. It has been reported that up to 25% of individual actinic keratoses spontaneously resolve over a 12-month period, although new lesions tend to develop continually. The risk of malignant transformation from a given actinic keratosis is only 0.24% per year, but over extended follow-up, a person with multiple actinic keratoses has a 12%–16% incidence of squamous cell carcinoma. Squamous cell carcinomas arising from actinic keratoses are thought to be less aggressive than those developing de novo.

For lesions arising in the periocular region, incisional or excisional biopsy is recommended. Extensive lesions may be treated with topical 5-fluorouracil or imiquimod cream.

Gupta AK, Davey V, Mcphail H. Evaluation of the effectiveness of imiquimod and 5-fluorouracil for the treatment of actinic keratosis: critical review and meta-analysis of efficacy studies. *J Cutan Med Surg.* 2005;9(5):209–214.

## In Situ Epithelial Malignancies

### *Squamous cell carcinoma in situ*

The term *Bowen disease* refers to squamous cell carcinoma in situ of the skin. These lesions typically appear as elevated, nonhealing, erythematous lesions. They may present with scaling, crusting, or pigmented keratotic plaques. Pathologically, the lesions demonstrate full-thickness epidermal atypia without dermal invasion. In 5% of patients, Bowen disease may progress to vertically invasive squamous cell carcinoma; therefore, complete surgical excision is advised. Alternatively, cryotherapy of Bowen disease may be used, especially in larger areas of involvement.

### *Keratoacanthoma*

Although keratoacanthoma was previously considered to be a benign, self-limiting lesion, many authors now regard this entity as a low-grade squamous cell carcinoma. The lesion usually begins as a flesh-colored papule on the lower eyelid that develops rapidly into a dome-shaped nodule with a central keratin-filled crater and elevated rolled margins (Fig 10-26). Keratoacanthomas typically occur in middle-aged and elderly patients and show an increased incidence in immunosuppressed patients. Gradual involution over the course of 3–6 months has often been observed. The abundant keratin production in the center of the lesion may incite a surrounding inflammatory reaction, which may play a

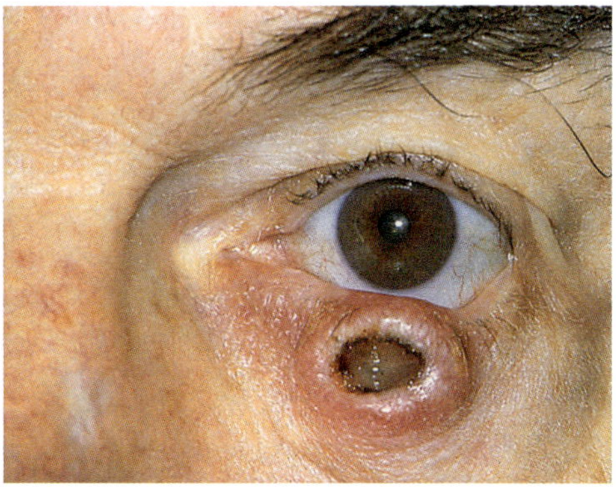

**Figure 10-26** Keratoacanthoma.

role in ultimate resolution. At present, incisional biopsy followed by complete surgical excision is recommended.

Grossniklaus HE, Wojno TH, Yanoff M, Font RL. Invasive keratoacanthoma of the eyelid and ocular adnexa. *Ophthalmology.* 1996;103(6):937–941.

## Premalignant Melanocytic Lesions: Lentigo Maligna

Also known as *Hutchinson melanotic freckle* or *precancerous melanosis,* lentigo maligna is a flat, irregularly shaped, unevenly pigmented, slowly enlarging lesion that typically occurs on the malar regions in older white persons. Unlike senile or solar lentigo, lentigo maligna is characterized by significant pigmentary variation, irregular borders, and progressive enlargement. These characteristics reflect a radial, intraepidermal, uncontrolled growth phase of melanocytes, which in 30%–50% of patients eventually progresses to nodules of vertically invasive melanoma.

The area of histologic abnormality frequently extends beyond the visible pigmented borders of the lesion; in the periocular region, cutaneous lentigo maligna of the eyelid may extend onto the conjunctival surface, where the lesion appears identical to primary acquired melanosis. Excision with adequate surgical margins is recommended with permanent sections for final monitoring. Close observation for recurrence is warranted.

## Malignant Eyelid Tumors

### *Basal cell carcinoma*

Basal cell carcinoma, the most common eyelid malignancy, accounts for approximately 90%–95% of malignant eyelid tumors. Basal cell carcinomas are often located on the lower eyelid margin (50%–60%) and near the medial canthus (25%–30%). Less commonly, they may occur on the upper eyelid (15%) and lateral canthus (5%). Basal cell carcinomas may have many different clinical manifestations in the eyelid (Fig 10-27).

Patients at highest risk for basal cell carcinoma are fair-skinned, blue-eyed, red-haired or blond, middle-aged and elderly persons with English, Irish, Scottish, or Scandinavian ancestry. They may have a history of prolonged sun exposure during the first 2 decades of life. A history of cigarette smoking also increases the risk of basal cell carcinoma. Patients

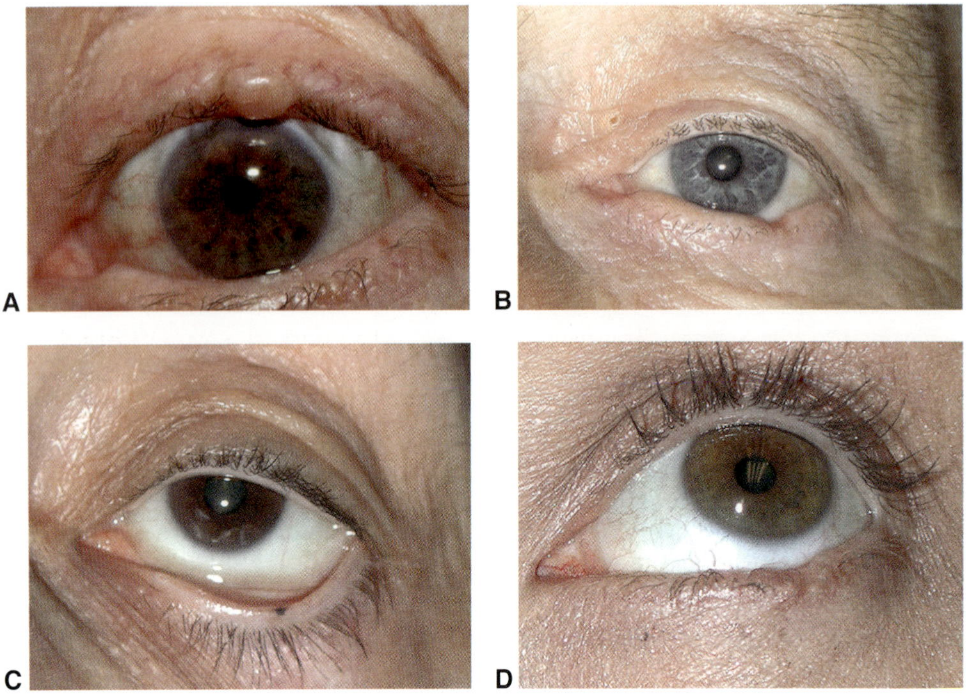

**Figure 10-27** Basal cell carcinoma. **A,** Nodular. **B,** Ulcerative. **C,** Pigmented. **D,** Morpheaform. *(Courtesy of Jill Foster, MD.)*

with prior basal cell carcinomas have a higher probability of developing additional skin cancers.

Basal cell carcinoma is being seen with increasing frequency in younger patients, and discovery of malignant eyelid lesions in these patients or those with a positive family history should prompt inquiry into possible systemic associations such as basal cell nevus syndrome or xeroderma pigmentosum. *Basal cell nevus syndrome (Gorlin syndrome)* is an uncommon autosomal dominant, multisystem disorder characterized by multiple nevoid basal cell carcinomas, which appear early in life and are associated with skeletal anomalies, especially of the mandible, maxilla, and vertebrae. *Xeroderma pigmentosum* is a rare autosomal recessive disorder characterized by extreme sun sensitivity and a defective repair mechanism for UV light–induced DNA damage in skin cells.

*Nodular basal cell carcinoma,* the most common clinical appearance of basal cell carcinoma, is a firm, raised, pearly nodule that may be associated with telangiectasia and central ulceration. Histologically, tumors of this form demonstrate nests of basal cells that originate from the basal cell layer of the epithelium and may show peripheral palisading. As the nests of atypical cells break through to the surface of the epithelium, central necrosis and ulceration may occur.

The *morpheaform* tumor type is less common, and behaves more aggressively, than the nodular form of basal cell carcinoma. Morpheaform lesions may be firm and slightly elevated, with margins that may be indeterminate on clinical examination. Histologically, these lesions do not show peripheral palisading but rather occur in thin cords that radiate peripherally. The surrounding stroma may show proliferation of connective tissue into a pattern of fibrosis.

Basal cell carcinoma may simulate chronic inflammation of the eyelid margin and is frequently associated with loss of eyelashes *(madarosis). Multicentric* or *superficial* basal cell carcinoma may be mistaken for chronic blepharitis and can silently extend along the eyelid margin.

Carneiro RC, de Macedo EM, Matayoshi S. Imiquimod 5% cream for the treatment of periocular basal cell carcinoma. *Ophthal Plast Reconstr Surg.* 2010;26(2):100–102.

Margo CE, Waltz K. Basal cell carcinoma of the eyelid and periocular skin. *Surv Ophthalmol.* 1993;38(2):169–192.

**Management** A biopsy is necessary to confirm any clinical suspicion of basal cell carcinoma (Fig 10-28). The most accurate diagnosis can be ensured if every incisional biopsy provides tissue that

- is representative of the clinically evident lesion
- is of adequate size for histologic processing
- is not excessively traumatized or crushed
- contains normal tissue at the margin to show the transitional area

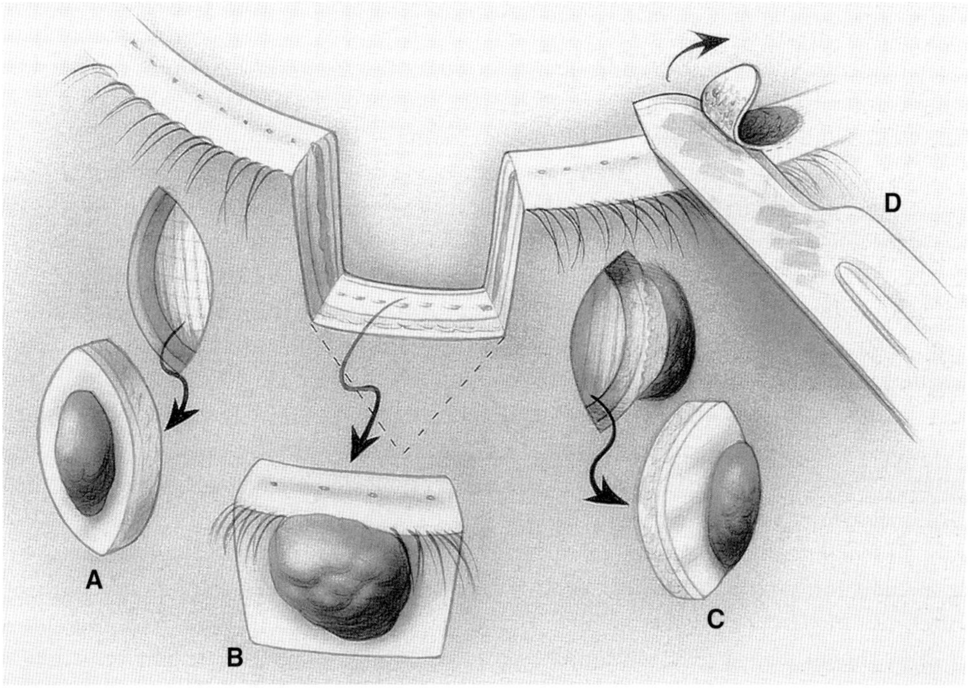


**Figure 10-28** Techniques of eyelid biopsy. **A,** Excisional biopsy. **B,** Full-thickness eyelid biopsy. **C,** Incisional or punch biopsy including normal skin. **D,** Shave biopsy of eyelid margin lesion. *(Illustration by Christine Gralapp.)*

An *incisional biopsy* can be used as a confirmatory office procedure for suspected malignant tumors. The site of the incisional biopsy should be photographed because the site may heal so well that the original location of the tumor becomes difficult to find for subsequent tumor removal.

An *excisional biopsy* is reasonable when eyelid lesions are small and do not involve the eyelid margin or when eyelid margin lesions are centrally located, away from the lateral canthus or lacrimal punctum. However, histologic monitoring of tumor borders to ensure complete excision is mandatory. The borders of any excisional biopsy should be marked in case the excision is incomplete and further resection is necessary. Excisional biopsies should be oriented vertically so that closure does not put vertical traction on the eyelid. If the margins of the excised portion of the eyelid are positive for residual tumor cells, the involved area of the eyelid should be reexcised, with surgical monitoring of the margins by Mohs micrographic technique or by frozen section technique.

Surgery is the treatment of choice for all basal cell carcinomas of the eyelid. Surgical excision affords the advantages of complete tumor removal with histologic control of the margins. The recurrence rate is lower with excision than with any other treatment modality. Surgical excision also offers superior cosmetic results in most cases.

When basal cell carcinomas involve the medial canthal area, the lacrimal drainage system may have to be removed in order to completely eradicate the tumor. If the lacrimal drainage system has been removed for tumor eradication, reconstruction of the lacrimal outflow system is not undertaken until it is established that the patient is tumor free.

Orbital invasion of basal cell carcinoma is particularly common in cases that have been inadequately treated, in clinically neglected tumors, or in morpheaform tumors. Orbital exenteration may be required in such cases. Retrospective studies show that the mortality rate from ocular adnexal basal cell carcinoma is 3%. The vast majority of patients who have died from basal cell carcinoma had disease that started in the canthal areas, had undergone prior radiation therapy, or had clinically neglected tumors.

Histologic examination of the margins of an excised malignant tumor should be performed to check for complete tumor excision. Frozen section techniques permit such examination during the course of surgery. The surgeon excises the clinically apparent tumor along with 1–2 mm margins, and then sends the entire specimen, oriented on a drawing, to the pathologist for frozen section evaluation.

Reconstruction is undertaken when all margins are found to be free of tumor. Some tumors have subcutaneous extensions that are not recognized preoperatively. Consequently, the surgeon must always be prepared to do a much larger reconstruction than originally anticipated from the clinical appearance of the tumor.

To facilitate complete removal of recurrent, deeply infiltrated, or morpheaform tumors and tumors in the medial canthal region, dermatologists with special training often use *Mohs micrographic surgery.* Tissue may be removed in thin layers that allow 3-dimensional mapping of the tumor excision. Mohs micrographic tumor resection is most commonly used in the excision of morpheaform basal cell carcinoma and squamous cell carcinoma.

Micrographic excision preserves the maximal amount of healthy tissue while providing the best assurance of complete cancer removal. Preoperative planning between the micrographic surgeon and oculoplastic surgeon allows for the most efficient patient care. In some cases, micrographic excision may allow the preservation of a globe, whereas conventional surgical techniques might indicate the need for exenteration. However, a limitation of Mohs micrographic surgery is in identifying margins of the tumor when the tumor has invaded orbital fat.

Following Mohs tumor resection, the eyelid should be reconstructed by the ophthalmologist. (Reconstruction techniques are reviewed later in this chapter.) Urgent reconstruction is not critical, but surgery should be performed expeditiously. Early surgery affords maximum protection for the globe and allows reconstruction to take place while the remaining eyelid margins are still fresh. If immediate reconstruction is not possible, the cornea should be protected by patching or temporarily suturing the remaining eyelid closed over the globe. If defects are small, spontaneous granulation may be a treatment alternative.

The recurrence rate following *cryotherapy* is higher than that following surgical therapy for well-circumscribed nodular lesions. When cryotherapy is used to treat more diffuse sclerosing lesions, the recurrence rate is unacceptably high. In addition, histologic margins cannot be evaluated with cryotherapy. Consequently, this treatment modality is avoided for canthal lesions, recurrent lesions, lesions greater than 1 cm in diameter, and morpheaform lesions. Furthermore, because cryotherapy may lead to depigmentation and tissue atrophy, it should not be used when final cosmesis is important. Accordingly, cryotherapy for eyelid basal cell carcinoma is generally reserved for patients who are poor surgical candidates.

*Radiation therapy* should also be considered only a palliative treatment that should generally be avoided for periorbital lesions. In particular, it should not be used for canthal lesions because of the risk of orbital recurrence. As with cryotherapy, histologic margins cannot be evaluated with radiation treatment. The recurrence rate following radiation treatment is higher than that following surgical treatment. Moreover, recurrence after radiation is more difficult to detect, occurs at a longer interval after initial treatment, and is more difficult to manage surgically because of the altered healing of previously irradiated tissues.

Complications of radiation therapy include cicatricial changes in the eyelids, lacrimal drainage scarring with obstruction, keratitis sicca, and radiation-induced malignancy. Radiation-induced injury to the globe may also occur if the globe is not shielded during treatment. See also BCSC Section 4, *Ophthalmic Pathology and Intraocular Tumors.*

Oral vismodegib may be a useful treatment for advanced orbital infiltrative basal cell carcinoma that is not amenable to surgical resection or radiation. Initial studies show that this drug is well tolerated and effective, although patients need to be carefully monitored for squamous cell carcinomas at uninvolved sites.

Gill HS, Moscato EE, Chang AL, Soon S, Silkiss RZ. Vismodegib for periocular and orbital basal cell carcinoma. *JAMA Ophthal.* 2013;131(12)1591–1594.

Howard GR, Nerad JA, Carter KD, Whitaker DC. Clinical characteristics associated with orbital invasion of cutaneous basal cell and squamous cell tumors of the eyelid. *Am J Ophthalmol.* 1992;113(2):123–133.

Leshin B, Yeatts P, Ansher M, Montano G, Dutton JJ. Management of periocular basal cell carcinoma: Mohs' micrographic surgery versus radiotherapy. *Surv Ophthalmol.* 1993;38(2): 193–212.

Mohs FE. Micrographic surgery for the microscopically controlled excision of eyelid cancers. *Arch Ophthalmol.* 1986;104(6):901–909.

Waltz K, Margo CE. Mohs' micrographic surgery. *Ophthalmol Clin North Am.* 1991;4(1): 153–163.

### *Squamous cell carcinoma*

Squamous cell carcinoma of the eyelid is 40 times less common than basal cell carcinoma, but it is more aggressive (Fig 10-29). Tumors can arise spontaneously or from areas of solar injury and actinic keratosis, and they may be potentiated by immunodeficiency. The treatment modalities available for squamous cell carcinoma are similar to those for basal cell carcinoma. Mohs micrographic resection or surgical excision with wide margins and frozen sections is preferred because of the potentially lethal nature of this tumor. Squamous cell carcinoma may metastasize through lymphatic transmission, blood-borne transmission, or direct extension, often along nerves. Recurrences of squamous cell carcinoma should be treated with wide surgical resection, possibly including orbital exenteration or neck dissection, and may require collaboration with a head and neck cancer surgeon. Targeted therapy using hedgehog pathway and epidermal growth factor receptor (EGFR) inhibitors has shown promise in the treatment of orbital and periocular basal cell carcinoma and cutaneous squamous cell carcinoma in patients who are not candidates for surgery.

Reifler DM, Hornblass A. Squamous cell carcinoma of the eyelid. *Surv Ophthalmol.* 1986; 30(6):349–365.

Yin VT, Pfeiffer ML, Esmali B. Targeted therapy for orbital and periocular basal cell carcinoma and squamous cell carcinoma. *Ophthal Plast Reconstr Surg.* 2013;29(2):87–92.

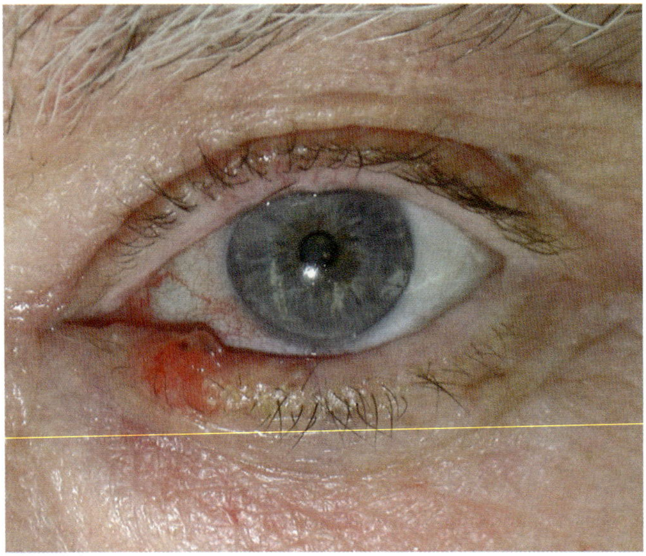

**Figure 10-29** Squamous cell carcinoma, left lower eyelid. *(Courtesy of Jill Foster, MD.)*

***Sebaceous adenocarcinoma***

Carcinoma of the sebaceous glands is a highly malignant and potentially lethal tumor that arises from the meibomian glands of the tarsal plate; from the glands of Zeis associated with the eyelashes; or from the sebaceous glands of the caruncle, eyebrow, or facial skin. Unlike basal cell or squamous cell carcinoma, sebaceous gland carcinoma occurs more frequently in females and originates twice as often in the upper than in the lower eyelid, reflecting the greater numbers of meibomian and Zeis glands in the upper eyelid. Multicentric origin is common, and separate upper and lower eyelid tumors occur in 6%–8% of patients. The tumor often appears yellow as a result of lipid material within the neoplastic cells. Patients are commonly older than 50 years, but these tumors have been reported in younger patients as well.

These tumors often masquerade as benign eyelid diseases. Clinically, they may simulate chalazia, chronic blepharitis, basal cell or squamous cell carcinoma, mucous membrane (ocular cicatricial) pemphigoid, superior limbic keratoconjunctivitis, or pannus associated with adult inclusion conjunctivitis. Typically, effacement of the meibomian gland orifices with destruction of follicles of the cilia occurs, leading to loss of eyelashes (Fig 10-30).

In sebaceous carcinoma, the tumor within the tarsal plate tends to progress to an intraepidermal growth phase, which may extend over the palpebral and bulbar conjunctiva. A fine papillary elevation of the tarsal conjunctiva may indicate pagetoid spread of tumor cells; intraepithelial growth may replace corneal epithelium as well. Marked conjunctival inflammation and hyperemia may be present.

A nodule that initially simulates a chalazion but later causes loss of eyelashes and destruction of the meibomian gland orifices warrants a biopsy, as this presentation is

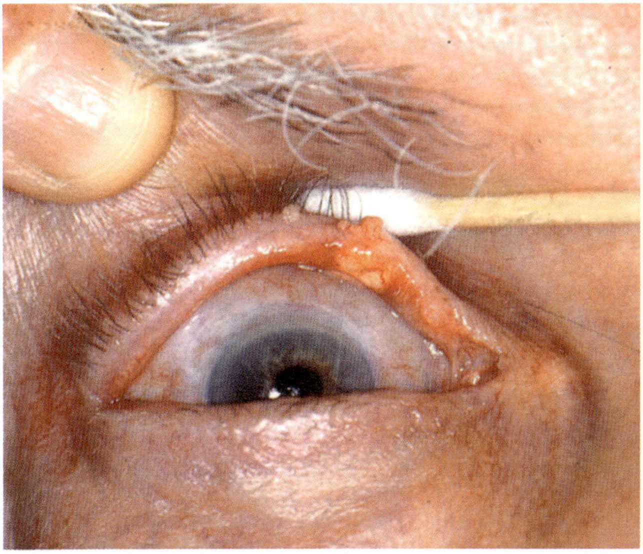

**Figure 10-30** Sebaceous gland carcinoma. *(Courtesy of John B. Holds, MD.)*

characteristic of sebaceous gland carcinoma. Solid material from a chalazion that has been surgically excised more than once should be submitted for histologic examination. Because the rate of histologic misdiagnosis is high among general pathologists, the clinician should maintain suspicion based on clinical findings and request special stains (lipid) or outside consultation. Any chronic unilateral blepharitis could also raise the possibility of sebaceous gland carcinoma.

Because eyelid margin sebaceous carcinomas originate in the tarsal plate or the eyelash margin, superficial shave biopsies may reveal chronic inflammation but miss the underlying tumor. A full-thickness eyelid biopsy with permanent sections may be necessary to obtain the correct diagnosis. Alternatively, full-thickness punch biopsy of the tarsal plate may be diagnostic.

Wide surgical excision is mandatory for adequate treatment of sebaceous adenocarcinoma. Mohs micrographic surgery has been used in some cases; however, considerable caution is required because of the skip areas, pagetoid spread, and polycentricity characteristic of these tumors. Map biopsies of the conjunctiva are helpful to eliminate the potential of pagetoid spread. If pagetoid spread is present, adjunctive cryotherapy may be used. Orbital exenteration (see Chapter 8) may be considered for recurrent or large tumors invading through the orbital septum. These tumors usually metastasize to regional lymph nodes but may rarely spread hematogenously or through direct extension. Radiation therapy is usually not appropriate, as sebaceous carcinomas are relatively radioresistant.

Sentinel lymph node (SLN) biopsy is considered for patients with eyelid sebaceous cell carcinoma with high-risk features (recurrent lesions or extensive involvement of the eyelid or orbit), conjunctival or cutaneous melanoma with a Breslow thickness greater than 1 mm, or Merkel cell carcinoma of the eyelid. With the exception of basal cell carcinoma, cancers of the eyelid and conjunctiva typically metastasize to the regional lymph nodes, and regional metastasis commonly occurs before metastasis to distant sites. The identification of microscopic regional nodal metastases may indicate that more extensive therapy is warranted. It can also provide prognostic information to the physician and the patient.

Ho VH, Ross MI, Prieto VG, Khaleeq A, Kim S, Esmaeli B. Sentinel lymph node biopsy for sebaceous cell carcinoma and melanoma of the ocular adnexa. *Arch Otolaryngol Head Neck Surg.* 2007;133(8):820–826.

Khan JA, Doane JF, Grove AS Jr. Sebaceous and meibomian carcinomas of the eyelid: recognition, diagnosis, and management. *Ophthal Plast Reconstr Surg.* 1991;7(1):61–66.

Nijhawan N, Ross MI, Diba R, Ahmadi MA, Esmaeli B. Experience with sentinel lymph node biopsy for eyelid and conjunctival malignancies at a cancer center. *Ophthal Plast Reconstr Surg.* 2004;20(4):291–295.

Shields JA, Demirci H, Marr BP, Eagle RC Jr, Shields CL. Sebaceous carcinoma of the eyelids: personal experience with 60 cases. *Ophthalmology.* 2004;111(12):2151–2157.

### *Melanoma*

Melanoma accounts for approximately 5% of cutaneous cancers, but about 75% of skin cancer deaths are due to melanoma. The incidence of melanoma in the United States has been steadily increasing over the past 30 years. Multiple factors, including sunlight exposure, genetic predisposition, and environmental mutagens, have been implicated in this increase. Cutaneous melanomas may develop de novo or from preexisting melanocytic nevi or lentigo maligna. Primary cutaneous melanoma of the eyelid skin is rare (<0.1% of eyelid malignancies). Melanomas should be suspected in any patient with an acquired pigmented lesion beyond the first 2 decades of life. Melanomas typically have variable pigmentation and irregular borders, and they may ulcerate and bleed.

There are 4 clinicopathologic forms of cutaneous melanoma: (1) lentigo maligna melanoma, (2) nodular melanoma, (3) superficial spreading melanoma, and (4) acrolentiginous melanoma. The eyelid is most often involved by either lentigo maligna melanoma or nodular melanoma.

*Lentigo maligna melanoma* represents the invasive vertical malignant growth phase that occurs in 10%–20% of patients with a lentigo maligna. It accounts for 90% of head and neck melanomas. Clinically, the invasive areas are marked by nodule formation within the broader, flat, tan to brown irregular macule. The eyelid is usually involved by secondary extension from the malar region, and pigmentation may progress over the eyelid margin and onto the conjunctival surface. Surgical excision is recommended for a premalignant lentigo maligna and is mandatory in patients with lentigo maligna melanoma.

*Nodular melanoma* accounts for approximately 10% of cutaneous melanomas but is extremely rare on the eyelids (Fig 10-31). These tumors may be amelanotic. The vertical invasive growth phase is the initial presentation of these lesions; thus, they are likely to have extended deeply by the time of diagnosis.

Treatment of cutaneous melanoma includes wide surgical excision with histologic assurance (by means of permanent sections) of complete tumor removal. Randomized trials have so far provided insufficient information to address optimal excision margins for primary cutaneous melanoma. In the periocular regions, margins less than 1 cm are often used to help preserve tissue needed for reconstruction and protection of the eye. Regional lymph node dissection or SLN biopsy may be performed in patients with melanomas that show microscopic evidence of vascular or lymphatic involvement or Breslow thickness greater than 1 mm. Complete preoperative metastatic workup is indicated for

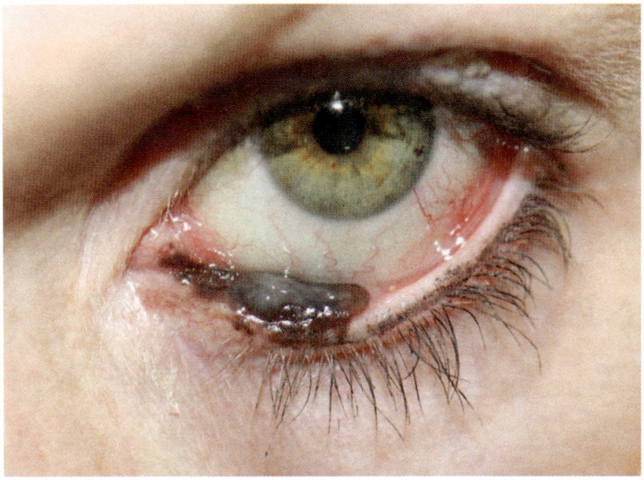

**Figure 10-31** Lower eyelid melanoma spreading to the conjunctiva and caruncle. *(Courtesy of Jill Foster, MD.)*

tumors with thickness greater than 1.5 mm. Thin lesions (<0.75 mm) confer a 5-year survival rate of 98%; thicker lesions (>4 mm) with ulceration confer a survival rate of less than 50%. Because tumor thickness has strong prognostic implications, a biopsy should be performed on these lesions—specifically, a biopsy with a disposable punch that allows a core to be taken through the full depth of the tumor. Biopsy of these lesions does not increase the risk of metastatic spread. Although cryotherapy may have a role in the treatment of acquired melanomas in the conjunctiva, it should not be considered for treatment of cutaneous melanoma.

Boulos PR, Rubin PA. Cutaneous melanomas of the eyelid. *Semin Ophthalmol.* 2006;21(3): 195–206.

Demirci H, Johnson T, Frueh BR, Musch DC, Fullen D, Nelson CC. Management of periocular cutaneous melanoma with a staged excision technique and permanent sections: the square procedure. *Ophthalmology.* 2008;115(12):2295–2300.

Linos E, Swetter S, Cockburn MG, Colditz GA, Clarke CA. Increasing burden of melanoma in the United States. *J Invest Dermatol.* 2009;129(7):1666–1674.

Sladden MJ, Balch C, Barzilai DA, et al. Surgical excision margins for primary cutaneous melanoma. *Cochrane Database Syst Rev.* 2009;4:CD004835.

Sober AJ, Chuang TY, Duvic M, et al; Guidelines/Outcome Committee. Guidelines of care for primary cutaneous melanoma. *J Am Acad Dermatol.* 2001;45(4):579–586.

### *Kaposi sarcoma*

This previously rare tumor presents as a chronic reddish dermal mass and is a frequent manifestation of AIDS (Fig 10-32). The conjunctival lesions can be mistaken for foreign-body granuloma or cavernous hemangioma. The lesion is composed of spindle cells of probable endothelial origin. It may be treated with cryotherapy, excision, radiation, or intralesional chemotherapeutic agents. Kaposi sarcoma may regress with adequate antiviral treatment of the HIV infection.

Shuler JD, Holland GN, Miles SA, Miller BJ, Grossman I. Kaposi sarcoma of the conjunctiva and eyelids associated with the acquired immunodeficiency syndrome. *Arch Ophthalmol.* 1989;107(6):858–862.

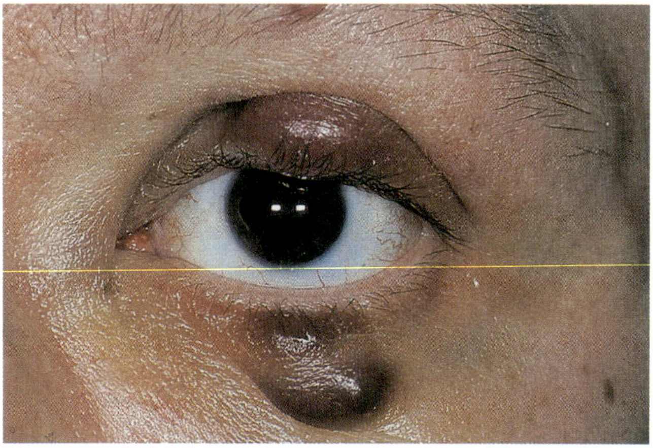

**Figure 10-32** Kaposi sarcoma.

#### *Merkel cell carcinoma*

The Merkel cell is part of the dendritic (neuroendocrine) cell population of the skin. Studies suggest that it has a role in mediating the sense of touch. Merkel cells can give rise to malignant neoplasms, 10% of which occur in the eyelid and periocular area and manifest as painless, erythematous nodules with overlying telangiectatic blood vessels. Merkel cell carcinoma can mimic other malignant lesions; thus, the diagnosis can be difficult. One-third of the tumors recur after excision, and there is a high rate of metastasis. The estimated 5-year survival rate is 50%. Initial treatment should be aggressive and include wide surgical resection, with consideration of postoperative radiation and/or chemotherapy.

Herbert HM, Sun MT, Selva D, et al. Merkel cell carcinoma of the eyelid: management and prognosis. *JAMA Ophthalmol.* 2014;132(2):197–204.

Peters GB 3rd, Meyer DR, Shields JA, et al. Management and prognosis of Merkel cell carcinoma of the eyelid. *Ophthalmology.* 2001;108(9):1575–1579.

## Eyelid Trauma

Injuries of the eyelid may be divided into 2 categories: blunt trauma and penetrating trauma. Cardinal rules in the management of eyelid trauma include the following:

- Take a careful history.
- Record the best visual acuity for each eye.
- Thoroughly evaluate the globe and orbit.
- Obtain appropriate radiologic studies.
- Have a detailed knowledge of eyelid and orbital anatomy.
- Ensure the best possible primary repair.

### Blunt Trauma

Ecchymosis and edema are the most common presenting signs of blunt trauma. Patients should be evaluated for intraocular injury with a thorough biomicroscopic evaluation and a dilated fundus examination. Computed tomography may be necessary to determine whether an orbital fracture is present. See Chapter 6 for further discussion of orbital fractures.

### Penetrating Trauma

Detailed knowledge of eyelid anatomy helps the surgeon in repairing a penetrating eyelid injury and often reduces the need for secondary repairs. Generally, the treatment of eyelid lacerations depends on the depth and location of the injury.

#### *Lacerations not involving the eyelid margin*

Superficial eyelid lacerations involving just the skin and orbicularis oculi muscle usually require only skin sutures. Unnecessary scarring can be avoided by following the basic principles of plastic repair. These include conservative debridement of the wound, use of small-caliber sutures, eversion of the wound edges, and early suture removal.

The presence of orbital fat in the wound means that the orbital septum has been violated. Superficial or deep foreign bodies should be searched for meticulously, in addition to copious irrigation, before these deeper eyelid lacerations are repaired. Orbital fat prolapse in an upper eyelid wound is an indication for exploration of the levator muscle and aponeurosis. A lacerated levator muscle or aponeurosis must be carefully repaired to enable the levator muscle to function as normally as possible. Upper eyelid lagophthalmos and tethering to the superior orbital rim are common if the orbital septum is inadvertently incorporated into the laceration repair. Orbital septum lacerations should not be sutured. Meticulous closure of overlying eyelid skin and orbicularis muscle is adequate in all cases and minimizes the risk of vertical shortening of the sutured orbital septum.

### *Lacerations involving the eyelid margin*

Repair of eyelid margin lacerations requires precise suture placement and critical suture tension to minimize notching of the eyelid margin. It is important that tarsal approximation be made in a meticulous, direct manner (Fig 10-33) and that the eyelid margin be

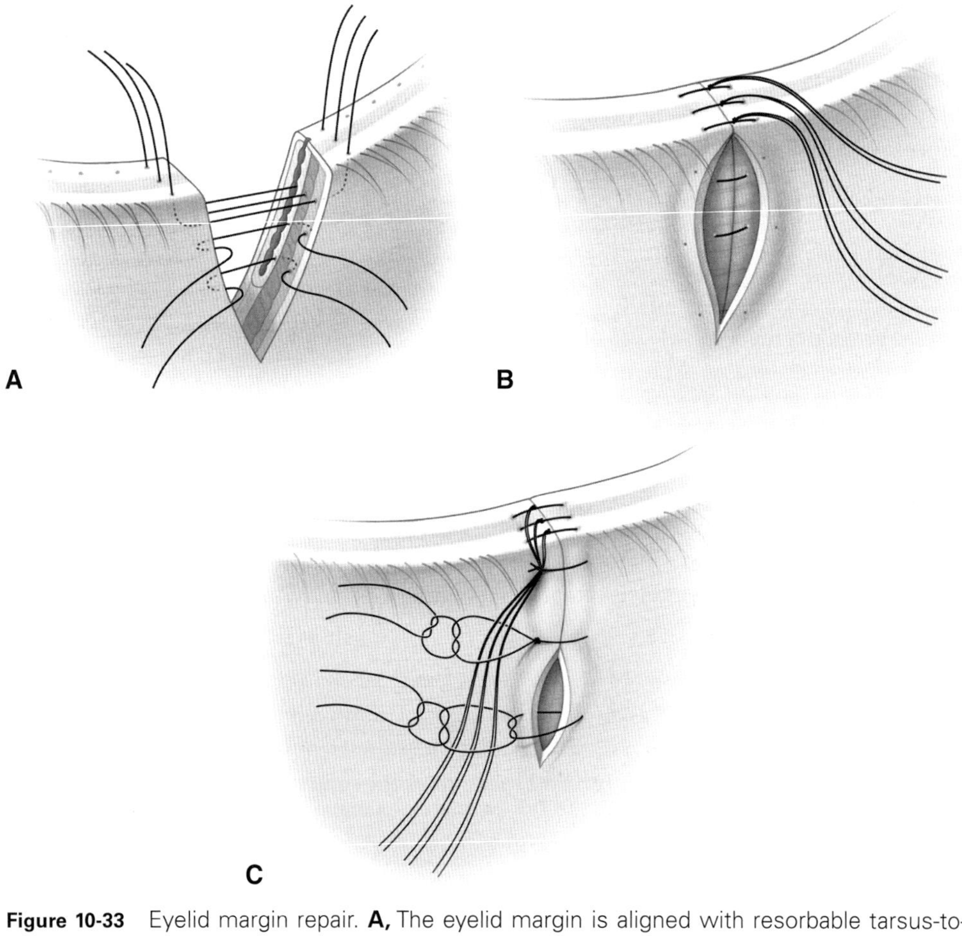


**Figure 10-33** Eyelid margin repair. **A,** The eyelid margin is aligned with resorbable tarsus-to-tarsus sutures, and the lash line, gray line, and mucocutaneous junction are aligned with eyelid margin sutures. **B,** The tarsal sutures are tied and cut; the eyelid margin sutures are tied and left long. **C,** The skin surface of the eyelid is sewn closed, with the skin sutures used to tie down the tails of the margin sutures. *(Illustration by Christine Gralapp.)*

precisely anatomically aligned. Eyelid margin closure may be accomplished by placing 2 or 3 sutures for alignment through the lash line, the meibomian gland plane, and (optionally) the gray line. Surgeons differ as to whether they place the tarsal or the eyelid margin sutures first, and many variations of the suturing technique are acceptable. To prevent corneal epithelial disruption, the tarsal sutures should not extend through the conjunctival surface. The eyelid margin closure should result in a moderate eversion of the well-approximated wound edges. Resorbable buried sutures may be used in the margin as an alternative to permanent externally tied sutures.

#### *Trauma involving the canthal soft tissue*

Trauma to the medial or lateral canthal areas is usually the result of horizontal traction on the eyelid, which causes avulsion of the eyelid at its weakest points, the medial or lateral canthal tendon. Careful review of the patient's history often confirms that an object or finger engaged the eyelid soft tissue in the central aspect of the eyelid, with subsequent horizontal traction of the eyelid. Thus, lacerations in the medial canthal area demand evaluation of the lacrimal drainage apparatus. Canalicular involvement is usually confirmed by inspection and gentle probing. The examiner can assess the integrity of the inferior and superior limbs of the medial or lateral canthal tendon by grasping each eyelid with toothed forceps and tugging away from the injury while palpating the insertion of the tendon.

Medial canthal tendon avulsion should be suspected when there is rounding of the medial canthal angle and acquired telecanthus. Attention to the posterior portion of the tendon's attachment to the posterior lacrimal crest is critical.

Treatment of medial canthal tendon avulsions depends on the nature of the avulsion. If the upper or lower limb is avulsed but the posterior attachment of the tendon is intact, the avulsed limb may be sutured to its stump or to the periosteum overlying the anterior lacrimal crest. If the entire tendon, including the posterior portion, is avulsed but there is no naso-orbital fracture, the avulsed tendon may be wired through small drill holes in the ipsilateral posterior lacrimal crest. If the entire tendon is avulsed and there is a naso-orbital fracture, transnasal wiring or plating is necessary after reduction of the fracture. A Y-shaped miniplate may be fixed anteriorly on the nasal bone, with posterior extension into the orbit. The suture is sewn through the severed tendons and passed through the holes in the miniplate. This technique is particularly helpful when the bone of the posterior lacrimal crest is missing.

Devoto MH, Kersten RC, Teske SA, Kulwin DR. Simplified technique for eyelid margin repair. *Arch Ophthalmol.* 1997;115(4):566–567.

Goldenberg DC, Bastos EO, Alonso N, Friedhofer J, Ferreira MC. The role of micro-anchor devices in medial canthopexy. *Ann Plast Surg.* 2008;61(1):47–51.

Howard GR, Nerad JA, Kersten RC. Medial canthoplasty with microplate fixation. *Arch Ophthalmol.* 1992;110(12):1793–1797.

### Secondary Repair

Secondary repair of eyelid trauma usually requires treatment of cicatricial changes that resulted from either the initial trauma or the subsequent surgical repair. Revision of scars may require simple excision with primary closure or a more complex rearrangement of tissue. The location of a particular scar in relation to the relaxed skin tension lines determines the best technique or combination of techniques to use. An elliptical excision of the scar is most useful for revision of scars that follow the relaxed skin tension lines. Single Z-plasty or multiple Z-plasty reconstructive techniques can be used for the revision of scars that do not conform to relaxed skin tension lines.

Free skin grafts alone or in combination with various flaps are used when tissue has been lost. Although any non–hair-bearing skin can be used, full-thickness postauricular or preauricular skin is the most common donor site for eyelid reconstruction. Ipsilateral or contralateral upper eyelid, supraclavicular or subclavicular areas, and even brachial or inner thigh areas are all potential donor sites.

Tarsoconjunctival grafts are good substitutes for posterior lamella eyelid defects when both the tarsal plate and the conjunctiva are deficient. Buccal mucosa may be used when only the conjunctiva is missing. Hard palate composite grafts have also become increasingly popular for posterior lamella defects in the lower eyelid. However, they should be avoided as a tarsal replacement in the upper eyelid because of the presence of keratinized epithelium, which can irritate the cornea.

Before treatment is considered for traumatic ptosis, the patient should be observed for 6 months to allow for spontaneous return of function. An exception to this rule may be in a young child, in whom the possibility of deprivation amblyopia may necessitate early surgery to clear the visual axis.

### Dog and Human Bites

Tearing and crushing injuries occur secondary to dog or human bites. Partial-thickness and full-thickness eyelid lacerations, canthal avulsions, and canalicular lacerations are common. Irrigation and early wound repair are mandatory, and tetanus and rabies protocols should be observed. Systemic antibiotics are recommended.

Bartley GB. Periorbital animal bites. *Focal Points: Clinical Modules for Ophthalmologists.* San Francisco: American Academy of Ophthalmology; 1992, module 3.

### Burns

Burns of the eyelid are rare and generally are seen in patients who have sustained significant burns over large areas of the body. Often, these patients are semiconscious or heavily sedated and require ocular surface protection to prevent corneal exposure, ulceration, and infection. Lubricating antibiotic eyedrops and ointments, moisture chambers, and frequent evaluation of both the globes and the eyelids are part of the early treatment of these patients. Once cicatricial changes begin in the eyelids, relentless and rapid deterioration of the patient's ocular status often ensues secondary to cicatricial eyelid retraction, lagophthalmos, and corneal exposure. If tarsorrhaphies are used, they should always be more extensive than seems to be immediately necessary. Unfortunately, with progression of the cicatricial traction, even the most aggressive eyelid adhesions may dehisce. In the past, skin grafting was usually delayed until the cicatricial changes stabilized, but the early use of full-thickness skin grafts, amniotic membrane, and various types of flaps can effectively reduce ocular morbidity in selected patients.

## Eyelid and Canthal Reconstruction

The following discussion of eyelid reconstruction applies to defects resulting from tumor resection as well as congenital and traumatic defects. Several methods may be appropriate for reconstruction of a particular eyelid defect. The surgeon's choice of procedure depends on the age of the patient, the condition of the eyelids, the size and position of the defect, and personal experience and preference. Priorities in eyelid reconstruction are

- development of a stable eyelid margin
- provision of adequate vertical eyelid height
- adequate eyelid closure
- smooth, epithelialized internal surface
- maximum cosmesis and symmetry

The following general principles guide the practice of eyelid reconstruction:

- One may reconstruct either the anterior or the posterior eyelid lamella, but not both, with a graft; 1 of the layers must provide the blood supply *(pedicle flap).*
- Maximize horizontal tension and minimize vertical tension.
- Maintain sufficient and anatomical canthal fixation.
- Match like tissue to like tissue.
- Narrow the defect as much as possible before sizing a graft.
- Get help from a subspecialist if you need it.

### Eyelid Defects Not Involving the Eyelid Margin

Defects not involving the eyelid margins can be repaired by direct closure if this procedure does not distort the eyelid margin. If undermining does not allow direct closure, advancement or transposition of flaps of skin may be used. Tension of closure should be directed horizontally because vertical tension may cause eyelid retraction or ectropion. Avoidance of vertical tension requires placement of vertically oriented incision lines.

If the defect is too large to be closed primarily, several advancement or transposition techniques of local skin flaps may be used. The flaps most commonly used are rectangular advancement, rotation, and transposition. Flaps usually provide the best tissue match and aesthetic result but require planning in order to minimize secondary deformities. Although skin-grafting procedures are generally easier to perform, the final texture, contour, and cosmesis are typically better with flaps.

Anterior lamella upper eyelid defects are best repaired with full-thickness skin grafts from the contralateral upper eyelid. Preauricular or postauricular skin grafts may be used, but their greater thickness may limit upper eyelid mobility. Lower eyelid defects are best filled with preauricular or postauricular skin grafts. If skin is not available from the upper eyelids or auricular areas, full-thickness grafts may be obtained from the supraclavicular fossa or the inner upper arm. It is important to avoid placement of hair-bearing skin grafts near the eyes.

Use of split-thickness grafts should be avoided in eyelid reconstruction. They are recommended only in the treatment of severe burns of the face when adequate full-thickness skin is not available.

Patrinely JR, Marines HM, Anderson RL. Skin flaps in periorbital reconstruction. *Surv Ophthalmol.* 1987;31(4):249–261.

Teske SA, Kersten RC, Devoto MH, Kulwin DR. The modified rhomboid transposition flap in periocular reconstruction. *Ophthal Plast Reconstr Surg.* 1998;14(5):360–366.

## Eyelid Defects Involving the Eyelid Margin

### *Small upper eyelid defects*

Small defects involving the upper eyelid margin can be repaired by primary closure if this technique does not place too much tension on the wound (Fig 10-34). Primary closure is usually employed when one-third or less of the eyelid margin is involved; if a larger area is involved, advancement of adjacent tissue or grafting of distant tissue may be required. The surgeon can cut the superior limb of the lateral canthal tendon to allow 3–5 mm of medial mobilization of the remaining lateral eyelid margin, taking care to avoid the lacrimal ductules in the lateral third of the upper eyelid. Removal or destruction of these ductules may lead to dry eye problems. Postoperatively, the eyelid appears tight and ptotic because of traction, but it relaxes over several weeks.

### *Moderate upper eyelid defects*

Moderate defects of the upper eyelid margin (33%–50% involvement) can be repaired by advancement of the lateral segment of the eyelid. The lateral canthal tendon is incised, and a semicircular skin flap is made below the lateral portion of the eyebrow and canthus to allow for further mobilization of the eyelid. Tarsal-sharing procedures involving the lower eyelid may also be employed.

### *Large upper eyelid defects*

Upper eyelid defects involving more than half of the upper eyelid margin are likely to require advancement of adjacent tissues. With an incision below the lower eyelid tarsus, a full-thickness lower eyelid flap is moved into the defect of the upper eyelid by advancement of the flap behind the remaining lower eyelid margin *(Cutler-Beard procedure).* This procedure, however, results in a thick and relatively immobile upper eyelid. Alternatively, a free tarsoconjunctival graft taken from the contralateral upper eyelid can be positioned and covered with a skin–muscle flap if adequate redundant upper eyelid skin is present.

### *Small lower eyelid defects*

Small defects (involvement of less than one-third) of the lower eyelid can be repaired by primary closure (Fig 10-35). In addition, the inferior crus of the lateral canthal tendon can be internally or externally released so that there is an additional 3–5 mm of medial mobilization of the remaining lateral eyelid margin.

### *Moderate lower eyelid defects*

Semicircular advancement or rotation flaps, which have been described for upper eyelid repair, can be used for reconstruction of moderate defects in the lower eyelid as well. The most commonly used flap in such cases is a modification of the Tenzel semicircular rotation flap. Tarsoconjunctival autografts harvested from the underside of the upper eyelid may be transplanted into the lower eyelid defect for reconstruction of the posterior

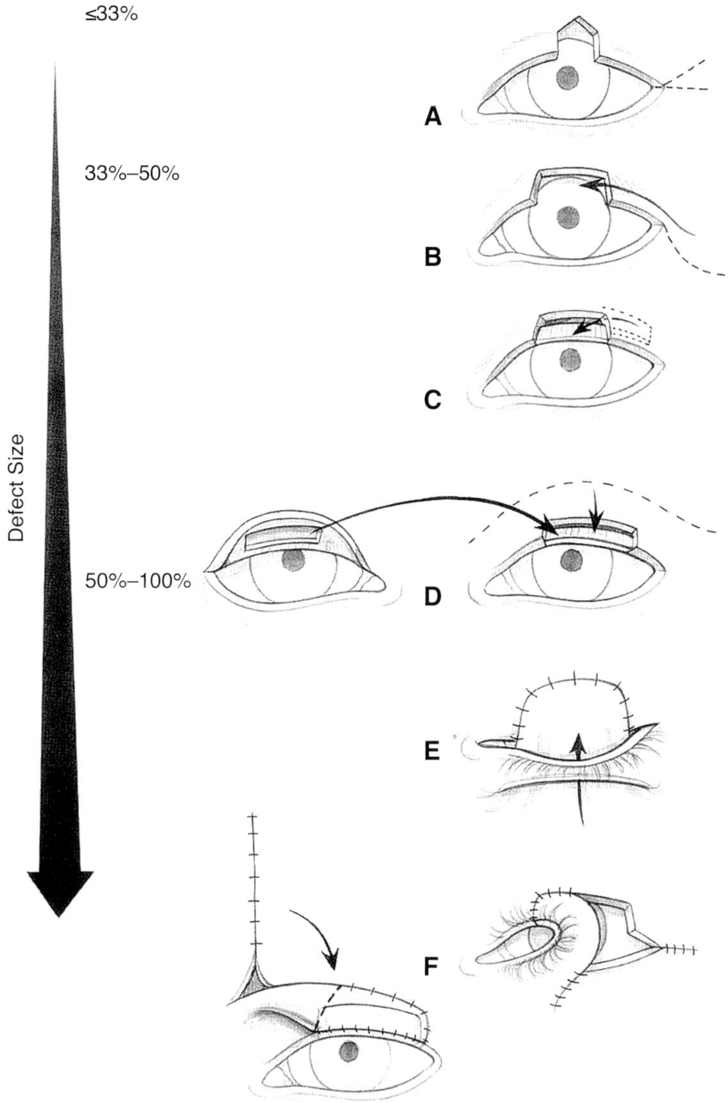


**Figure 10-34** Reconstructive ladder for upper eyelid defect. **A,** Primary closure with or without lateral canthotomy or superior cantholysis. **B,** Semicircular flap. **C,** Adjacent tarsoconjunctival flap and full-thickness skin graft. **D,** Free tarsoconjunctival graft and skin flap. **E,** Full-thickness lower eyelid advancement flap *(Cutler-Beard procedure).* **F,** Lower eyelid switch flap or median forehead flap. *(Illustration by Christine Gralapp.)*

lamella of the eyelid. When tarsal grafts are being harvested, the marginal 4–5 mm height of the tarsus is preserved to prevent distortion of the donor eyelid margin. Tarsoconjunctival autografts may be covered with skin flaps of various types. Cheek elevation may also be required so that vertical traction on the eyelid and ectropion can be avoided. Alternatively, a tarsoconjunctival flap developed from the upper eyelid and a full-thickness skin graft can also be used (discussed in the next subsection).

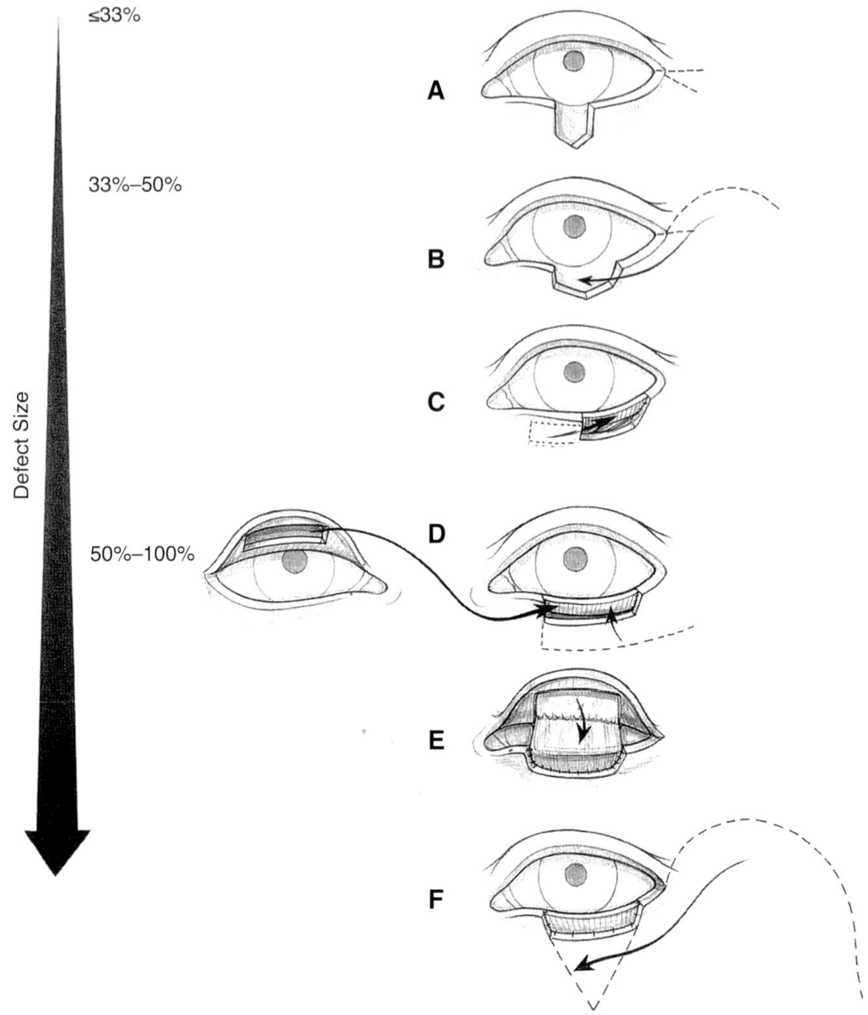


**Figure 10-35** Reconstructive ladder for lower eyelid defect. **A,** Primary closure with or without lateral canthotomy or superior cantholysis. **B,** Semicircular flap. **C,** Adjacent tarsoconjunctival flap and full-thickness skin graft. **D,** Free tarsoconjunctival graft and skin flap. **E,** Tarsoconjunctival flap from upper eyelid and skin graft *(modified Hughes procedure).* **F,** Composite graft with cheek advancement flap *(Mustardé flap). (Illustration by Christine Gralapp.)*

### *Large lower eyelid defects*

Defects involving more than half of the lower eyelid margin can be repaired by advancement of a tarsoconjunctival flap from the upper eyelid into the posterior lamellar defect of the lower eyelid. The anterior lamella of the reconstructed eyelid is then created with an advancement skin flap or, in most cases, a free skin graft taken from the preauricular or postauricular area *(modified Hughes procedure).* The modified Hughes procedure therefore results in placement of a bridge of conjunctiva from the upper eyelid across the pupil for several weeks. The vascularized pedicle of conjunctiva is then released in a staged, second procedure once the lower eyelid flap is revascularized. Eyelid-sharing techniques should be avoided in children, as these patients may develop deprivation amblyopia. Large rotating cheek flaps *(Mustardé procedure)* can work well for repair of large anterior lamellar defects, but they require some tarsal substitute such as a free tarsoconjunctival autograft, hard-palate mucosa, or a Hughes flap for posterior lamella replacement. Both the Mustardé cheek rotation flap and the Tenzel semicircular rotation flap frequently result in a rounded lateral canthus. The surgeon can mitigate this problem by creating a very high incision toward the lateral end of the eyebrow where the incision emanates from the lateral commissure. Free tarsoconjunctival autografts from the upper eyelid covered with a vascularized skin flap have been used to repair large defects as well. This type of procedure has the advantage of requiring only 1 surgical stage and prevents even temporary occlusion of the visual axis.

## Lateral Canthal Defects

Laterally based transposition flaps of upper eyelid tarsus and conjunctiva can be used for large lower eyelid defects extending to the lateral canthus. These flaps can be covered with free skin grafts. Semicircular advancement flaps of skin can also be used to repair defects extending to the lateral canthal area. Sometimes, strips of periosteum and/or deep temporal fascia left attached at the lateral orbital rim can be swung over and attached to the remaining lateral eyelid margins for reconstruction of the entire lateral canthal posterior lamella. A Y-shaped pedicle flap of periosteum is optimal for reconstruction of the entire lateral canthal posterior lamella.

## Medial Canthal Defects

The medial canthal area is amenable to various reconstructive methods. Spontaneous granulation of anterior lamellar defects has been used with varying success. Full-thickness skin grafting or flap reconstructions are more widely accepted repair techniques for medial canthal defects. When full-thickness medial eyelid defects are present, the medial canthal attachments of the remaining eyelid margin must be fixed to firm periosteum or bone. This fixation may be accomplished with heavy permanent suture, wire, or titanium miniplates. Defects involving the lacrimal drainage apparatus are more complex and require simultaneous microsurgical reconstruction and possible silicone intubation or marsupialization. If extensive sacrifice of the canaliculi has occurred in the resection of a tumor, the patient may have to tolerate epiphora until recurrence of the tumor is no longer a risk. Until tumor recurrence is ruled out, it is critical to avoid lacrimal surgery that could create a pathway for the tumor to spread into the nose or sinuses. After a recurrence-free period of 5 years (based on clinical judgment), the patient may undergo a conjunctivodacryocystorhinostomy with a Jones tube (see Chapter 13).

Full-thickness skin grafts offer an excellent way to reconstruct the medial canthus compared with the cicatrix resulting from spontaneous granulation. The full-thickness grafts are thin enough to allow for early detection of tumor recurrence. However, the clinician should make every effort at the time of tumor resection to minimize the risk of recurrent medial canthal tumors. Frozen sections and wide margins or Mohs micrographic resection techniques minimize the risk of recurrent medial canthal tumors and the risk of orbital or lacrimal extension of these tumors. Large medial canthal defects of anterior lamellar structures may be reconstructed through the transposition of forehead or glabellar flaps. However, such flaps have the disadvantage of being thick, thereby making early detection of recurrences difficult. In addition, they often require second-stage thinning in order to achieve the best cosmetic result. Mohs micrographic resection of tumors offers the highest cure rates for eradication of medial canthal epithelial malignancies.

Lowry JC, Bartley GB, Garrity JA. The role of second-intention healing in periocular reconstruction. *Ophthal Plast Reconstr Surg.* 1997;13(3):174–188.

Spinelli HM, Jelks GW. Periocular reconstruction: a systematic approach. *Plast Reconstr Surg.* 1993;91(6):1017–1024; discussion 1025–1026.

CHAPTER 11

# Periocular Malpositions and Involutional Changes

*This chapter includes related videos, which can be accessed by scanning the QR codes provided in the text or going to www.aao.org/bcscvideo_section07.*

## History and Examination

Whether young or old, presenting for medical (functional) or cosmetic concerns, patients with eyelid malpositions require careful evaluation. A history of the presenting concerns, as well as a general medical history, is essential. The presenting morphology must be compared with normal, and any deviations noted. The eye is evaluated, including visual acuity, ocular motility, corneal assessment (slit-lamp examination), and tests of tearing and protective mechanisms. Photographs documenting the preoperative state are taken, with specialized testing of visual function, visual field, and other parameters as appropriate. For a general discussion of the perioperative management of ocular surgery, see BCSC Section 1, *Update on General Medicine.*

## Ectropion

Ectropion (Fig 11-1) is an outward turning of the eyelid margin and may be classified as

- congenital
- involutional
- paralytic
- cicatricial
- mechanical

Most cases seen in a general ophthalmology practice are involutional, with horizontal eyelid laxity being the primary cause. Horizontal lower lid tightening is the common component in surgical repair of the various types of ectropion (see "Horizontal eyelid tightening" section). Congenital ectropion of the eyelid is rare and is discussed in Chapter 10 of this volume and in BCSC Section 6, *Pediatric Ophthalmology and Strabismus.*

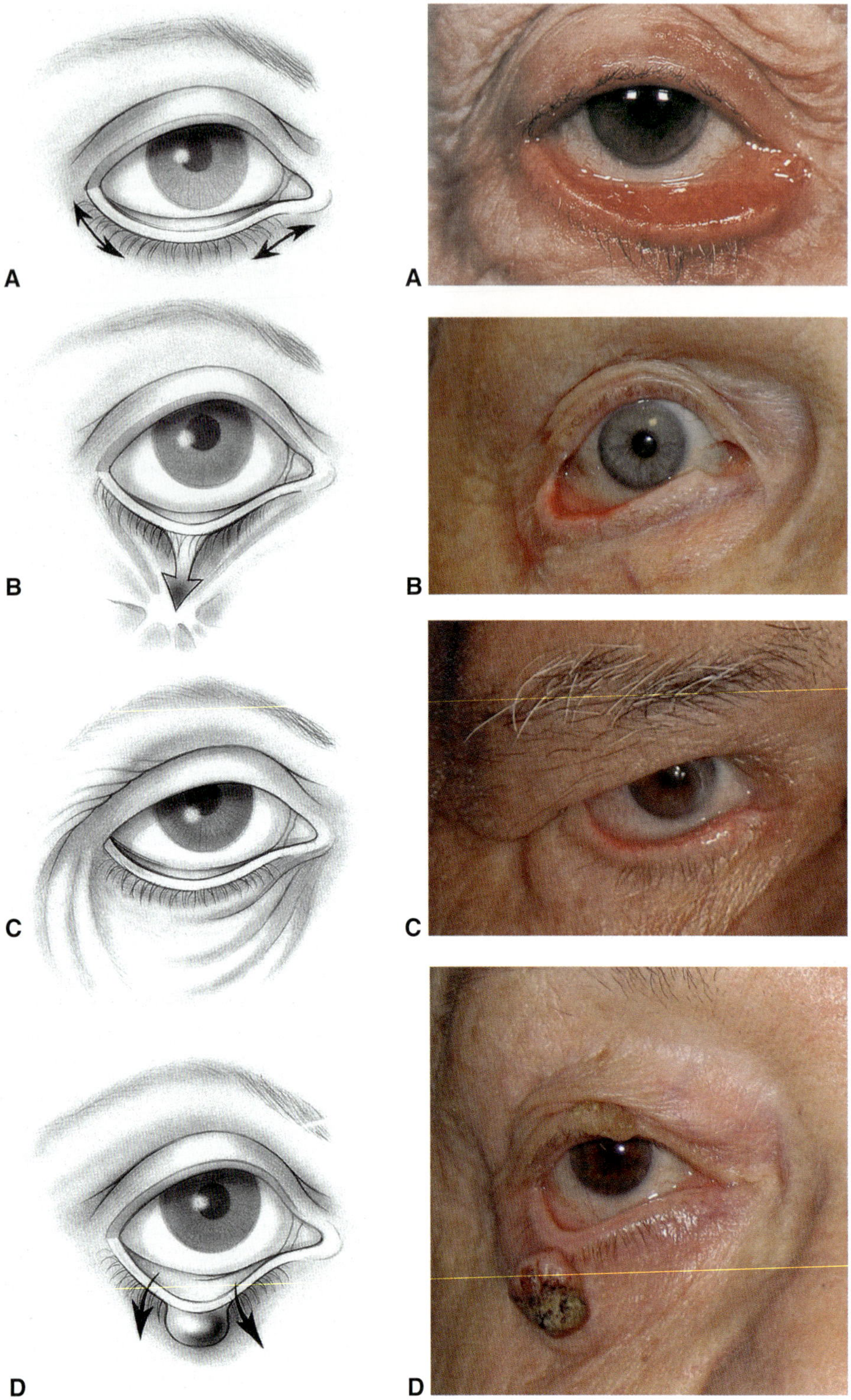

**Figure 11-1** Types of ectropion. **A,** Involutional. **B,** Cicatricial. **C,** Paralytic. **D,** Mechanical. *(Illustrations by Christine Gralapp. Photographs courtesy of James R. Patrinely, MD [part A]; Bobby S. Korn, MD, PhD [parts B, C]; Morris E. Hartstein, MD [part D].)*

## Involutional Ectropion

Involutional ectropion results from horizontal eyelid laxity in the medial or lateral canthal tendons or both. Untreated, this condition leads to loss of eyelid apposition to the globe with eversion of the eyelid margin. Chronic conjunctival inflammation with hypertrophy and keratinization results from mechanical irritation and drying of the conjunctival surface. Involutional ectropion usually occurs in the lower eyelid because of the effects of gravity on a horizontally lax lower eyelid.

### *Horizontal eyelid tightening*

The *lateral tarsal strip procedure* is the classic procedure for treatment of horizontal lower eyelid laxity. Horizontal laxity can be detected by poor orbicularis tone *(snapback test)* and by the ability to pull the eyelid more than 6 mm from the globe *(distraction test)*. Lateral stretching of the eyelid at the time of the preoperative evaluation helps the surgeon assess whether lateral canthal resuspension would return the eyelid to its normal anatomical position (Fig 11-2A). In this procedure, the lateral tarsus is sutured (and when appropriate, shortened) and reattached to the lateral orbital rim periosteum (Fig 11-2B). The goal of this procedure is to correct the position of the eyelid while maintaining the horizontal dimension of the palpebral fissure and a sharp, correctly positioned lateral canthal angle (Video 11-1).

**VIDEO 11-1** Lateral tarsal strip procedure (02:43).
*Courtesy of Bobby S. Korn, MD, PhD.*
Scan the QR code or access Section 7 videos at www.aao.org/bcscvideo_section07.

One alternative used for achieving horizontal eyelid tightening is a full-thickness excision of the eyelid just medial to the lateral canthal angle *(Bick procedure)*. Repair of the eyelid defect following full-thickness resection is similar to that described in Chapter 10 for a full-thickness eyelid margin laceration (see Fig 10-33). Inappropriate resection of the eyelid in this location may cause rounding and medial displacement of the lateral canthal angle.

Laxity of the lower limb of the medial canthal tendon can be diagnosed by demonstration of excessive lateral movement of the lower punctum with lateral eyelid traction. Repair of medial canthal laxity is more challenging than repair of horizontal lower eyelid laxity, as the anterior and posterior limbs of the medial canthal tendon surround the lacrimal sac. The repair may be complicated by a kinking of the canaliculus or distraction of the punctum away from the globe, with resultant epiphora.

### *Medial spindle procedure*

In cases of mild medial ectropion with punctal eversion, horizontal fusiform excision of conjunctiva and eyelid retractors 4 mm inferior to the puncta, with closure performed with inverting sutures (*medial spindle procedure*, Fig 11-2C), predictably corrects the punctal malposition. In cases with associated horizontal eyelid laxity, lateral canthal tightening (see Fig 11-2B) may be used in conjunction with this operation.

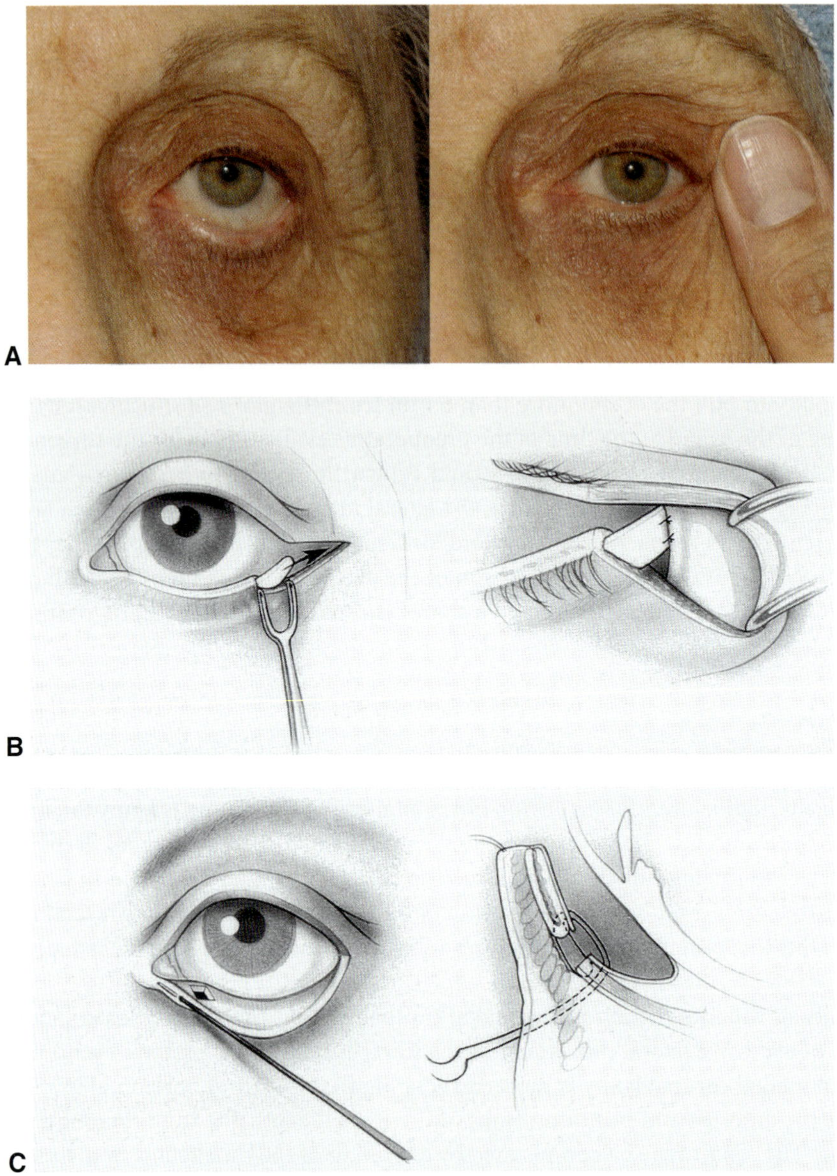

**Figure 11-2** **A,** Lateral stretching of the eyelid demonstrates the potential of lower lid tightening. **B,** Lateral tarsal strip procedure: anchoring of tarsal strip to periosteum inside the lateral orbital rim. **C,** Medial spindle procedure: outline of excision of conjunctiva and retractors. *(Part A courtesy of Bobby S. Korn, MD, PhD; illustrations by Christine Gralapp.)*

### *Repair of lower eyelid retractors*

Retractor laxity, disinsertion, or dehiscence may be associated with ectropion, especially when the eyelid is completely everted, a condition known as *tarsal ectropion.* Attenuation or disinsertion of the inferior retractors may occur as an isolated defect or may accompany horizontal laxity in involutional ectropion. When both defects are present, repair of the retractors is combined with horizontal tightening of the eyelid. Reattachment of the retractors is performed to advance the lower eyelid retractors to the inferior border of the tarsus.

Jordan DR, Anderson RL. The lateral tarsal strip revisited. The enhanced tarsal strip. *Arch Ophthalmol.* 1989;107(4):604–606.

Korn BS. Ectropion and entropion. *Focal Points: Clinical Modules for Ophthalmologists.* San Francisco: American Academy of Ophthalmology; 2014, module 2.

Nowinski TS, Anderson RL. The medial spindle procedure for involutional medial ectropion. *Arch Ophthalmol.* 1985;103(11):1750–1753.

Tse DT, Kronish JW, Buus D. Surgical correction of lower-eyelid tarsal ectropion by reinsertion of the retractors. *Arch Ophthalmol.* 1991;109(3):427–431.

## Paralytic Ectropion

See discussion under Facial Paralysis later in this chapter.

## Cicatricial Ectropion

Cicatricial ectropion of the upper or lower eyelid occurs when there is a deficiency of skin secondary to thermal or chemical burns, mechanical trauma, surgical trauma, or chronic actinic skin damage. Cicatricial ectropion can also be caused by chronic inflammation of the eyelid from dermatologic conditions such as rosacea, atopic dermatitis, or eczematoid dermatitis or by scarring from herpes zoster infections. Treatment of the underlying cause, along with conservative medical protection of the cornea, is essential as primary management. Cicatricial ectropion of the lower eyelid is usually treated in a 3-step procedure (Fig 11-3):

1. Vertical cicatricial traction is surgically released.
2. The eyelid is horizontally tightened with a lateral tarsal strip procedure.
3. The anterior lamella is vertically lengthened via a midface-lift or full-thickness skin graft. If a full-thickness skin graft is used, the eyelid may be placed on superior traction with a Frost suture.

Treatment of cicatricial ectropion or retraction of the upper eyelid usually requires only release of traction and augmentation of the vertically shortened anterior lamella with a full-thickness skin graft.

Although skin from the opposite upper eyelid is the ideal match for skin grafting, this source is usually inadequate except in patients with significant dermatochalasis. The postauricular, preauricular, supraclavicular, and medial upper arm areas are other potential donor sites.

## Mechanical Ectropion

Mechanical ectropion is usually caused by the effect of gravity or mass effect induced by bulky tumors of the eyelid. Fluid accumulation, herniated orbital fat, or poorly fitted spectacles may also be mechanical factors in lower eyelid ectropion.

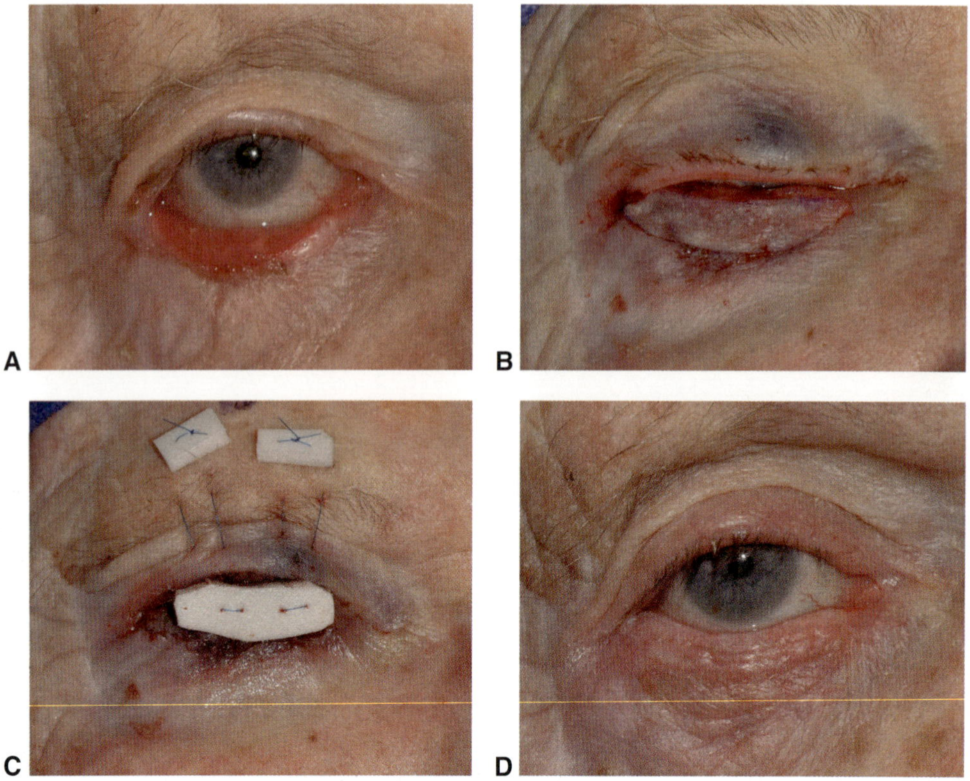

**Figure 11-3** **A,** Cicatricial ectropion. **B,** Release of vertical cicatricial traction and placement of full-thickness skin graft in association with lateral canthal resuspension. **C,** Immobilization of skin graft with Frost suture. **D,** Final appearance after skin graft placement and lateral tarsal strip. *(Courtesy of Bobby S. Korn, MD, PhD.)*

## Entropion

Entropion is an inversion of the eyelid margin. Lower eyelid entropion (usually involutional) is much more common than upper eyelid entropion (usually cicatricial). Entropion may be unilateral or bilateral and is often classified as follows:

- congenital
- involutional
- acute spastic
- cicatricial

### Congenital Entropion

Congenital entropion is discussed in Chapter 10.

### Involutional Entropion

Involutional entropion occurs in the lower eyelids (Fig 11-4). Causative factors include horizontal laxity of the eyelid, attenuation or disinsertion of eyelid retractors, and

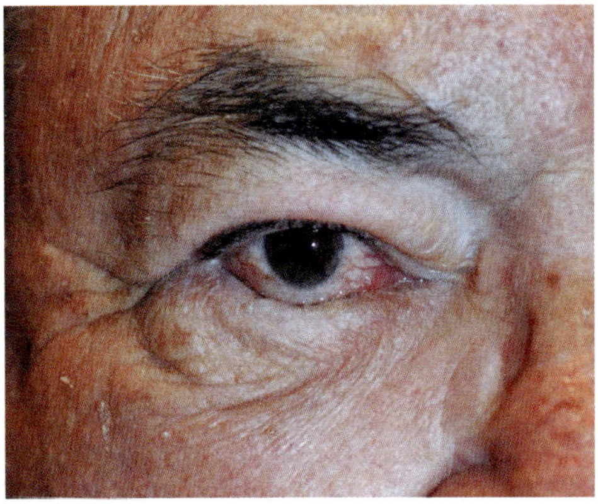

**Figure 11-4** Involutional entropion of the right lower eyelid. *(Courtesy of Bobby S. Korn, MD, PhD.)*

overriding by the preseptal orbicularis oculi muscle. Horizontal laxity can be assessed with snapback and distraction testing, as described above for involutional ectropion. Such laxity is a result of involutional stretching of the eyelid and canthal tendons. Normally, the lower eyelid retractors maintain the lower eyelid margin in proper orientation. However, attenuation of the eyelid retractors (capsulopalpebral fascia and inferior tarsal muscle), in conjunction with preseptal orbicularis override, allows the inferior border of the tarsus to ride forward and superiorly, with the eyelid margin rotating inward. Several clinical clues may be present to indicate disinsertion of the retractors:

- a white subconjunctival line several millimeters below the inferior tarsal border caused by the leading edge of the detached retractors
- a deeper-than-normal inferior fornix
- reverse ptosis of the lower eyelid (lower eyelid margin sits higher than normal)
- little or no inferior movement of the lower eyelid on downgaze (diminished lower eyelid excursion)

Superior override of the preseptal orbicularis is detected by observation of the preseptal orbicularis as the patient squeezes his or her eyes closed after the entropic eyelid has been placed in its normal position. This maneuver is thought to accentuate the inward rotation of the lower eyelid margin. Procedures to repair involutional entropion of the lower eyelid fall into 3 groups—temporizing measures, horizontal tightening procedures, and retractor repair—and are discussed in the following subsections. Often, a combination of procedures is necessary. Trichiasis (misdirected lashes) may require specific treatment, either in conjunction with the entropion repair or subsequently, if lashes remain misdirected after proper positioning of the eyelid margin (see Trichiasis section).

#### *Temporizing measures for acute intervention*

Lubrication and a bandage contact lens may be used to protect the cornea from mechanical abrasion by the misdirected eyelashes. Suture techniques (Quickert sutures; Fig 11-5) are occasionally helpful as temporizing measures in involutional entropion; but, when used as an isolated intervention, recurrence is anticipated. An example of the use of this suture technique would be spastic entropion that resolves once the source of irritation is treated.

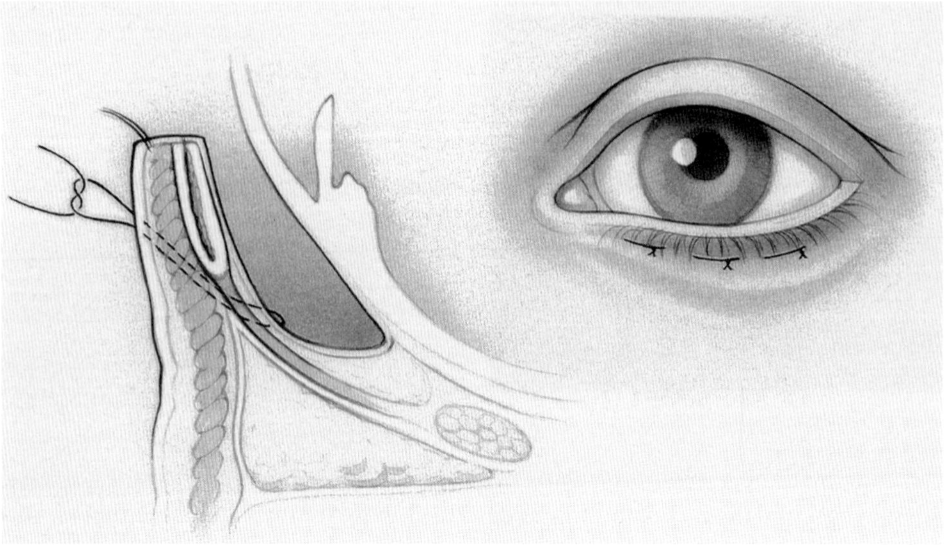

**Figure 11-5** Quickert suture repair of spastic entropion. *(Illustration by Christine Gralapp.)*

***Surgical techniques for repair of lower eyelid involutional entropion***

Direct exploration and repair of lower eyelid retractor defects through a skin incision (Fig 11-6A) or transconjunctival approach (Fig 11-6B) can be performed to stabilize the inferior border of the tarsus. In addition, a small amount of preseptal orbicularis oculi muscle can be removed in selected patients who have preseptal orbicularis overriding the pretarsal orbicularis. Reinsertion of the eyelid retractors and limited myectomy of the orbicularis in conjunction with a lower eyelid shortening procedure such as a lateral tarsal strip operation or wedge resection (see Fig 11-2B) correct all 3 etiologic factors in involutional entropion (Video 11-2).

**VIDEO 11-2** Transconjunctival lower eyelid entropion repair (05:24).
*Courtesy of Bobby S. Korn, MD, PhD.*

Barnes JA, Bunce C, Olver JM. Simple effective surgery for involutional entropion suitable for the general ophthalmologist. *Ophthalmology.* 2006;113(1):92–96.

Ben Simon GJ, Molina M, Schwarcz RM, McCann JD, Goldberg RA. External (subciliary) vs internal (transconjunctival) involutional entropion repair. *Am J Ophthalmol.* 2005;139(3): 482–487.

Erb MH, Uzcategui N, Dresner SC. Efficacy and complications of the transconjunctival entropion repair for lower eyelid involutional entropion. *Ophthalmology.* 2006;113(12): 2351–2356.

Michels KS, Czyz CN, Cahill KV, Foster JA, Burns JA, Everman KR. Age-matched, case-controlled comparison of clinical indicators for development of entropion and ectropion. *J Ophthalmol.* 2014;231487. Epub 2014 March 5.

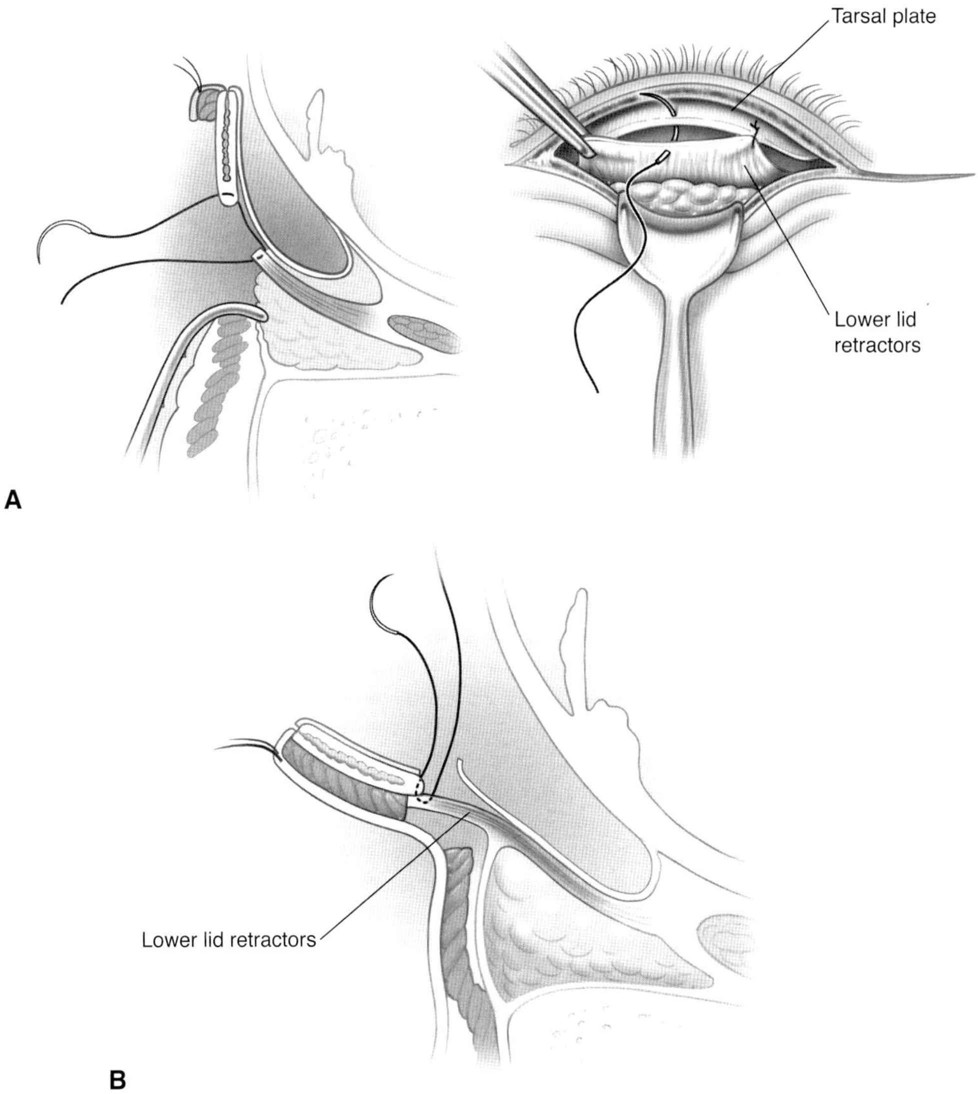


**Figure 11-6** Retractor repair of involutional entropion. **A,** Transcutaneous approach. **B,** Transconjunctival approach. *(Illustration by Christine Gralapp.)*

## Acute Spastic Entropion

This condition arises following ocular irritation or inflammation. It occurs most commonly after intraocular surgery in patients who had unrecognized or mild involutional eyelid changes preoperatively. Sustained orbicularis oculi muscle contraction causes inward rotation of the eyelid margin. A cycle of increasing frequency of orbicularis muscle spasm caused by corneal irritation perpetuates the problem. The acute entropion usually resolves when the irritation–entropion cycle is broken by treatment of the underlying cause.

Taping of the inturned eyelid to evert the margin, cautery, or various suture techniques afford temporary relief for most patients (eg, Quickert sutures; see Fig 11-5). In selected cases, botulinum toxin injection can be used to temporarily paralyze the overriding preseptal orbicularis muscle. However, because underlying involutional changes are often present in the eyelid, additional definitive surgical repair may be required for permanent correction of the entropion.

## Cicatricial Entropion

Cicatricial entropion is caused by vertical tarsoconjunctival contracture and internal rotation of the eyelid margin, with resulting irritation of the globe from inturned cilia or the keratinized eyelid margin (Fig 11-7). Various conditions may lead to cicatricial entropion, including *autoimmune* (mucous membrane [ocular cicatricial] pemphigoid), *inflammatory* (Stevens-Johnson syndrome), *infectious* (trachoma, herpes zoster), *surgical* (enucleation, posterior-approach ptosis correction, transconjunctival surgery), and *traumatic* (thermal or chemical burns, scarring) conditions. The long-term use of topical glaucoma medications, especially miotics, may cause chronic conjunctivitis with vertical conjunctival shortening and secondary cicatricial entropion.

The patient's history, along with a simple diagnostic test (digital eversion), usually distinguishes cicatricial entropion from involutional entropion. Attempting to return the eyelid to a normal anatomical position using digital traction will correct the abnormal margin position in involutional entropion but not in cicatricial entropion. In addition, inspection of the posterior lamella reveals subtle to severe scarring of the tarsal conjunctiva in cases of cicatricial entropion.

Effectiveness of treatment in cicatricial entropion depends primarily on the cause and severity. When the cause is autoimmune or inflammatory disease, the prognosis is guarded because of frequent disease progression; when the cause is prior surgery or trauma, the prognosis is generally good because the process tends to be localized and reversible. Infectious causes fall somewhere in between.

Successful management of cicatricial entropion depends on thoughtful preoperative evaluation to determine the cause, severity, and prominent features in each patient. Cicatricial

A 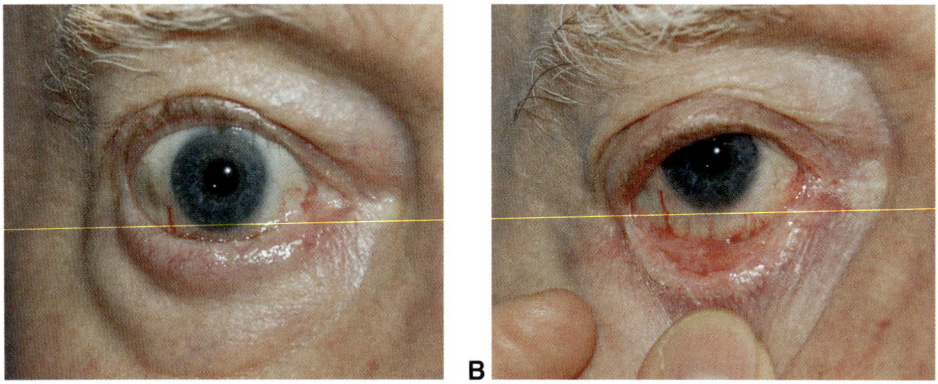 B

**Figure 11-7** **A,** Cicatricial entropion of the right lower eyelid. **B,** Eyelid everted showing conjunctival scarring and shortening of the fornix. *(Courtesy of Don O. Kikkawa, MD.)*

entropion usually requires surgery, but lubricating drops and ointments, barriers to symblepharon formation, and eyelash ablation with lash cautery or cryotherapy are sometimes useful adjuncts. Indeed, surgery is contraindicated during the acute phase of autoimmune diseases, and topical and systemic medications are more appropriate until the disease stabilizes.

The *tarsal fracture operation* is useful in cases of mild to moderate cicatricial entropion (marginal entropion) of the upper or lower eyelid (Fig 11-8). In this situation, lashes abrade the cornea, and careful examination shows that the eyelid margin has lost its square edges and is rotated posteriorly. A posterior horizontal tarsal incision is made 2 mm distal to the eyelid margin. This incision through the full thickness of the tarsus allows the eyelid margin to be rotated away from the globe in an everted position. The eyelid position is stabilized with everting sutures.

For margin rotation to be effective, the tarsus should be intact and of reasonably good quality. Because it is advisable not to violate the conjunctiva in patients with active autoimmune disease, medical management of the inflammatory condition with systemic and topical anti-inflammatory agents is desirable. When surgery is indicated, maximal inflammatory suppression is achieved with pulsed systemic anti-inflammatory medications (corticosteroids and immunosuppressive agents).

Because it is usually scarred and distorted in patients with severe cicatricial entropion, the involved tarsus generally needs to be replaced. In the upper eyelid, tarsoconjunctival and other mucosal grafts are useful tarsal substitutes; in the lower eyelid, autogenous ear cartilage, preserved scleral grafts, and hard-palate mucosa have been used.

Bleyen I, Dolman PJ. The Wies procedure for management of trichiasis or cicatricial entropion of either upper or lower eyelids. *Br J Ophthalmol.* 2009;93(12):1612–1615.

Heiligenhaus A, Shore JW, Rubin PA, Foster CS. Long-term results of mucous membrane grafting in ocular cicatricial pemphigoid: implications for patient selection and surgical considerations. *Ophthalmology.* 1993;100(9):1283–1288.

Kersten RC, Kleiner FP, Kulwin DR. Tarsotomy for the treatment of cicatricial entropion with trichiasis. *Arch Ophthalmol.* 1992;110(5):714–717.

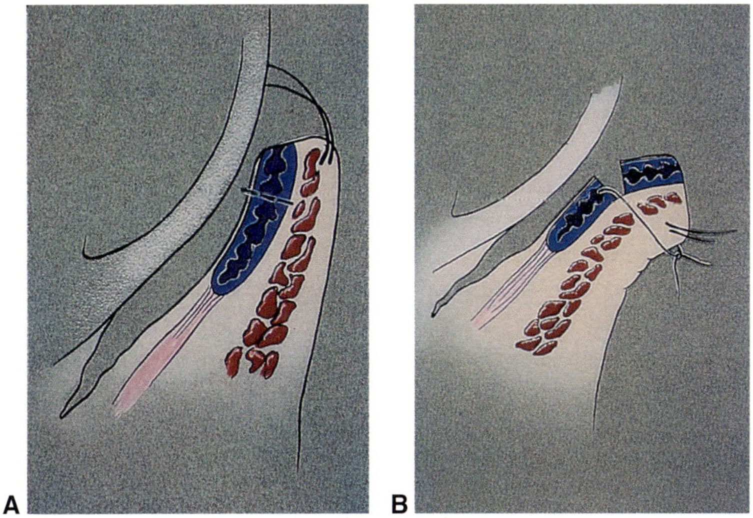


**Figure 11-8** Tarsal fracture operation. **A,** Tarsotomy. **B,** Margin rotation for cicatricial entropion.

## Symblepharon

Symblepharon is an adhesion between conjunctival surfaces. Symblepharon can occur as a result of inflammation, infection, trauma, or previous surgery. Conjunctival Z-plasties are sometimes effective for localized contracted linear adhesions when vertical lengthening of the involved tissue is the primary objective. More extensive symblepharon formation requires a full-thickness conjunctival graft or flap, a partial-thickness buccal mucous membrane graft, or amniotic membrane graft.

## Trichiasis

Trichiasis is an acquired misdirection of the eyelashes. The method used for treating trichiasis is usually dictated by the pattern (segmental or diffuse) of the misdirected lashes and the quality of the posterior lamella of the involved eyelid. Inturned lashes not associated with involutional entropion are usually seen in cases of posterior lamellar scarring (marginal cicatricial entropion). If the eyelid margin is misdirected, treatment should be directed at correcting the entropion.

### Management

Trichiasis may be initially treated using *mechanical epilation,* removing misdirected lashes with forceps at the slit lamp. Because of eyelash regrowth, recurrence can be expected 3–8 weeks after epilation. Broken cilia are often more irritating to the cornea than mature longer lashes.

Standard *electrolysis* or radiofrequency ablation is used for definitive treatment of trichiasis. The energy is delivered with an insulated needle to destroy the hair follicle. When the needle tip is removed, the lash is easily extracted. However, the recurrence rate is high, adjacent normal lashes may be damaged, and scarring of the adjacent eyelid margin tissue can worsen the problem.

Segmental trichiasis can be treated with *cryotherapy* in an office procedure that requires only local infiltrative anesthesia. The involved area is frozen for approximately 25 seconds, allowed to thaw, and then refrozen for 20 seconds *(double freeze–thaw technique).* The lashes are mechanically removed with forceps after treatment. Edema lasting several days, loss of skin pigmentation, notching of the eyelid margin, and possible interference with goblet cell function are disadvantages of cryotherapy. This method may be combined with various surgical techniques and repeated if offending lashes persist or recur.

*Argon laser* treatment of trichiasis can be useful when only a few scattered eyelashes require ablation or when the stimulation of larger areas of inflammation is undesirable. Some pigment is required in the base of the lash to absorb the laser energy and ablate the lash, making this technique sensitive to hair color.

In all these procedures, success rates vary, and additional treatment sessions are commonly necessary. *Full-thickness pentagonal resection* with primary closure may be considered when trichiasis is confined to a segment of the eyelid.

Dutton JJ, Tawfik HA, DeBacker CM, Lipham WJ. Direct internal eyelash bulb extirpation for trichiasis. *Ophthal Plast Reconstr Surg.* 2000;16(2):142–145.

Rosner M, Bourla N, Rosen N. Eyelid splitting and extirpation of hair follicles using a radiosurgical technique for treatment of trichiasis. *Ophthalmic Surg Lasers Imaging.* 2004;35(2):116–122.

Wilcsek GA, Francis IC. Argon laser and trichiasis. *Br J Ophthalmol.* 2003;87(3):375.

## Blepharoptosis

The shortened form, *ptosis,* is frequently used in place of the more accurate term, *blepharoptosis,* to describe drooping or inferior displacement of the upper eyelid. Ptosis is a common cause of reversible peripheral vision loss. Although the superior visual field is most often involved, central vision can also be affected. Many patients with ptosis report difficulty with reading because the ptosis worsens in downgaze. Ptosis has also been shown to decrease the overall amount of light reaching the macula and, therefore, can reduce visual acuity, especially at night.

Two classification systems are used to describe upper eyelid ptosis. It may be categorized by onset: congenital or acquired. In addition, it may be classified by the cause: myogenic, aponeurotic, neurogenic, mechanical, or traumatic. The most common type of *congenital* ptosis results from a poorly developed levator muscle (myogenic cause); the most common type of *acquired* ptosis is caused by stretching or disinsertion of the levator aponeurosis (aponeurotic cause).

Cahill KV, Bradley EA, Meyer DR, et al. Functional indications for upper eyelid ptosis and blepharoplasty surgery: a report by the American Academy of Ophthalmology. *Ophthalmology.* 2011;118(12):2510–2517.

### Evaluation

The patient's history usually distinguishes congenital from acquired ptosis. Patients with congenital or acquired blepharoptosis may be aware of a family history of the condition. Marked variability in the degree of ptosis during the day and complaints of diplopia should suggest ocular myasthenia gravis (MG). Complaints of dysphonia, dyspnea, dysphagia, or proximal muscle weakness suggest systemic MG.

### Physical Examination

Physical examination of the ptosis patient begins with 5 clinical measurements:

- margin–reflex distance
- vertical palpebral fissure height
- upper eyelid crease position
- levator function (upper eyelid excursion)
- presence of lagophthalmos

The physician can record these data by using a drawing showing the cornea, the pupil size, and the position of the upper and lower eyelids in relation to these structures (Fig 11-9).

The *margin–reflex distance 1 ($MRD_1$),* which is the distance from the upper eyelid margin to the corneal light reflex in primary position, is probably the single most important measurement in describing the amount of ptosis. In severe ptosis, the light reflex may

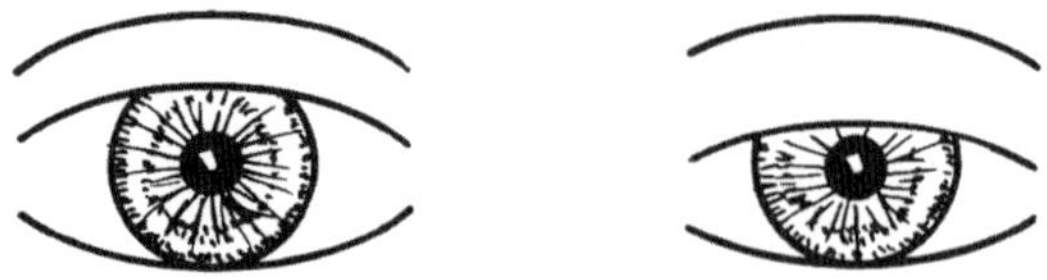

| | | |
|---|---|---|
| Margin–reflex distance 1 | +4 | +2 |
| Palpebral fissure height | 9.5 | 7.5 |
| Upper eyelid crease | 8 | 11 |
| Levator function | 15 | 14 |
| Lagophthalmos | 0 | 0 |

**Figure 11-9** Example of ptosis data collection sheet.

be obstructed by the eyelid and therefore have a zero or negative value. If the patient reports visual obstruction while reading, the $MRD_1$ is also checked in the reading position. Lower eyelid retraction (or scleral show) should be noted separately as the *margin–reflex distance 2 ($MRD_2$).* The $MRD_2$ is the distance from the corneal light reflex to the lower eyelid margin. The sum of the $MRD_1$ and the $MRD_2$ should equal the vertical palpebral fissure height.

The *vertical palpebral fissure* is measured at the widest point between the lower eyelid and the upper eyelid. This measurement is taken with the patient fixating on a distant object in primary gaze.

The distance from the *upper eyelid crease* to the eyelid margin is measured. Because the insertion of fibers from the levator muscle into the skin contributes to formation of the upper eyelid crease, high, duplicated, or asymmetric creases may indicate an abnormal position of the levator aponeurosis. In the typical Occidental eyelid, the upper eyelid crease is 8–9 mm in males and 9–11 mm in females. The crease is usually elevated in patients with involutional ptosis and is often shallow or absent in patients with congenital ptosis. As a normal anatomical finding, the upper eyelid crease is typically lower or obscured in the Asian eyelid, with or without ptosis.

*Levator function* is estimated by measuring the upper eyelid excursion, or ULE, from downgaze to upgaze with frontalis muscle function negated and with the head positioned in the frontal or Frankfort plane (defined as the plane determined when the line intersecting the highest point on the upper margin of each external auditory canal and the lowest point on the lower margin of the left orbit is parallel to the ground) (Fig 11-10). Fixating the brow with digital pressure minimizes contributions from accessory elevators of the eyelids such as the frontalis muscle. Failure to negate the influence of the frontalis muscle results in overestimation of levator function, which may affect the diagnosis and treatment plan.

Finally, the patient should be assessed for *lagophthalmos;* if it is present, the gap between the eyelids should be measured and the amount noted (in millimeters). Lagophthalmos and poor tear film quantity or quality may predispose the patient to complications of ptosis repair such as dryness and exposure keratopathy.

Baroody M, Holds JB, Vick VL. Advances in the diagnosis and treatment of ptosis. *Curr Opin Ophthalmol.* 2005;16(6):351–355.

A

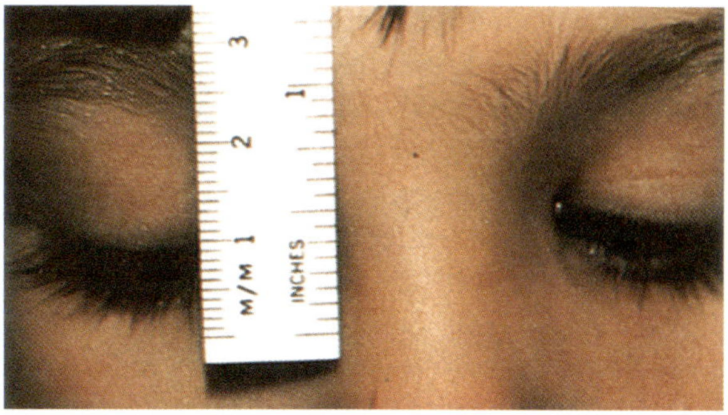


B

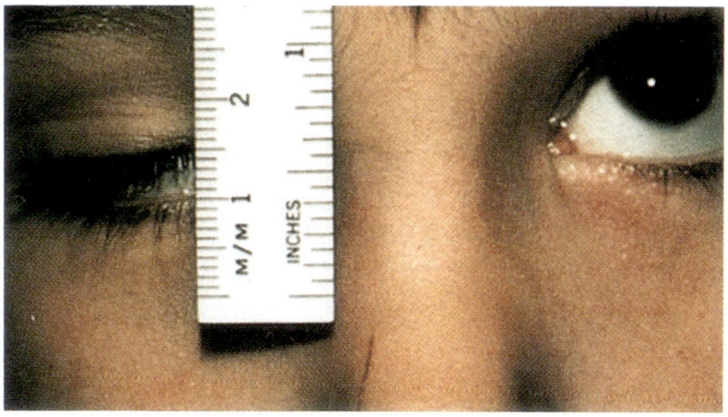


**Figure 11-10** Measurement of levator excursion. **A,** Downgaze. **B,** Upgaze.

#### *Additional considerations*

Physical examination also includes checking head position, chin elevation, brow position, and brow action in attempted upgaze. These features help to show the patient how ptosis affects function. Quantity and quality of the tear film is documented in the initial examination. The examiner should also note the presence or absence of supraduction of the globe with eyelid closure (Bell phenomenon) and assess whether corneal sensation is normal; these factors may also affect the treatment plan.

Variation in the amount of ptosis with extraocular muscle or jaw muscle movements *(synkinesis)* is identified. Synkinesis may be seen in Marcus Gunn jaw-winking ptosis, aberrant regeneration of the oculomotor nerve or the facial nerve, and some types of Duane retraction syndrome. The examiner should attempt to elicit synkinesis as part of the evaluation of patients with congenital blepharoptosis or those with possible aberrant regeneration.

The *position of the ptotic eyelid in downgaze* (palpebral fissure in downgaze) can help differentiate between congenital and acquired causes. The congenitally ptotic eyelid is typically higher in downgaze than the contralateral normal eyelid. The congenitally ptotic eyelid may also manifest lagophthalmos. By contrast, in acquired involutional ptosis the affected eyelid remains ptotic in all positions of gaze and may even worsen in downgaze with relaxation of the frontalis muscle.

The ophthalmologist must assess *visual function and refractive error* in all cases of congenital or childhood ptosis in order to identify and treat the child with concomitant amblyopia resulting from anisometropia, high astigmatism, strabismus, or occlusion of the pupil. Amblyopia occurs in approximately 20% of patients with congenital ptosis. *Extraocular muscle function* should also be assessed because extraocular muscle dysfunction associated with ptosis occurs in various congenital conditions (combined superior rectus/levator muscle maldevelopment, congenital oculomotor palsy) and acquired conditions (ocular or systemic MG, chronic progressive external ophthalmoplegia, oculopharyngeal dystrophy, and oculomotor palsy with or without aberrant regeneration).

In addition, *pupillary examination* is important in the evaluation of ptosis. Pupil abnormalities are present in some acquired and congenital conditions associated with ptosis (eg, Horner syndrome, cranial nerve III palsy). Miosis that is most apparent in dim illumination is a finding in Horner syndrome; mydriasis is seen in some cases of oculomotor nerve palsy.

*External examination* may reveal other abnormalities as well. For example, severe bilateral congenital ptosis may be associated with telecanthus, epicanthus inversus, hypoplasia of the superior orbital rims, horizontal shortening of the eyelids, ear deformities, hypertelorism, and hypoplasia of the nasal bridge. These findings characterize an autosomal dominant condition known as *blepharophimosis–ptosis–epicanthus inversus syndrome (BPES)* (discussed in Chapter 10).

### Ancillary Tests

*Visual field testing* with the eyelids untaped (in the natural, ptotic state) and taped (artificially elevated) helps determine the patient's level of functional visual impairment. Comparison of the taped and untaped visual fields gives an estimate of the superior visual field improvement that can be anticipated following surgery. Visual field testing and external full-face photography are required by third-party payers as a part of the initial evaluation in order to distinguish *functional* from *cosmetic* blepharoptosis repair.

*Pharmacologic testing, pupillary evaluation in light and dark,* and *the presence of reverse ptosis of the lower eyelid (smaller* $MRD_2$*)* may be helpful in confirming the clinical diagnosis of *Horner syndrome* and in localizing the causative lesion (see BCSC Section 5, *Neuro-Ophthalmology*). Although the differentiation among first-, second-, and third-order neuron dysfunction in the cause of Horner syndrome is important in the patient's general medical assessment, this information seldom alters treatment of the ptosis. Third-order neuron dysfunction resulting in Horner syndrome is typically benign. However, neuron dysfunction of the first or second order is sometimes associated with malignant neoplasms such as an apical lung (Pancoast) tumor, aneurysm, or dissection of the carotid artery.

Pharmacologic testing may also be used in the diagnosis of MG, a disease in which ptosis is the most common presenting sign. Fluctuating ptosis that seems to worsen with fatigue or prolonged upgaze, especially when accompanied by diplopia or other clinical signs of systemic MG, is an indication for further diagnostic evaluation with the edrophonium chloride, ice-pack, or acetylcholine receptor antibody tests. These tests are discussed later in this chapter under Neurogenic ptosis.

## Classification

### *Myogenic ptosis*

The patient's history usually distinguishes congenital from acquired ptosis. *Congenital myogenic ptosis* results from dysgenesis of the levator muscle. Instead of normal muscle fibers, fibrous or adipose tissue is present in the muscle belly, diminishing the ability of the levator to contract and relax. Therefore, most congenital ptosis caused by maldevelopment of the levator muscle is characterized by decreased levator function, lid lag, and, sometimes, lagophthalmos (Fig 11-11). The amount of levator function is an indication of the amount of normal muscle. The upper eyelid crease is often absent or poorly formed, especially in cases of more severe ptosis. Congenital myogenic ptosis associated with a poor Bell phenomenon (supraduction of globe with eyelid closure) or with vertical strabismus may indicate concomitant maldevelopment of the superior rectus and levator muscles *(monocular elevation deficiency, formerly, double-elevator palsy).*

*Acquired myogenic ptosis* results from localized or diffuse muscular disease such as muscular dystrophy, chronic progressive external ophthalmoplegia, MG, or oculopharyngeal dystrophy. Because of the underlying muscle dysfunction, surgical correction may be difficult, requiring frontalis sling procedures and/or procedures to repair lower eyelid retraction and improve corneal protection.

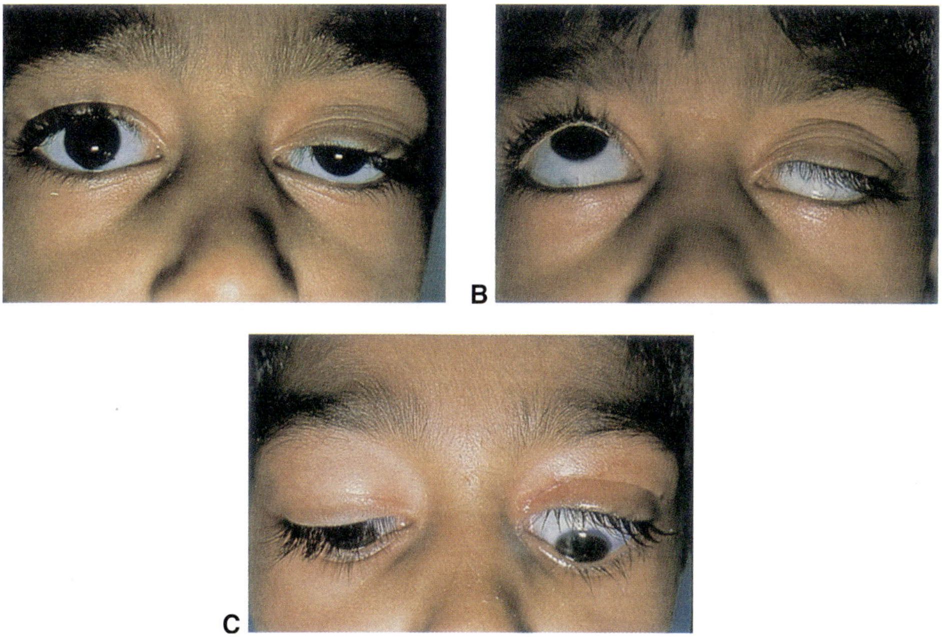

**Figure 11-11** Left congenital ptosis. **A,** Note margin–reflex distance ($MRD_1$ = 5.0 mm OD, 1.0 mm OS). Normal = 4.5 mm. **B,** Upgaze accentuates ptosis. **C,** Downgaze reveals lid lag. *(Courtesy of Robert C. Kersten, MD.)*

Allen RC, Zimmerman MB, Watterberg EA, Morrison LA, Carter KD. Primary bilateral silicone frontalis suspension for good levator function ptosis in oculopharyngeal muscular dystrophy. *Br J Ophthalmol.* 2012;96(6):841–845.

Demartelaere SL, Blaydon SM, Shore JW. Tarsal switch levator resection for the treatment of blepharoptosis in patients with poor eye protective mechanisms. *Ophthalmology.* 2006;113(12):2357–2363.

#### *Aponeurotic ptosis*

The levator aponeurosis transmits levator force to the eyelid. Thus, any disruption in its anatomy or function can lead to ptosis.

*Acquired aponeurotic ptosis* is the most common form of ptosis. It results from stretching or dehiscence of the levator aponeurosis or disinsertion from its normal position. Common causes are involutional attenuation or repetitive traction on the eyelid, which may occur with frequent eye rubbing or prolonged use of rigid contact lenses. Aponeurotic ptosis may also be caused or exacerbated by intraocular surgery or eyelid surgery (Fig 11-12).

Eyelids with aponeurotic defects characteristically have a high or an absent upper eyelid crease secondary to upward displacement or loss of the insertion of levator fibers into the skin. Thinning of the eyelid superior to the upper tarsal plate is often an associated finding. Because the levator muscle itself is healthy, levator function in aponeurotic ptosis is usually normal (12–15 mm). Acquired aponeurotic ptosis may worsen in downgaze and therefore interfere with the patient's ability to read as well as limit the superior visual field. Table 11-1 compares acquired aponeurotic ptosis with congenital myogenic ptosis.

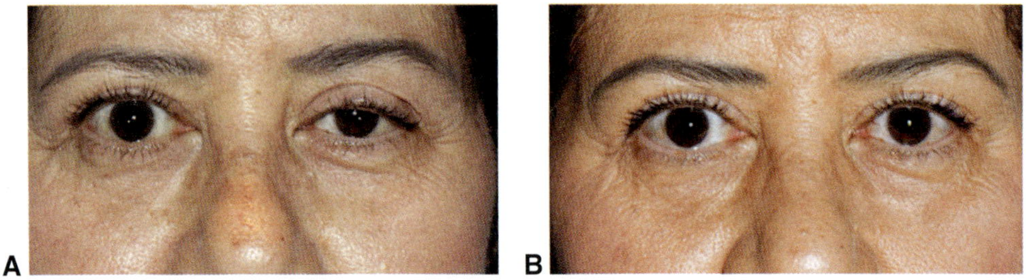

**Figure 11-12** **A,** Aponeurotic ptosis of the left upper eyelid after cataract surgery. Similar aponeurotic ptosis can occur following various other intraocular and eyelid surgical procedures. **B,** After aponeurotic ptosis repair of the left upper eyelid; note the improvement in the symmetry of the eyelid crease and the eyelid fold in addition to the elevation of the eyelid margin. *(Courtesy of Bobby S. Korn, MD, PhD.)*

**Table 11-1 Blepharoptosis Comparison**

| | Congenital Myogenic Ptosis | Acquired Aponeurotic Ptosis |
|---|---|---|
| Margin–reflex distance 1 | Mild to severe ptosis | Mild to severe ptosis |
| Upper eyelid crease | Poorly formed | Higher than normal or absent |
| Levator function | Reduced | Near normal |
| Downgaze | Lid lag | Eyelid drop |

### *Neurogenic ptosis*

**Congenital conditions** Congenital neurogenic ptosis is caused by innervational defects that occur during embryonic development. This condition is relatively rare and is most commonly associated with congenital cranial nerve III (CN III) palsy, congenital Horner syndrome, or the Marcus Gunn jaw-winking syndrome.

*Congenital oculomotor nerve (CN III) palsy* is manifested as ptosis together with inability to elevate, depress, or adduct the globe. The pupils may also be dilated. This palsy may be partial or complete, but ptosis is very rarely an isolated finding in CN III palsy. It is uncommon to find aberrant innervation in congenital CN III palsies. Management of strabismus and amblyopia is difficult in many cases of congenital third nerve palsy. Treatment of the associated ptosis is also complicated, usually requiring a frontalis suspension procedure, which often leads to some degree of lagophthalmos. As a result of lagophthalmos, poor ocular motility, and poor postoperative eyelid excursion, postoperative management may be complicated by diplopia, exposure keratopathy, and corneal ulceration.

*Congenital Horner syndrome* is a manifestation of an interrupted sympathetic nervous chain and may cause mild ptosis associated with miosis, anhidrosis, and decreased pigmentation of the iris on the involved side. The mild ptosis of Horner syndrome is due to an innervational deficit to the sympathetic Müller muscle, an eyelid elevator second in importance to the levator muscle. Decreased sympathetic tone to the inferior tarsal muscle in the lower eyelid, the analogue of the Müller muscle in the upper eyelid, results in elevation of the lower eyelid, also known as *lower eyelid reverse ptosis.* The combined upper and lower eyelid ptosis decreases the vertical palpebral fissure and may falsely suggest enophthalmos. The pupillary miosis is most apparent in dim illumination, when the contralateral pupil dilates more.

Congenital neurogenic ptosis may also be synkinetic. *Marcus Gunn jaw-winking syndrome* is the most common form of congenital synkinetic neurogenic ptosis (Fig 11-13). In this synkinetic syndrome, the unilaterally ptotic eyelid elevates with jaw movements. The movement that most commonly causes elevation of the ptotic eyelid is lateral mandibular movement to the contralateral side. This phenomenon is usually first noticed by the mother when she is feeding or nursing the baby. This synkinesis is thought to be caused by aberrant connections between the motor division of CN V and the levator muscle. Infrequently, this syndrome is associated with abnormal connections between CN III and other cranial nerves. Some forms of Duane retraction syndrome also cause elevation of a ptotic eyelid with movement of the globe. This congenital syndrome is also thought to result from aberrant nerve connections.

Demirci H, Frueh BR, Nelson CC. Marcus Gunn jaw-winking synkinesis: clinical features and management. *Ophthalmology.* 2010;117(7):1447–1452.

**Acquired conditions** *Acquired neurogenic ptosis* results from interruption of normally developed innervation and is most often secondary to an acquired CN III palsy, to an acquired Horner syndrome, or MG.

Delineation of the cause of acquired oculomotor nerve palsy is important. Distinction must be made between *ischemic* and *compressive* etiologies. Most acquired oculomotor palsies are *ischemic* and associated with diabetes mellitus, hypertension, or arteriosclerotic

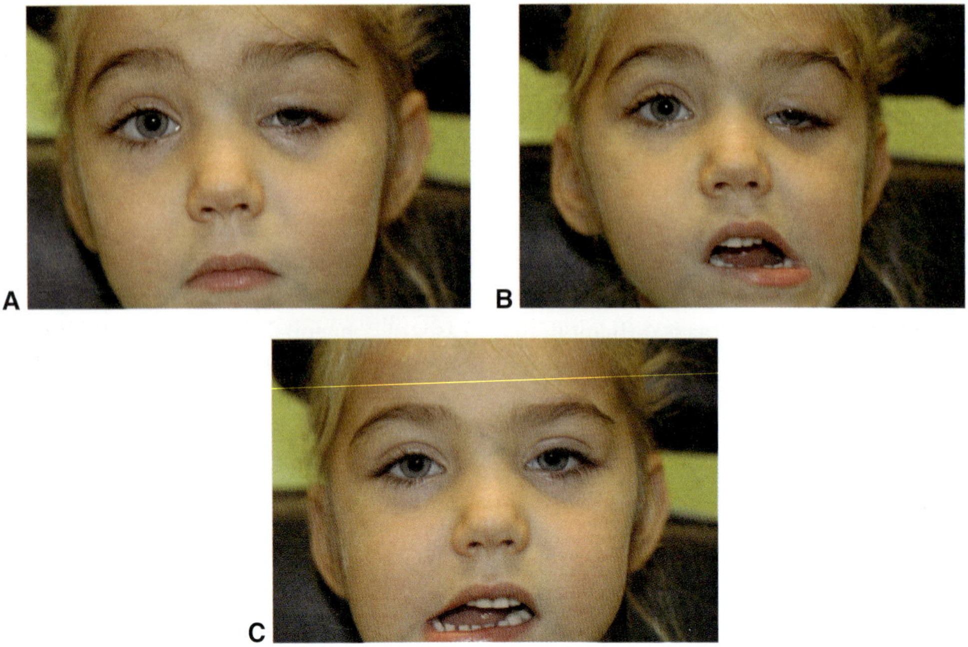

**Figure 11-13** Marcus Gunn jaw-winking ptosis (synkinesis linking cranial nerve V to cranial nerve III). **A,** Relaxed position with ptosis of the left upper eyelid. **B,** Moving mandible to the left, the eyelid position remains low. **C,** Moving mandible to the right with elevation of the left upper eyelid. *(Courtesy of Jill Foster, MD.)*

disease. Typically, *ischemic* acquired CN III palsies do not include pupillary abnormalities, they may be associated with pain, and they resolve spontaneously with satisfactory levator function within 3 months. If a pupil-sparing CN III palsy fails to resolve spontaneously within 3–6 months, further workup for a compressive lesion is indicated. However, if a patient presents with a CN III palsy involving the pupil, an immediate workup (including neuroimaging) should commence in order to rule out a compressive neoplastic or aneurysmal lesion. Surgical correction of ptosis related to CN III palsy usually requires frontalis suspension and should be reserved for patients in whom strabismus surgery allows single binocular vision in a useful field of gaze.

Less common causes of acquired neurogenic ptosis include myotonic dystrophy, chronic progressive external ophthalmoplegia, Guillain-Barré syndrome, oculopharyngeal dystrophy, and iatrogenic botulism. Botulinum toxin injection in the forehead or orbital region to ameliorate benign essential blepharospasm or to reduce facial rhytids may result in diffusion of the neurotoxin into the levator muscle complex. The resultant neurogenic ptosis is temporary, usually resolving after a few weeks.

**Myasthenia gravis** Myasthenia gravis is an autoimmune disorder in which autoantibodies attack the acetylcholine receptors of the neuromuscular junction. MG is most often generalized and systemic. Approximately 10% of patients with generalized MG have an associated thymoma; thus, chest computed tomography (CT) scanning should be considered for all patients with MG to rule out this lesion. Surgical thymectomy results in clinical improvement in 75% of cases of generalized MG and complete remission in 35% of cases. Early manifestations of MG are often ophthalmic, with ptosis being the most common presenting sign; diplopia is often present as well. When the effects of MG are isolated to the periocular musculature, the condition is called *ocular myasthenia gravis.* Marked variability in the degree of ptosis during the day and complaints of diplopia should suggest ocular MG. Other autoimmune disorders may occur in myasthenic patients; for example, thyroid eye disease occurs in 5%–10% of patients with MG.

No single test for MG will detect all cases. The *acetylcholine receptor antibody test* is a serum assay designed to detect the autoimmune antibody responsible for destruction of the motor end-plate receptors in patients with MG. Binding antibodies are detectable in about 90% of patients with systemic MG and in about 70% of patients with ocular MG. The ophthalmologist should be aware that some laboratories set their reference ranges artificially high, assessing for systemic MG. The antibody levels are lower in ocular MG. Therefore, acetylcholine receptor antibody levels below the abnormal reference range may be suggestive of ocular MG.

*Edrophonium chloride,* an acetylcholinesterase inhibitor, is used in diagnostic testing for MG. In the myasthenic patient, whose acetylcholine receptors have been compromised through autoimmune destruction, the infusion of edrophonium chloride typically causes a brief improvement in ptosis or ocular motility. Clinicians administering this test should be aware of potential adverse effects of edrophonium and should be prepared to administer atropine and other appropriate care in case of adverse reactions. The *ice-pack test* is an alternative approach that has fewer side effects. An ice pack is applied to the patient's eyelid(s) for 3 minutes. If MG is present, the ptosis often improves because of the enhancement of neuromuscular transmission that occurs with inhibition of acetylcholinesterase under cold conditions. Some clinicians use a sleep or rest test as well. For this test, the patient lies (with eyes closed) in a darkened room for approximately 20 minutes. Immediately after the patient's eyes open, the upper eyelid position is assessed to see whether it is higher than the prerest position. Rest or sleep briefly improves myasthenic ptosis. *Single-fiber electromyography* may also be used to detect MG.

The ptosis of ocular MG often responds poorly to systemic anticholinesterase medication alone, but response may improve with the addition of corticosteroids. Neuro-ophthalmologic consultation is useful in the evaluation and treatment of difficult cases. Surgical treatment of ptosis in the myasthenic patient should be delayed until medical management is maximized. Because of the variability of levator function, frontalis suspension may be considered. See BCSC Section 5, *Neuro-Ophthalmology,* for further discussion.

Gilbert ME, Savino PJ. Ocular myasthenia gravis. *Int Ophthalmol Clin.* 2007;47(4):93–103, ix.

Smith KH. Myasthenia gravis. *Focal Points: Clinical Modules for Ophthalmologists.* San Francisco: American Academy of Ophthalmology; 2003, module 4.

### *Mechanical ptosis*

Mechanical ptosis usually refers to the condition in which an eyelid or orbital mass weighs or pulls down the upper eyelid, resulting in inferior displacement. It may be caused by a *congenital abnormality,* such as a plexiform neurofibroma or hemangioma, or by an *acquired neoplasm,* such as a large chalazion or skin carcinoma. Postsurgical or posttraumatic edema may also cause temporary mechanical ptosis.

#### *Traumatic ptosis*

Trauma to the levator aponeurosis or the levator muscle may also cause ptosis through myogenic, aponeurotic, neurogenic, or mechanical defects. Eyelid lacerations exposing preaponeurotic fat indicate that the orbital septum has been transected and suggest possible damage to the levator aponeurosis. Exploration of the levator muscle or aponeurosis may be indicated in these patients if levator function is diminished or ptosis is present. Orbital and neurosurgical procedures may also lead to traumatic ptosis. Because such ptosis may resolve or improve spontaneously, the ophthalmologist normally observes the patient for 6 months before considering surgical intervention.

#### *Pseudoptosis*

Pseudoptosis—apparent eyelid drooping—should be differentiated from true ptosis. An eyelid may appear to be abnormally low in various conditions, including hypertropia, enophthalmos, microphthalmia, anophthalmia, phthisis bulbi, or a superior sulcus defect secondary to trauma or other causes. Contralateral upper eyelid retraction may also simulate ptosis. The term *pseudoptosis* is also sometimes used to describe *dermatochalasis,* the condition in which excess upper eyelid skin overhangs the eyelid margin, transects the pupil, and gives the appearance of a true ptosis of the eyelid margin (Fig 11-14).

### Treatment of Ptosis

Ptosis repair is a challenging oculoplastic surgical procedure that requires correct diagnosis, thoughtful planning, thorough understanding of eyelid anatomy, experience, and good surgical technique. The patient's ocular, medical, and surgical history help determine whether surgical repair of ptosis is appropriate for that individual. The surgeon should be aware of any history of symptoms of dry eye and should temper blepharoptosis repair in the presence of significant dry eye problems. Other pertinent historical queries should include the presence of thyroid eye disease, previous eye or eyelid surgery, and prior periorbital trauma.

Ptosis that causes significant superior visual field loss or difficulty with reading is considered to be a *functional* problem, and correction of this defect often improves a patient's

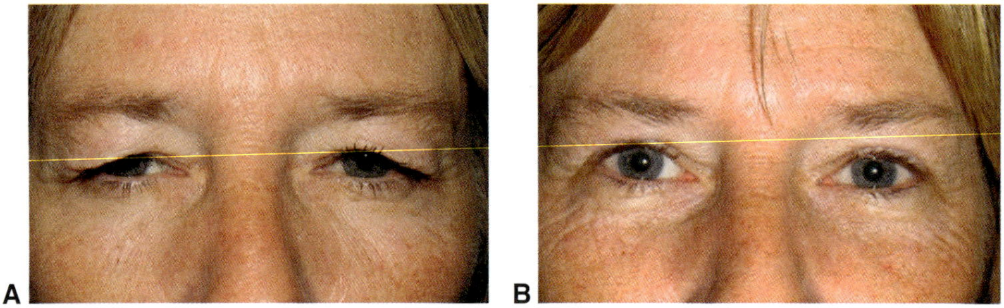

**Figure 11-14** **A,** Patient with dermatochalasis and pseudoptosis of both upper eyelids. **B,** Clearance of the visual axis is achieved following blepharoplasty alone. *(Courtesy of Bobby S. Korn, MD, PhD.)*

ability to perform the activities of daily living. In other instances, ptosis is considered to be a *cosmetic* issue, causing a tired or sleepy appearance in the absence of a visual function deficit. Because ptosis repair is an elective surgical procedure, it is particularly important for the surgeon to have a preoperative discussion with the patient to communicate the potential risks, benefits, and alternatives to treatment.

Surgical procedures designed to correct ptosis should be directed toward correction of the underlying pathologic condition. The 3 categories of surgical procedures most commonly used in ptosis repair are

- external (transcutaneous) levator advancement
- internal (transconjunctival) levator/tarsus/Müller muscle resection approaches
- frontalis muscle suspensions

The amount and type of ptosis and the degree of levator function are the most common determining factors in the choice of surgical procedure for ptosis repair. The surgeon's comfort level and experience with various procedures is also an important factor. In patients with good levator function, surgical correction is generally directed toward the levator aponeurosis: the levator muscle is the most potent elevator of the eyelid in most patients. However, if levator function is poor or absent, frontalis muscle suspension techniques are the preferred repair procedures.

*External (transcutaneous)* levator advancement surgery is most commonly used when levator function is normal and the upper eyelid crease is high (Video 11-3). In this setting, the levator muscle itself is normal, but the levator aponeurosis (its tendinous attachment to the tarsal plate) is stretched or disinserted (see Fig 11-15A), thus requiring advancement. The surgery is ideally performed under local anesthesia with monitored care. The levator aponeurosis is approached externally through an upper eyelid crease incision. The levator aponeurosis is advanced to the superior tarsal border (Fig 11-15), and patient cooperation is elicited to obtain optimal lid height and contour. Reinsertion of the aponeurosis usually produces an excellent result. In some cases, the distal end of the aponeurosis may be found to be higher than its normal position on the lower anterior surface of the tarsus.

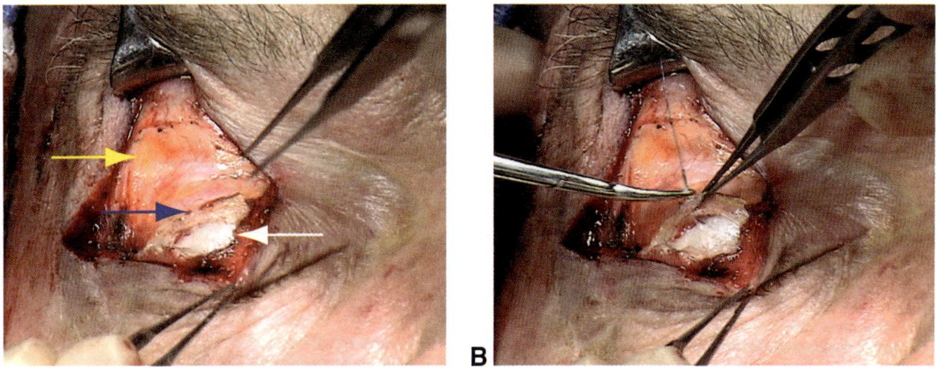

A B

**Figure 11-15** **A,** External levator advancement surgery showing the preaponeurotic fat *(yellow arrow)*, disinserted edge of levator aponeurosis *(blue arrow)*, and tarsal plate *(white arrow)*. **B,** Advancement of the levator muscle to the tarsal plate. *(Courtesy of Bobby S. Korn, MD, PhD.)*

**VIDEO 11-3** External levator advancement ptosis repair (01:48).
*Courtesy of Jill Foster, MD; Dan Straka, MD; and Craig Czyz, DO.*

The *internal (transconjunctival)* approach to ptosis repair may be directed toward the Müller muscle, the tarsus, or the levator aponeurosis or muscle. *Müller muscle–conjunctival resections (MMCRs)* (Video 11-4) are used in patients who have an adequate upper eyelid position following instillation of a drop of 2.5% phenylephrine hydrochloride (Figs 11-16A, B). MMCRs are typically used for repair of minimal ptosis (2 mm or less) and are generally considered useful for maintaining preoperative eyelid contour (Figs 11-16C, D). The *Fasanella-Servat* ptosis repair procedure, which is also used for small amounts of ptosis, includes removal of the superior tarsus with the conjunctiva and Müller muscle.

**VIDEO 11-4** Müller muscle–conjunctival resection (01:42).
*Courtesy of Jill Foster, MD; Dan Straka, MD; and Craig Czyz, DO.*

Most patients with significant ptosis automatically use the frontalis muscle in an attempt to raise the eyelid and clear the visual axis. In *frontalis suspension surgery* (Fig 11-17), which is performed when levator function is poor or absent, the eyelid is suspended directly from the frontalis muscle so that movement of the brow is efficiently transmitted to the eyelid. Thus, the patient is able to elevate the eyelid by using the frontalis muscle to lift the brow. Autogenous tensor fascia lata, banked fascia lata, and synthetic materials have

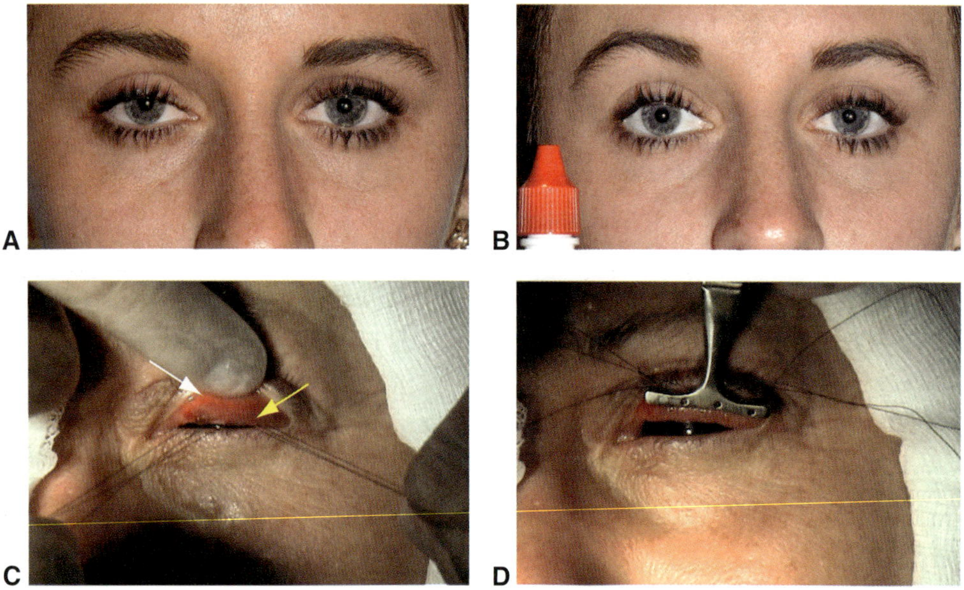


**Figure 11-16** **A,** Patient with ptosis of the right upper eyelid. **B,** Improvement of right upper eyelid ptosis after instillation of 2.5% phenylephrine hydrochloride. **C,** Intraoperative photograph showing tarsus *(white arrow)*, conjunctiva, and Müller muscle *(yellow arrow)*. **D,** Ptosis clamp securing conjunctiva and Müller muscle prior to excision. *(Courtesy of Bobby S. Korn, MD, PhD.)*

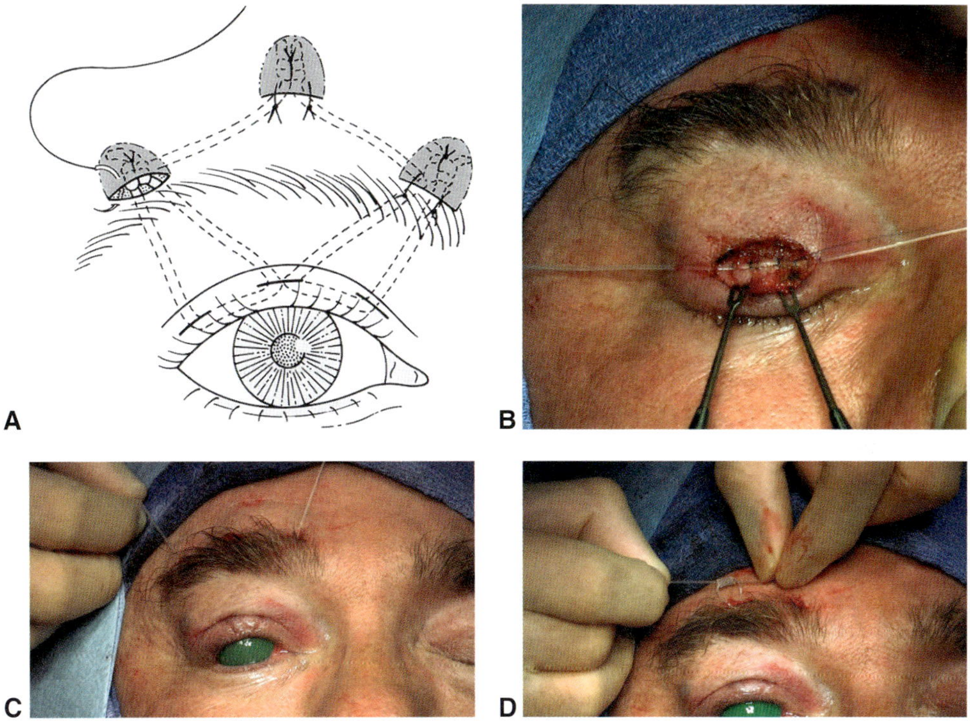

**Figure 11-17** **A,** Frontalis suspension: Crawford method. **B,** Fixation of silicone rod to tarsal plate. **C,** Passage of silicone rod through nasal and temporal brow incisions. **D,** Fixation of silicone rod through central brow incision over Watzke sleeve. *(Part A reprinted from Stewart WB.* Surgery of the Eyelid, Orbit, and Lacrimal System. *Ophthalmology Monograph 8, vol 2. San Francisco: American Academy of Ophthalmology; 1994:120. Parts B–D courtesy of Bobby S. Korn, MD, PhD.)*

been used for this purpose. *Autogenous fascia lata* has shown the best long-term results but requires harvesting and additional surgery. Generally, autogenous fascia lata can be used in patients who are at least 3 years old or weigh 35 pounds or more. *Banked fascia lata* may be obtained from a variety of sources and obviates the need for additional operative sites and harvesting. However, this material may incite inflammation, it has the theoretic potential to transmit infectious agents, and it has poorer long-term outcomes than does autogenous tissue. *Synthetic materials* such as silicone rods are commonly used. They do not require a second harvest site, and they allow easier adjustment or removal if necessary.

There is some controversy about whether bilateral frontalis suspension should be performed in patients with unilateral congenital ptosis. A bilateral procedure may improve the patient's symmetry and stimulate the need to utilize the frontalis muscle to lift the eyelids, but it subjects the normal eyelid to surgical risks. The decision of whether to modify a normal eyelid in an attempt to gain symmetry must be discussed by the surgeon and patient (or the patient's caregiver, if the patient is a child).

Lee MJ, Oh JY, Choung HK, Kim NJ, Sung MS, Khwarg SI. Frontalis sling operation using silicone rod compared with preserved fascia lata for congenital ptosis a three-year follow-up study. *Ophthalmology.* 2009;116(1):123–129.

### *Complications*

Creating symmetry between the two eyelids is the most difficult aspect of ptosis repair. This has led some ptosis surgeons to use adjustable suture techniques or to advocate early adjustment in the office during the first 2 postoperative weeks when indicated. Undercorrection is the most common complication of ptosis repair, and judgment is required to differentiate true undercorrection from apparent undercorrection resulting from postoperative edema. Other potential complications include overcorrection, unsatisfactory eyelid contour, scarring, wound dehiscence, eyelid crease asymmetry, conjunctival prolapse, tarsal eversion, and lagophthalmos with exposure keratopathy. Lagophthalmos following ptosis repair is most common in patients with decreased levator function. This condition is usually temporary, but it requires treatment with lubricating drops or ointments until it resolves.

Fagien S, Putterman AM, eds. *Putterman's Cosmetic Oculoplastic Surgery.* 4th ed. Philadelphia: Saunders; 2008.

Hakimbashi M, Kikkawa DO, Korn BS. Complications of ptosis repair: prevention and management. In: Cohen AJ, Weinberg DA, eds. *Evaluation and Management of Blepharoptosis.* New York: Springer; 2011:275–288.

## Eyelid Retraction

Eyelid retraction is present when the upper eyelid is displaced superiorly or the lower eyelid, inferiorly, exposing sclera between the limbus and the eyelid margin (Fig 11-18). Lower eyelid retraction may also be a normal anatomical variant in patients with shallow orbits or certain genetic orbital or eyelid characteristics. Retraction of the eyelids often leads to lagophthalmos and exposure keratopathy. The effects of these conditions can range from ocular irritation and discomfort to vision-threatening corneal decompensation.

Eyelid retraction can have local, systemic, or central nervous system causes. The most common causes of eyelid retraction are thyroid eye disease (TED), recession of the vertical rectus muscles, aggressive skin excision in blepharoplasty, and overcompensation for a contralateral ptosis (in accordance with Hering's law).

TED is the most common cause of both upper and lower eyelid retraction, as well as the most common cause of unilateral or bilateral proptosis. Because proptosis commonly coexists with and may mimic eyelid retraction in patients with TED, these conditions are evaluated through eyelid measurements and exophthalmometry. A common finding in

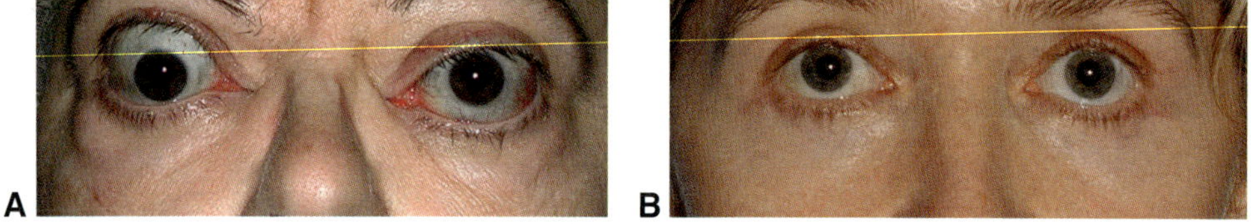


**Figure 11-18** **A,** Upper and lower eyelid retraction secondary to thyroid eye disease. **B,** Upper and lower eyelid retraction resulting from excessive skin removal and middle lamellar scarring after cosmetic blepharoplasty. *(Part A courtesy of Jill Foster, MD; part B courtesy of Bobby S. Korn, MD, PhD.)*

thyroid-related eyelid retraction is temporal flare. In this condition, the eyelid retraction is more severe laterally than medially, resulting in an abnormal upper eyelid contour that appears to flare upward along the lateral half of the eyelid margin. The histologic changes in the eyelid in TED are secondary to inflammatory infiltration and fibrous contraction of the eyelid retractors. The sympathetically innervated eyelid retractor muscles (the Müller muscle in the upper eyelid and the analogous eyelid retractor muscle in the lower eyelid) are preferentially affected by the inflammation and fibrosis of TED. See Chapter 4 for a more extensive discussion of TED.

Eyelid retraction may be iatrogenically induced by recession of the vertical rectus muscles, owing to anatomical connections between the superior rectus and the levator muscles in the upper eyelid and between the inferior rectus muscle and capsulopalpebral fascia in the lower eyelid.

Another cause of eyelid retraction, especially of the lower eyelids, is excessive resection of skin, middle lamellar scarring, and untreated lower eyelid laxity during cosmetic lower blepharoplasty. Midface-lifting, full-thickness skin grafting, or spacer grafting may be required to correct this iatrogenic deformity. Conservative excision of skin in lower blepharoplasty, along with concomitant correction of any lower eyelid laxity, minimizes the risk of this problem.

Overcompensation for a contralateral ptosis (Hering's law) may also give the appearance of upper eyelid retraction. The surgeon must distinguish this condition from true eyelid retraction by observing the position of the supposedly retracted eyelid while the contralateral, presumably ptotic, eyelid is either manually elevated or occluded.

*Parinaud syndrome* is an example of eyelid retraction caused by a central nervous system lesion. Congenital eyelid retraction occurs as a rare, isolated entity.

Lelli GJ Jr, Duong JK, Kazim M. Levator excursion as a predictor of both eyelid lag and lagophthalmos in thyroid eye disease. *Ophthal Plast Reconstr Surg.* 2010;26(1):7–10.

Meyer DR, Wobig JL. Detection of contralateral eyelid retraction associated with blepharoptosis. *Ophthalmology.* 1992;99(3):366–375.

## Treatment of Eyelid Retraction

Treatment of eyelid retraction is based on the underlying etiologic factors. Artificial tears, lubricants, and ointments may be sufficient to protect the cornea and minimize symptoms in cases of mild eyelid retraction. Mild eyelid retraction following lower blepharoplasty or in TED often resolves spontaneously with time. A variety of surgical techniques have been developed to correct eyelid retraction that persists or that causes an immediate threat to vision or the cornea. Unless there is severe exposure keratopathy, surgical intervention is indicated only after serial measurements have established stability of the disease over at least 6 months. Upper eyelid retraction can be corrected by excision or recession of the Müller muscle (anterior or posterior approach), recession of the levator aponeurosis with or without hang-back sutures or other spacer, measured myotomy of the levator muscle, or full-thickness transverse blepharotomy. Upper eyelid spacers include fascia lata, donor sclera, ear cartilage, or alloplastic materials.

If the patient has lateral flare (common in TED), a small eyelid-splitting lateral tarsorrhaphy combined with recession of the upper and lower eyelid retractors can improve the upper eyelid contour. This technique may limit the patient's lateral visual field.

As with correction of the upper eyelids, surgical correction of lower eyelid retraction is directed by the underlying etiologic factors. *Anterior lamellar deficiency* (eg, excess skin resection from blepharoplasty) requires recruitment of vertical skin by means of a midface-lift or addition of skin with a full-thickness skin graft. *Middle lamellar deficiency* (eg, posttraumatic septal scarring) requires scar release and possible placement of a spacer graft. *Posterior lamellar deficiency* from congenital scarring or conjunctival shortage (eg, mucous membrane pemphigoid) may require a full-thickness mucous membrane graft. In TED, the etiology of lower eyelid retraction is multifactorial.

Severe retraction of the lower eyelids, common in patients with TED, may require a spacer graft between the lower eyelid retractors and the inferior tarsal border. Autogenous auricular cartilage, hard-palate mucosa, and dermis fat are good spacer materials for this type of surgery. Preserved sclera and fascia lata have also been used, as well as materials such as processed collagens. Some form of horizontal eyelid or lateral canthal tightening or elevation is also often necessary. However, because horizontal tightening of the lower eyelid in a patient with proptosis may exacerbate the eyelid retraction, this technique requires caution.

Bartley GB. The differential diagnosis and classification of eyelid retraction. *Ophthalmology.* 1996;103(1):168–176.

Ben Simon GJ, Mansury AM, Schwarcz RM, Modjtahedi S, McCann JD, Goldberg RA. Transconjunctival Müller muscle recession with levator disinsertion for correction of eyelid retraction associated with thyroid-related orbitopathy. *Am J Ophthalmol.* 2005;140(1):94–99 [comment in *Am J Ophthalmol.* 2006;141(1):233; author reply 233–234].

Demirci H, Hassan AS, Reck SD, Frueh BR, Elner VM. Graded full-thickness anterior blepharotomy for correction of upper eyelid retraction not associated with thyroid eye disease. *Ophthal Plast Reconstr Surg.* 2007;23(1):39–45.

Kersten RC, Kulwin DR, Levartovsky S, Tiradellis H, Tse DT. Management of lower-lid retraction with hard-palate mucosa grafting. *Arch Ophthalmol.* 1990;108(9):1339–1343.

Korn BS, Kikkawa DO, Cohen SR, Hartstein M, Annunziata CC. Treatment of lower eyelid malposition with dermis fat grafting. *Ophthalmology.* 2008;115(4):744–751.

## Facial Paralysis

### Paralytic Ectropion

Paralytic ectropion usually follows CN VII paralysis or palsy. Concomitant upper eyelid lagophthalmos is usually present secondary to paralytic upper eyelid orbicularis dysfunction. Poor blinking and eyelid closure lead to chronic ocular surface irritation from corneal exposure, as well as poor tear film replenishment and distribution. Chronically stimulated reflex tear secretion along with atonic eyelids and lacrimal pump failure account for the frequent report of tearing in these patients.

Neurologic evaluation may be indicated to determine the cause of the CN VII paralysis. In cases resulting from stroke or intracranial surgery, clinical evaluation of corneal sensation is indicated because neurotrophic keratopathy combined with paralytic lagophthalmos results in increased risk of corneal decompensation.

Lubricating drops, viscous tear supplementation, ointments, taping of the temporal half of the lower eyelid, or moisture chambers may be used alone or in combination. Such measures may be the only treatment necessary, especially for temporary paralysis. For cases of long-term or permanent paralysis of the lower eyelid, tarsorrhaphy, medial or lateral canthoplasties, skin grafts, suspension procedures, and horizontal tightening procedures are useful in selected patients.

Tarsorrhaphies can be performed either medially or laterally. An adequate temporary tarsorrhaphy (1–3 weeks) can be achieved with placement of nonabsorbable sutures between the upper and lower eyelid margins. A temporary tarsorrhaphy may also be created by injection of botulinum toxin to the levator muscle. A permanent tarsorrhaphy involves de-epithelialization of the upper and lower eyelid margins, with the lash follicles avoided. Absorbable or nonabsorbable sutures are then placed to unite the raw surfaces of the upper and lower eyelids (Fig 11-19). In general, patients dislike the permanent tarsorrhaphy from a functional and cosmetic perspective. This procedure should be avoided, except in patients with recalcitrant corneal disease from exposure. Placement of a gold

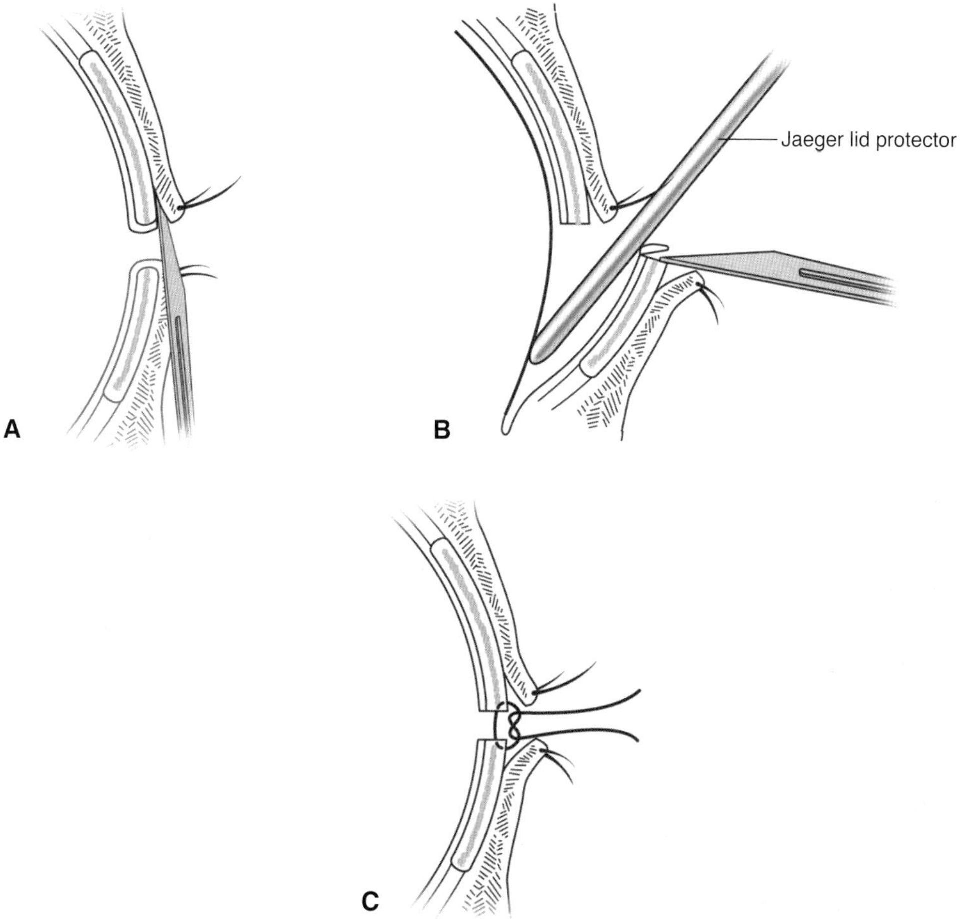


**Figure 11-19** Tarsorrhaphy. **A,** The eyelid is split 2–3 mm deep. **B,** Epithelium is carefully removed along the upper and lower eyelid margins; the lash follicles are avoided. **C,** The raw surfaces are then united with absorbable sutures. *(Illustration by Christine Gralapp.)*

weight in the upper eyelid and repair of horizontal eyelid laxity or ectropion of the lower lid may allow the patient to avoid permanent tarsorrhaphy.

Occasionally, a fascia lata or silicone suspension sling of the lower eyelid may be indicated. Vertical elevation of the lower eyelid is useful in reducing exposure of the inferior cornea. This elevation may be accomplished through recession of the lower lid retractors, combined with use of a spacer graft such as full-thickness hard-palate mucosal or ear cartilage graft. Surgical midface elevation can play an important role in lower eyelid support.

### Upper Eyelid Paralysis

Placement of a weight in the upper eyelid remains the most commonly performed procedure for the treatment of paralytic lagophthalmos. The appropriate weight can be selected through a process of preoperatively taping gold weights of different sizes to the upper eyelid skin to determine which one best achieves adequate relaxed eyelid closure with minimal eyelid ptosis in primary gaze. To implant the weight, the surgeon makes an upper eyelid crease incision through skin and orbicularis muscle. The gold weight is then sutured to the anterior surface of the tarsal plate. The gold weight implant (average weight, 0.8–1.6 g) reduces but does not usually eliminate lagophthalmos and corneal exposure. Should orbicularis function return, the weight is easily removed. A 1.2–2.2-g gold weight can also be placed behind the orbital septum, superior to the tarsus, to avoid thickening of the pretarsal area if cosmesis is a concern. Alternate materials such as platinum can also be used. Implanted eyelid springs, though initially useful to provide dynamic eyelid closure, are less commonly used because of long-term extrusion. Once ocular surface protection has been secured, brow ptosis repair and blepharoplasty may be indicated to clear the visual axis.

Tower RN, Dailey RA. Gold weight implantation: a better way? *Ophthal Plast Reconstr Surg.* 2004;20(3):202–206.

Townsend DJ. Eyelid reanimation for the treatment of paralytic lagophthalmos: historical perspectives and current applications of the gold weight implant. *Ophthal Plast Reconstr Surg.* 1992;8(3):196–201.

## Facial Dystonia

### Benign Essential Blepharospasm

Benign essential blepharospasm (BEB) is a bilateral focal dystonia that affects approximately 30 of every 100,000 people. The condition is characterized by increased blinking and involuntary spasms of the periocular protractor muscles. The spasms generally start as mild twitches and progress over time to forceful contractures. Other muscles of the face may also be involved with blepharospasm. Unlike hemifacial spasm, BEB spasms typically abate during sleep. The involuntary episodes of forced blinking or contracture may severely limit the patient's ability to drive, read, or perform activities of daily living. This condition can progress until the patient is functionally blind as a result of episodic inability to open the eyelids. Women are affected more frequently than men. The age of onset is usually older than 40 years. BEB is a clinical diagnosis, and neuroimaging is generally unrevealing and rarely indicated in the workup. Dry eye syndrome and other medical conditions may result in reflex blepharospasm and must be differentiated from BEB.

The cause of BEB is unknown; however, it is probably of central origin, in the basal ganglia. BEB can be managed by medical or surgical approaches. Medical treatment options may include devices called *eyelid crutches,* which are attached to eyeglass frames. Oral medications have some limited usefulness. Neurotoxin injections are the primary treatment for blepharospasm.

Anderson RL, Patel BC, Holds JB, Jordan DR. Blepharospasm: past, present, and future. *Ophthal Plast Reconstr Surg.* 1998;14(5):305–317.

Ross AH, Elston JS, Marion MH, Malhotra R. Review and update of involuntary facial movement disorders presenting in the ophthalmological setting. *Surv Ophthalmol.* 2011; 56(1):54–67.

#### *Botulinum toxin injection*

Repeated periodic injection of a botulinum toxin type A is the treatment of choice for BEB. Injection of these agents at therapeutic doses results in chemical denervation and localized muscle paralysis. Botulinum toxin injection is typically effective, but the improvement is temporary. Average onset of action is in 2–3 days, and average peak effect occurs at about 7–10 days following injection. Duration of effect also varies but is typically 3–4 months, at which point recurrence of the spasms and need for reinjection is anticipated (Fig 11-20). Complications associated with botulinum toxin injection include

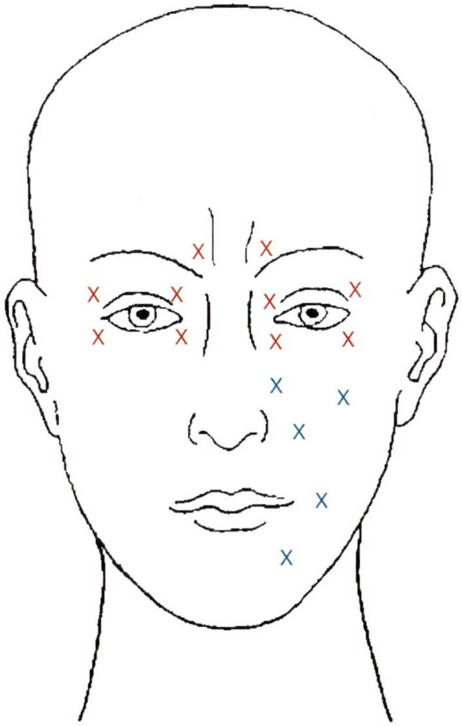

**Figure 11-20** Injection pattern of neurotoxin type A for benign essential blepharospasm *(red)* and hemifacial spasm *(unilateral red sites plus blue).* *(Modified from Dutton JJ, Fowler AM. Botulinum toxin in ophthalmology.* Focal Points: Clinical Modules for Ophthalmologists. *San Francisco: American Academy of Ophthalmology; 2007, module 3.)*

bruising, blepharoptosis, ectropion, epiphora, diplopia, lagophthalmos, and corneal exposure. These adverse reactions are usually transient and result from spread of the toxin to adjacent muscles.

Dutton JJ, Fowler AM. Botulinum toxin in ophthalmology. *Focal Points: Clinical Modules for Ophthalmologists.* San Francisco: American Academy of Ophthalmology; 2007, module 3.

#### *Surgical myectomy*

Treatment with surgical myectomy is reserved for patients who are poorly responsive to botulinum therapy and incapacitated by the spasms. Meticulous removal of the orbital and palpebral orbicularis muscle in the upper (and sometimes lower) eyelids is an effective and permanent treatment for blepharospasm. Complications of surgical myectomy include lagophthalmos, chronic lymphedema, recurrence of spasm, and periorbital contour deformities. More limited myectomy is helpful in patients with less severe disease and may result in improved responsiveness to botulinum toxin therapy.

Many patients with BEB have an associated dry eye condition that may be aggravated by any treatment modality that decreases eyelid closure. Artificial tears, ointments, punctal plugs or occlusion, moisture chamber shields, and tinted spectacle lenses may help minimize discomfort from ocular surface problems.

Pariseau B, Worley MW, Anderson RL. Myectomy for blepharospasm 2013. *Curr Opin Ophthalmol.* 2013;24(5):488–493.

#### *Surgical ablation of the facial nerve*

Though effective in treating BEB, selective facial neurectomy has been largely abandoned. Recurrence rates as high as 30% and frequent hemifacial paralysis from facial nerve dissection limit this treatment's appeal. The results obtained with facial nerve dissection are, therefore, less satisfactory than those of direct orbicularis oculi myectomy. Some surgeons have had greater success with microsurgical ablation of selected branches of the facial nerve.

Fante RG, Frueh BR. Differential section of the seventh nerve as a tertiary procedure for the treatment of benign essential blepharospasm. *Ophthal Plast Reconstr Surg.* 2001;17(4): 276–280.

#### *Muscle relaxants and sedatives*

Muscle relaxants and sedatives are rarely effective in the primary treatment of BEB. Oral medications such as orphenadrine, lorazepam, or clonazepam are sometimes effective in suppressing mild cases of BEB, prolonging the interval between botulinum toxin injections, or helping to dampen lower facial dystonia (Meige syndrome) associated with BEB. Psychotherapy has little or no value for the patient with blepharospasm.

### Hemifacial Spasm

Blepharospasm should be differentiated from hemifacial spasm (HFS). HFS is characterized by intermittent synchronous gross contractures of the entire side of the face and is rarely bilateral. HFS often begins in the periocular region and then progresses to involve the entire face. Unlike BEB, however, the spasms are present during sleep. HFS is often associated with ipsilateral facial nerve weakness. In most cases, the cause of HFS is a vascular compression of the facial nerve at the brain stem. Magnetic resonance imaging (MRI) often documents the ectatic vessel. MRI also helps rule out other cerebellopontine angle lesions that may be the cause in less than 1% of cases. Neurosurgical decompression of the facial nerve may be curative in HFS, but it exposes the patient to the relative risk of neurosurgical intervention. Periodic injection of botulinum toxin is a commonly used, effective treatment option for HFS. Oral medications, including drugs with membrane-stabilizing properties such as carbamazepine and clonazepam, are used less frequently because of their low efficacy.

Aberrant regeneration after facial nerve palsy also presents with hemifacial contracture and aberrant synkinetic facial movements. The history (eg, previous Bell palsy, trauma) and clinical examination are distinctive. Functionally troublesome synkinetic facial movements often respond well to botulinum toxin injection at very low doses to selected facial muscle groups.

## Involutional Periorbital Changes

### Dermatochalasis

Dermatochalasis refers to redundancy of eyelid skin and is often associated with orbital fat prolapse. Though more common in senescent patients, dermatochalasis also occurs in middle-aged persons, particularly if there is a familial predisposition. It may also accompany true ptosis of the upper eyelids (Fig 11-21).

Significant dermatochalasis of the upper eyelids leads to reports of a heavy feeling around the eyes, brow ache, eyelashes in the visual axis, and, eventually, reduction in the superior visual field. Dermatochalasis is often made worse by associated brow ptosis, especially if patients do not use their frontalis muscle to elevate the brows to relieve visual obscuration by the excess skin. Lower eyelid dermatochalasis is considered a cosmetic

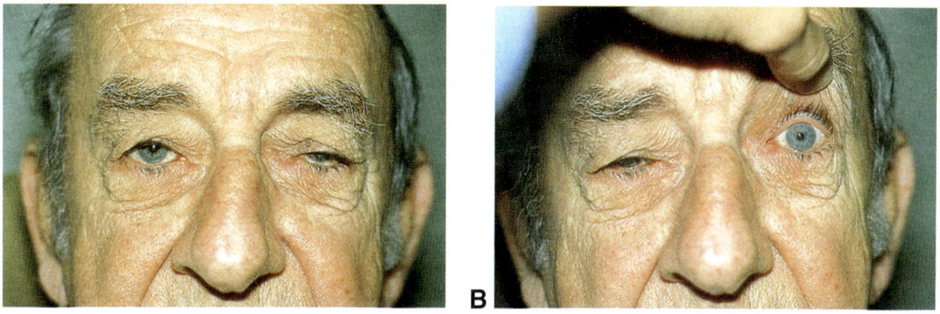

A B

**Figure 11-21** **A,** Patient with bilateral asymmetric drooping due to blepharoptosis and dermatochalasis. **B,** Elevation of more ptotic left upper eyelid reveals increased blepharoptosis on right, which had been masked by the effect of Hering's law of equal innervation to each levator muscle. *(Courtesy of Robert C. Kersten, MD.)*

issue unless the excess skin and prolapsed fat are so severe that the patient cannot be fitted with bifocals.

### Blepharochalasis

Although blepharochalasis is not an involutional change, it is included in this discussion because it can simulate, and must be differentiated from, dermatochalasis. Blepharochalasis is a rare familial variant of angioneurotic edema. It typically occurs in younger persons, most commonly young females, and is characterized by idiopathic episodes of inflammatory edema of the eyelids. As a result of recurrent bouts of inflammation and edema, the eyelid skin of a patient with blepharochalasis becomes thin and wrinkled, simulating the appearance of dermatochalasis. In addition, true ptosis, herniation of the orbital lobe of the lacrimal gland, atrophy of the orbital fat pads, and prominent eyelid vascularity may be associated with blepharochalasis. Surgical repair of the eyelid-skin changes and the ptosis that result from blepharochalasis may be complicated by repeated episodes of inflammation and edema, causing recurrence of the ptosis and other eyelid changes.

Koursh DM, Modjtahedi SP, Selva D, Leibovitch I. The blepharochalasis syndrome. *Surv Ophthalmol.* 2009;54(2):235–244.

## Blepharoplasty

### Upper Eyelid

Upper eyelid blepharoplasty is one of the most commonly performed *functional* as well as *cosmetic* oculoplastic surgical procedures (Video 11-5). Involutional skin and structural changes often begin in the periorbital area, and they can obstruct the superior visual field. Blepharoplasty is frequently performed to relieve this obstruction. Brow ptosis may also play a role and may need to be addressed. Functional indications for blepharoplasty are documented by means of external photography and visual field testing with and without manual eyelid elevation. Patients undergoing blepharoplasty for cosmetic reasons may have different expectations than patients undergoing functional blepharoplasty. Thus, a thorough preoperative discussion of the anticipated results is critical to preoperative planning.

**VIDEO 11-5** Upper eyelid blepharoplasty (01:53).
*Courtesy of Jill Foster, MD; Dan Straka, MD; and Craig Czyz, DO.*

### Lower Eyelid

Lower eyelid blepharoplasty is most commonly performed for cosmetic indications, although some patients undergo this procedure because of functional concerns such as difficulty reading, which can occur when prolapsed orbital fat and skin cover the bifocal spectacle segment. For cosmetic lower lid surgery, satisfactory results often require skin rejuvenation with skin removal, chemical peels, or laser resurfacing in addition to surgical alterations of periocular structure. In the preoperative discussion, the surgeon should clearly describe reasonable expectations as well as the risks of the procedure. Patients should understand that aggressive resection of lower eyelid skin and fat may lead to eyelid retraction; ectropion; or a sunken, aged periorbital appearance.

## Preoperative Evaluation for Blepharoplasty

Evaluation of any potential blepharoplasty patient should include the following:

- a complete ocular examination, including visual acuity testing and documentation
- a history of prior periocular surgery
- identification of amount and areas of excess skin, as well as the amount and contours of prolapsed orbital fat, in the upper and lower eyelids
- presence or absence of lagophthalmos, which can lead to postoperative dryness and exposure keratopathy
- assessment of orbital bone contours and discussion of findings with the patient
- evaluation of tear secretion or the tear film, which may be carried out through Schirmer testing, tear breakup time, or assessment of the adequacy of the tear meniscus
- detailed discussion of anticipated surgical results as well as possible surgical complications
- photographic documentation

### *Upper blepharoplasty*

In addition to the assessments previously discussed, physical examination before upper blepharoplasty should include the following elements:

- if needed for documentation, visual field testing to determine the presence and degree of superior visual field defects
- evaluation of the forehead and eyebrows (including brow height and contour) to detect forehead and eyebrow ptosis; the surgeon should make careful observations when the patient's facial and brow musculature is relaxed
- notation of the position of the upper eyelid crease

### *Lower blepharoplasty*

Preoperative examination for lower blepharoplasty should further include

- testing of the elasticity (snapback test) and distractibility of the lower eyelid; the surgeon should be alert to the need for possible horizontal tightening of the lower eyelids as part of the lower blepharoplasty procedure
- notation and discussion of prominent orbital rims, if present; malar hypoplasia or relative exophthalmos may predispose the patient to postoperative scleral show following lower blepharoplasty

Cahill KV, Bradley EA, Meyer DR, et al. Functional indications for upper eyelid ptosis and blepharoplasty surgery: a report by the American Academy of Ophthalmology. *Ophthalmology.* 2011;118(12):2510–2517.

## Techniques

A thorough working knowledge of periorbital and eyelid anatomy (discussed in Chapter 9) is essential for successful blepharoplasty. In addition, just as the brow and glabellar areas affect the upper eyelids, the midfacial structures are influential in the position, tone, contour, and function of the lower eyelid and must be considered in the planning of lower eyelid surgery.

Surgical preparation involves marking excess skin for excision prior to infiltration of local anesthetic. The surgeon may determine the amount of excess skin to be excised by grasping the upper eyelid skin with toothless forceps and identifying the amount of redundancy (pinch technique). To avoid excessive skin removal, the surgeon usually leaves at least 20 mm of skin remaining between the inferior border of the brow and the upper eyelid margin (Fig 11-22).

### *Upper blepharoplasty*

Upper blepharoplasty begins with the surgeon incising along the lines marked on the upper eyelid. The skin and underlying orbicularis oculi muscle can be excised as a single flap or in stages. In patients with dry eye syndrome, the surgeon should consider preservation of the orbicularis oculi muscle to minimize the development of lagophthalmos. The surgeon removes skin and then may selectively remove orbicularis and orbital fat to reshape the upper eyelid. Adjunctive procedures to re-form the eyelid crease and reposition the lacrimal gland may be necessary.

### *Lower blepharoplasty*

Lower eyelid blepharoplasty can be accomplished through a transconjunctival incision or a transcutaneous, infraciliary incision (Video 11-6). The transconjunctival approach offers a lower rate of postoperative eyelid retraction and absence of a postoperative scar. When skin removal is necessary, the infraciliary incision is used. The preoperative evaluation defines the extent and location of lower eyelid fat prolapse and thus determines the boundaries of surgical excision. During lower blepharoplasty, the surgeon is aware of the location of the inferior oblique muscle, which is between the nasal and central fat pads, to

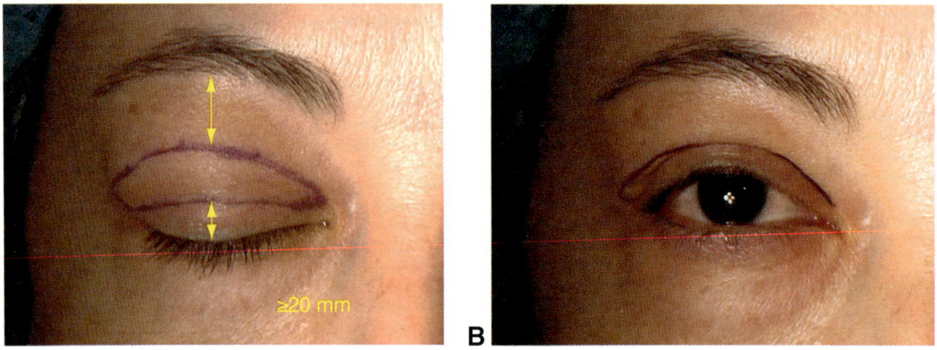


A B

**Figure 11-22** **A,** Typical skin marking for upper eyelid blepharoplasty. After skin marking, there should be at least 20 mm of remaining upper eyelid skin (sum of the distance indicated by the yellow arrows). **B,** With the eyes open, the upper and lower blepharoplasty markings are superimposed. *(Courtesy of Bobby S. Korn, MD, PhD.)*

avoid damaging this muscle. As in the upper eyelid, the medial fat pad of the lower eyelid is less yellow than the lateral fat pads. The central fat compartment is separated from the lateral fat compartment by the arcuate expansion of the inferior oblique muscle; removal or incision of this arcuate expansion may improve access to the lateral fat pad. The surgeon removes or repositions the fat. If the preoperative evaluation of lower lid horizontal laxity (see Fig 11-2A) has determined that tightening of the lower eyelid is required, surgical techniques for horizontal tightening or resuspension are employed (see Fig 11-2B). After structural alteration of the lower eyelid (eg, fat removal, fat transposition, midface resuspension, horizontal eyelid tightening), the need for conservative lower eyelid skin removal is addressed. The surgeon can ask the patient to open the eyes and mouth as far as possible and then assess the lower eyelid to see whether redundant skin is still present. Aggressive skin removal during lower blepharoplasty increases the risk of lower eyelid contour abnormalities, retraction, and ectropion. This risk can be minimized with conservative skin removal and lower eyelid tightening. Alternatively, excess skin can be tightened without excision through application of laser skin resurfacing or through chemical peeling.

**VIDEO 11-6** Lower lid blepharoplasty (08:43).
*Reproduced with permission from Korn BS, Kikkawa DO, eds.* Video Atlas of Oculofacial Plastic and Reconstructive Surgery. *Philadelphia: Elsevier/Saunders; 2011.*

Fagien S, Putterman AM, eds. *Putterman's Cosmetic Oculoplastic Surgery.* 4th ed. Philadelphia: Saunders; 2008.

Korn BS, Kikkawa DO, eds. *Video Atlas of Oculofacial Plastic and Reconstructive Surgery.* Philadelphia: Elsevier/Saunders; 2011.

## Complications

*Loss of vision* is the most dreaded complication of blepharoplasty. Almost every reported case of post blepharoplasty vision loss has been associated with *lower* blepharoplasty. Although blindness following eyelid surgery is rare, it has been reported. Such blindness is typically thought to occur secondary to postoperative retrobulbar hemorrhage, with the increased intraorbital pressure causing ischemic compression of the ciliary arteries supplying the optic nerve. Other mechanisms of injury may also be present, including ischemia caused by excessive surgical retraction or constriction of retrobulbar blood vessels in response to epinephrine in the local anesthetic. Orbital hemorrhage may result from injury to the deeper orbital blood vessels or from bleeding anteriorly. Risk factors for this complication are TED, blood dyscrasias, and anticoagulant use. Postoperative pressure dressings should be avoided: they increase orbital pressure and obscure underlying problems. Finally, patients should be observed immediately postoperatively so that orbital hemorrhage is detected. Patients reporting significant pain, marked asymmetric swelling, or proptosis following surgery are evaluated urgently. Visual dimming, darkness, or significant or asymmetric blurred vision following eyelid surgery may also be indicative of orbital hemorrhage and should be assessed and treated immediately.

Vision loss from orbital hemorrhage is an ophthalmic emergency. When compressive hemorrhage occurs in the orbit, the surgeon may decompress the orbit by opening the surgical wounds, performing lateral canthotomy with cantholysis, or performing peritomy, and by administering high doses of intravenous corticosteroids. Anterior chamber paracentesis has no role in the management of orbital hemorrhage. In addition, medical glaucoma management is not useful because the increased intra*ocular* pressure is caused by increased underlying intra*orbital* pressure. Lack of immediate response to these procedures may necessitate surgical decompression of the orbit.

*Diplopia* secondary to injury of extraocular muscles is another serious complication of blepharoplasty. Diplopia may result from injury to the inferior oblique, the inferior rectus, or the superior oblique muscle. The inferior oblique muscle originates in the anterior orbital floor lateral to the lacrimal sac and travels posterolaterally within the lower eyelid retractors. It separates the central and medial fat pads of the lower eyelid and courses across them; thus, the inferior oblique may be injured during removal of lower eyelid fatty tissue. The trochlea of the superior oblique muscle also may be injured by deep dissection in orbital fat in the superior nasal aspect of the upper eyelid.

*Excessive removal of skin* is a complication that can lead to lagophthalmos of the upper eyelids as well as cicatricial ectropion or retraction of the lower eyelids. Topical lubricants and massage may be helpful for managing mild postoperative lagophthalmos, retraction, or ectropion, all of which may resolve over time without further intervention. Injectable steroids or 5-fluorouracil can be used if a deep cicatrix contributes to the retraction. Severe cases require the use of free skin grafts, lateral canthoplasty, or release of scar tissue or eyelid retractors. Inferior scleral show can also result from septal scarring, orbicularis hematoma, and malar hypoplasia, even when no skin has been excised.

Mauriello JA. Upper blepharoplasty. In: Dunn JP, Langer PD, eds. *Basic Techniques of Ophthalmic Surgery.* San Francisco: American Academy of Ophthalmology; 2009:378–383.

Whipple KM, Korn BS, Kikkawa DO. Recognizing and managing complications in blepharoplasty. *Facial Plast Surg Clin North Am.* 2013;21(4):625–637.

## Brow Ptosis

Loss of elastic tissues and facial volume as well as involutional changes of the forehead skin lead to drooping of the forehead and eyebrows. This condition is known as *brow ptosis.* Severe brow ptosis may also result from facial nerve palsy. Brow ptosis frequently accompanies dermatochalasis and must be recognized as a factor that contributes to the appearance of aging in the periorbital area. Brow ptosis may become severe enough to affect the superior visual field. The patient often involuntarily compensates for this condition by using the frontalis muscle to elevate the eyebrows (Fig 11-23). Such chronic contracture of the frontalis muscle often leads to brow ache, headache, and prominent transverse forehead rhytids.

In most individuals, the brow is located above the superior orbital rim. Generally, the female brow is higher and more arched than is the typical male brow. The brow is considered ptotic when it falls below the superior orbital rim.

### Treatment of Functional Brow Ptosis

Brow ptosis should be recognized and treated prior to or concomitant with the surgical repair of coexisting dermatochalasis of the eyelids. Because brow elevation reduces the

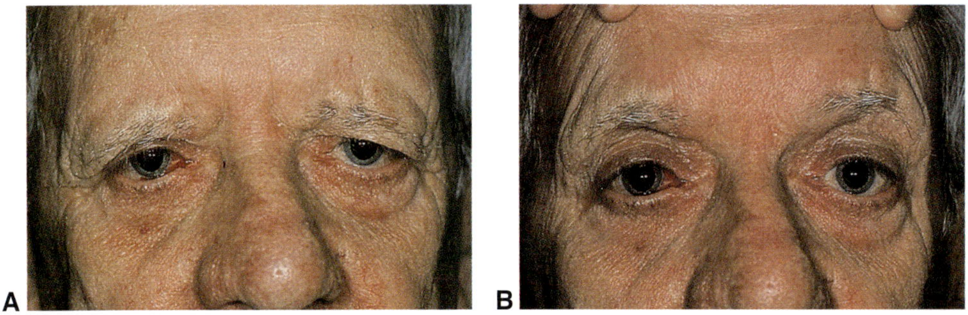

**Figure 11-23** Brow ptosis. **A,** Natural position of the brow below the superior orbital rim. **B,** With manual elevation to clear the visual axis.

amount of dermatochalasis present, it should be performed or simulated first when combined with upper blepharoplasty. Aggressive upper blepharoplasty alone in a patient with concomitant brow ptosis leads to further depression of the brow. Functional brow ptosis may be corrected with browpexy, direct brow-lift, or endoscopic or pretrichial brow-lift. (See the subsection titled "Pretrichial approach.")

### *Browpexy*

Browpexy is used for treatment of mild brow ptosis and is performed through an upper eyelid blepharoplasty incision. The sub-brow tissues are resuspended with sutures to the frontal bone periosteum above the orbital rim as part of a blepharoplasty. This procedure provides minimal improvement in brow position, but it may help prevent the retro-orbicularis oculi fat (ROOF) from descending into the eyelid.

McCord CD, Doxanas MT. Browplasty and browpexy: an adjunct to blepharoplasty. *Plast Reconstr Surg.* 1990;86(2):248–254.

### *Direct eyebrow elevation*

The eyebrows can be elevated with incisions placed at the upper edge of the eyebrow. This is an effective technique for treatment of functional brow ptosis and is particularly useful for men and women with lateral brow ptosis. When direct eyebrow elevation is used across the entire brow, it may result in an arch or scar. Sensory paresthesias may be an adverse effect of the direct brow procedure.

Booth AJ, Murray A, Tyers AG. The direct brow lift: efficacy, complications, and patient satisfaction. *Br J Ophthalmol.* 2004;88(5):688–691.

Miller TA, Rudkin G, Honig M, Elahi M, Adams J. Lateral subcutaneous brow lift and interbrow muscle resection: clinical experience and anatomic studies. *Plast Reconstr Surg.* 2000;105(3):1120–1127 [discussion, 1128].

## Facial Rejuvenation

The human face is an essential component of interpersonal communication. The face is composed of smaller cosmetic units of the forehead, eyelids, cheek, nose, and lips; and the neck is inextricably linked to facial appearance. As we age, one or more of these cosmetic units undergo changes that lead to facial imbalance, disharmony, and possibly miscommunication. The aging face may communicate fatigue, depression, anger, or fear in an otherwise well-rested, well-adjusted, fully functioning person.

Before a patient undergoes cosmetic facial surgery, the surgeon performs a comprehensive oculofacial evaluation that includes consideration of the upper, middle, and lower face. If only one subunit has aged out of proportion to the rest of the face, as in dermatochalasis, an isolated repair with a bilateral upper blepharoplasty can produce a nice result. On the other hand, if the patient has concomitant aging changes of the midface, lower face, and neck, these should be addressed in concert to ensure harmonious facial balance. In the United States, fellowship programs in oculofacial plastic surgery include training in all aspects of facial cosmetic and reconstructive surgery. While it is important for any eyelid surgeon to understand the surgical procedures discussed here, the performance of these procedures generally requires special training, experience, and expertise.

## Pathogenesis of the Aging Face

The facial contours and appearance are derived from soft tissue draped over underlying bone. The soft-tissue component is composed of skin, subcutaneous fat, muscle, deeper fat pads, and fascial layers. The underlying structural element is composed of bone, cartilage, and teeth.

As the face ages, the soft-tissue component moves inferiorly and the bone component loses mass. These changes leave relatively more soft tissue to hang from its attachments to the bone. Loss of subcutaneous fat, skin atrophy, and descent of facial fat pads compound this facial sagging. Around the eyes, the lateral brow typically descends more than the medial brow, which leads to temporal hooding. The orbital septum stretches, bulges, or dehisces, allowing fat to prolapse forward. In the lower eyelid, midface descent produces the skeletonization of the infraorbital rim and increases the prominence of the orbital fat. This has been described as a *double-convexity deformity,* and it also contributes to the increased prominence of the nasolabial fold. Sagging of the platysma muscle in the neck posterior to the mandibular ligament gives rise to jowling. The *turkey gobbler defect* in the neck is the result of redundant skin and separated medial borders of the platysma muscle at the midline.

## Physical Examination of the Aging Face

Much of the surgeon's appraisal of the aging face can be obtained through close observation of the patient during the introduction and history phase of the initial meeting. From the top, the surgeon should observe the hairstyle and hair thickness, the presence or absence of bangs, and the height of the hairline; the use of the frontalis; the position of the brow; the texture and quality of the facial skin; and the presence and location of rhytids, telangiectasias, pigmentary dyschromia, and expressive furrows.

If chemical peeling or laser skin resurfacing is being considered, the surgeon should also note the patient's Fitzpatrick skin type, which affects response to these procedures. There are 6 skin types in the Fitzpatrick classification system, which denotes skin color and reaction of the skin to sun exposure. The higher the number, the greater the amount of skin pigment. Thus, Fitzpatrick type I refers to persons with minimal skin pigment and very fair skin. These individuals always burn with sun exposure and do not tan. Type VI represents individuals with markedly pigmented black skin, typically persons of African ancestry.

In addition, the surgeon should assess eyelid skin and fat along with eyelid margin position relative to the pupil and cornea, presence or absence of horizontal lower lid laxity, midface position, presence of jowling, accumulation of subcutaneous fat in the neck, and chin position. He or she should note any nasal deformities and tip descent and broadening, as well as thinning of the lips. The surgeon may find a side view of the neck to be particularly helpful in determining the extent of aging. Preoperative photographs should be available in the operating room.

## Nonsurgical Facial Rejuvenation

Nonsurgical facial rejuvenation techniques such as laser resurfacing, soft tissue dermal fillers, neurotoxin injection, chemical peels, and microdermabrasion are used to treat involutional and actinic facial skin changes. These relatively superficial procedures may precede or be combined with surgical procedures that reposition deeper structures. It is important to remember that the upper eyelid appearance is inextricably linked to the position of the eyebrow. Similarly, the lower eyelid appearance is linked to the midface as well as the lower face and neck. Subunits of the facial cosmetic superstructure should not be viewed or manipulated individually but must be addressed in the context of the entire face and neck.

### Laser Skin Resurfacing

Laser skin resurfacing, a technology popularized in the early 1990s, is designed to reduce wrinkles and enhance the texture and appearance of the facial and periorbital skin. A variety of lasers have been developed to perform laser resurfacing; superpulsed or ultrapulsed $CO_2$ and erbium:YAG lasers are the most widely used. The development of superpulsed $CO_2$ lasers has allowed ablative skin resurfacing without excessive thermal damage. Superpulsed and ultrapulsed $CO_2$ lasers are designed to deliver small pulses of high-energy light to the skin. Pauses between the pulses allow cooling of the tissues in the treated area, minimizing the risk of thermal damage. The erbium:YAG laser has a nearly pure ablative effect on collagen and water-containing tissues, with a much smaller zone of thermal injury and much less heat transfer into the tissues than the $CO_2$ lasers. Safe and effective laser resurfacing requires special training. Additional understanding of the skin, skin anatomy, laser physics, and perioperative care is crucial to a successful outcome.

Laser resurfacing has been shown to be a useful adjunct to lower blepharoplasty. The skin-shrinking, collagen-tightening effect of laser skin resurfacing often allows the surgeon to avoid making an external incision and removing skin.

Selection of appropriate patients is also critical for successful laser skin resurfacing. Patients with a fair complexion and generally healthy, well-hydrated skin are ideal candidates. Patients with greater degrees of skin pigmentation can be safely treated, but additional care and caution are necessary. The darker the skin pigmentation, the greater the risk of postoperative inflammatory hyperpigmentation. Laser resurfacing is contraindicated in patients who have used isotretinoin within the past 12 months because re-epithelialization is inhibited. Other contraindications include inappropriate, unrealistic expectations, collagen vascular disease such as active systemic lupus erythematosus, and significant uncorrected lower eyelid laxity.

Most surgeons treat patients perioperatively with suppressing doses of antiviral agents as prophylaxis against outbreaks of herpes simplex virus on the laser-resurfaced skin. Herpes simplex virus infection after laser resurfacing may lead to scarring. Other complications of laser skin resurfacing may include a variety of ophthalmic problems such as lagophthalmos, exposure keratitis, corneal injury, ectropion, and lower eyelid retraction.

A desire to improve superficial skin characteristics and facial wrinkling without the prolonged period of healing and erythema seen with ablative laser skin resurfacing has led to the development of devices that use fractionated lasers, intense pulsed light, ultrasound or radiofrequency to deliver energy to the skin. These modalities can potentially even skin tone, remove cutaneous dyschromias or fine wrinkles, and even lift and smooth facial tissues. Each of these devices has its own list of risks and limitations, but they offer some improvement in aspects of facial aging, with fewer risks and shorter recovery times than with ablative laser skin resurfacing.

Aslam A, Alster TS. Evolution of laser skin resurfacing: from scanning to fractional technology. *Dermatol Surg.* 2014;40(11):1163–1172.

Sullivan SA, Dailey RA. Complications of laser resurfacing and their management. *Ophthal Plast Reconstr Surg.* 2000;16(6):417–426.

## Cosmetic Uses of Botulinum Toxin

The use of botulinum toxin in patients with blepharospasm and HFS led to the observation that botulinum toxin reduces or eliminates some facial wrinkles. The first neurotoxin available for aesthetic indications was onabotulinumtoxinA, which already had a long history of ophthalmic use in the treatment of blepharospasm and HFS. In 1992, it was approved by the US Food and Drug Administration (FDA) to temporarily reduce wrinkles in the glabellar area; more recently, it received FDA approval for lateral canthal lines (crow's-feet). AbobotulinumtoxinA, the second neurotoxin available in the US market, is also approved for the treatment of wrinkling in the glabellar area. IncobotulinumtoxinA, the most recent addition, is approved for both cosmetic and medical applications. A number of non–FDA-approved botulinum toxin products are available worldwide; however, US physicians should recognize the significant medicolegal risk of using a non–FDA-approved substance for injection. Also, unit dosing differs among all of these products, requiring that careful adjustments be made when they are used for treating various clinical characteristics

Apart from the glabella, the areas most amenable to neuromodulation are the forehead, lateral canthal lines, perioral rhytids, and platysmal bands. Use of botulinum toxins for cosmetic improvement of areas beyond the glabella and lateral canthus is currently considered off-label. The amount of botulinum toxin required and the location of injections in the forehead and platysmal bands vary significantly among patients and should be individualized.

The eyebrow can be chemically lifted when botulinum toxin is injected into the depressors of the eyebrow. The corners of the mouth can be elevated with injection into the depressor anguli oris muscle. The onset of action, peak effect, duration of effect, and complications of botulinum toxin for cosmetic purposes are the same as those noted earlier for botulinum toxin as therapy for benign essential blepharospasm.

Flynn TC. Botulinum toxin: examining duration of effect in facial aesthetic applications. *Am J Clin Dermatol.* 2010;11(3):183–199.

Lipham WJ. *Cosmetic and Clinical Applications of Botox and Dermal Fillers.* 2nd ed. Thorofare, NJ: SLACK, Inc; 2008.

Lorenc ZP, Kenkel JM, Fagien S, et al. Consensus panel's assessment and recommendations on the use of 3 botulinum toxin type A products in facial aesthetics. *Aesthet Surg J.* 2013; 33(1 Suppl):35S–40S.

## Soft Tissue Dermal Fillers

Many fillers are available for nonsurgical facial rejuvenation. Bovine collagen was initially approved by the FDA in 1995. However, its use required skin testing for allergic reaction to bovine-derived collagen; usage declined with the increased use of hyaluronic acid fillers derived from bacteria. These hyaluronic acid fillers do not require skin or allergy testing, and they have been FDA approved for treatment of wrinkles in the perioral region such as the nasolabial folds (Fig 11-24) and for lip augmentation. Off-label usage of hyaluronic acid fillers for the periocular region has been described extensively in the literature (Fig 11-25), but these fillers must be used with care. Complications from intravascular injection have been reported, including regional soft-tissue necrosis and central retinal artery occlusion. In the case of central retinal artery occlusion, inadvertent high-pressure injection of hyaluronic acid filler into an artery results in retrograde embolization into the central retinal artery (Fig 11-26).

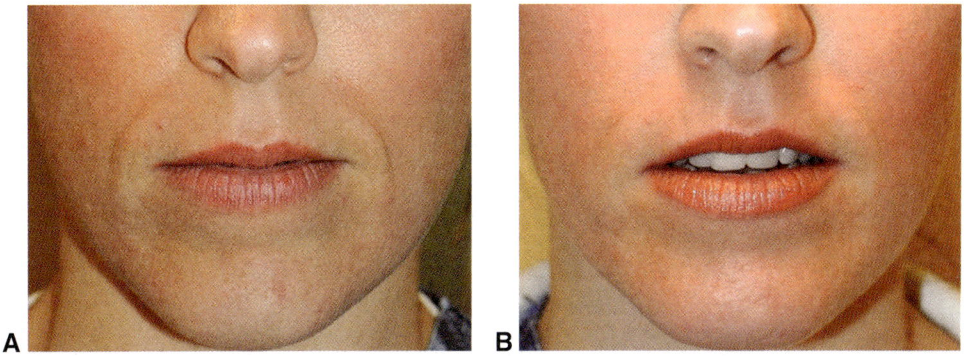


**Figure 11-24** Before **(A)** and after **(B)** injection of a hyaluronic acid filler to the nasolabial folds. *(Courtesy of Bobby S. Korn, MD, PhD.)*

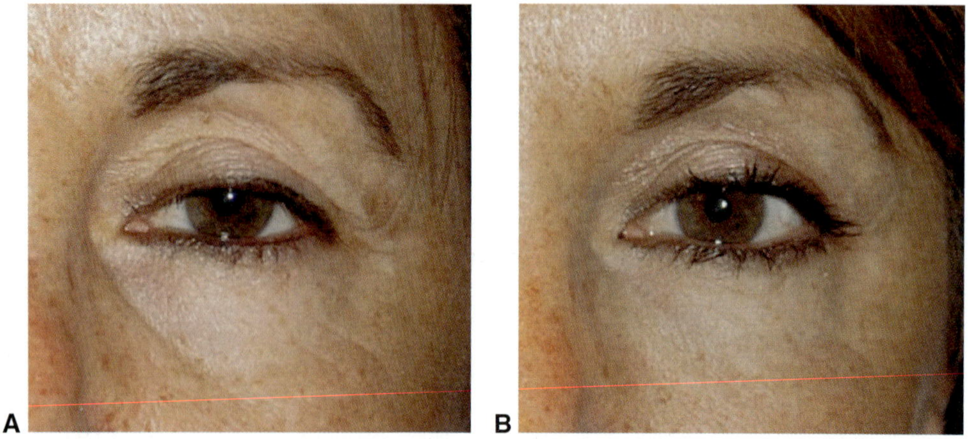

Figure 11-25 Before **(A)** and after **(B)** injection of a hyaluronic acid filler to improve the contour of the lower eyelid. *(Courtesy of Bobby S. Korn, MD, PhD.)*

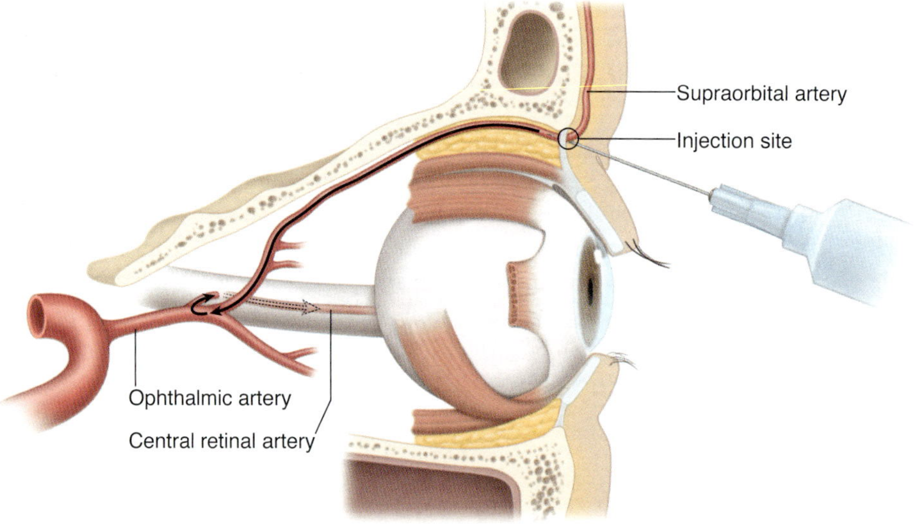


**Figure 11-26** Mechanism for retrograde embolization of the central retinal artery by filler injection. *(Adapted with permission from DeLorenzi C. Complications of injectable fillers, part 2: vascular complications.* Aesthet Surg J. *2014;34(4):584–600. Illustration by Mark M. Miller.)*

Duranti F, Salti G, Bovani B, Calandra M, Rosati ML. Injectable hyaluronic acid gel for soft tissue augmentation. A clinical and histological study. *Dermatol Surg.* 1998;24(12): 1317–1325.

Goldberg RA, Fiaschetti D. Filling the periorbital hollows with hyaluronic acid gel: initial experience with 244 injections. *Ophthal Plast Reconstr Surg.* 2006;22(5):335–341.

Peter S, Mennel S. Retinal branch artery occlusion following injection of hyaluronic acid (Restylane). *Clin Experiment Ophthalmol.* 2006;34(4):363–364.

## Facial Rejuvenation Surgery

Facial and eyelid surgery should be approached with care. Adequate preoperative preparation includes properly informing the patient of the proposed benefit as well as the potential complications of the procedure. Significant complications—including facial nerve paralysis, skin flap necrosis, and vision loss—are potential risks.

Patients should be encouraged to read, understand, and sign an operative consent in the relaxed atmosphere of the ophthalmologist's office, or they can take it home to read. It is preferable to obtain this consent before the day of surgery, as patient anxiety or preoperative medication may make informed consent on the day of surgery difficult or impossible. The patient must have an opportunity to discuss with the surgeon any concerns about the procedure or the operative permit.

Rejuvenation of the aging face requires a multitude of techniques. Chemical peeling, laser resurfacing, dermabrasion, liposculpting, and various other laser treatments can all augment the results following surgical intervention or even make incisional surgery unnecessary.

### Forehead Rejuvenation

Many options are available for forehead rejuvenation, but the following discussion focuses on 2 methods commonly used in cosmetic surgery: the standard endoscopic brow-lift and the pretrichial approach.

#### *Endoscopic brow- and forehead-lift*

Endoscopic techniques allow the surgeon to raise the brow and rejuvenate the forehead (foreheadplasty) through small incisions approximately 1 cm behind the hairline (Fig 11-27). Dissection is accomplished with an endoscopic periosteal elevator, sharp scissors, suction, and monopolar cautery. Key steps are the incisions, creation of an optical cavity, periosteal release at the orbital rim, and fixation of the elevated flap.

Berkowitz RL, Jacobs DI, Gorman PJ. Brow fixation with the Endotine Forehead device in endoscopic brow lift. *Plast Reconstr Surg.* 2005;116(6):1761–1767 [discussion 1768–1770].

Jones BM, Grover R. Endoscopic brow lift: a personal review of 538 patients and comparison of fixation techniques. *Plast Reconstr Surg.* 2004;113(4):1242–1250 [discussion, 1251–1252].

#### *Pretrichial approach*

The pretrichial approach is used in patients who have a high hairline. Access is gained through a pretrichial incision (Fig 11-28) instead of the small skin incisions used with the endoscopic approach. Dissection is performed in the subcutaneous layer. An appropriate amount of forehead skin is resected, and the underlying frontalis and galea are plicated with a subsequent layered closure. The advantages of shortening the forehead are balanced by the adverse effects of a more visible scar and increased scalp paresthesias.

### Midface Rejuvenation

The entire midface should be evaluated in a patient presenting for lower eyelid blepharoplasty. With age, cheek tissue descends and orbital fat herniates, creating the double-convexity

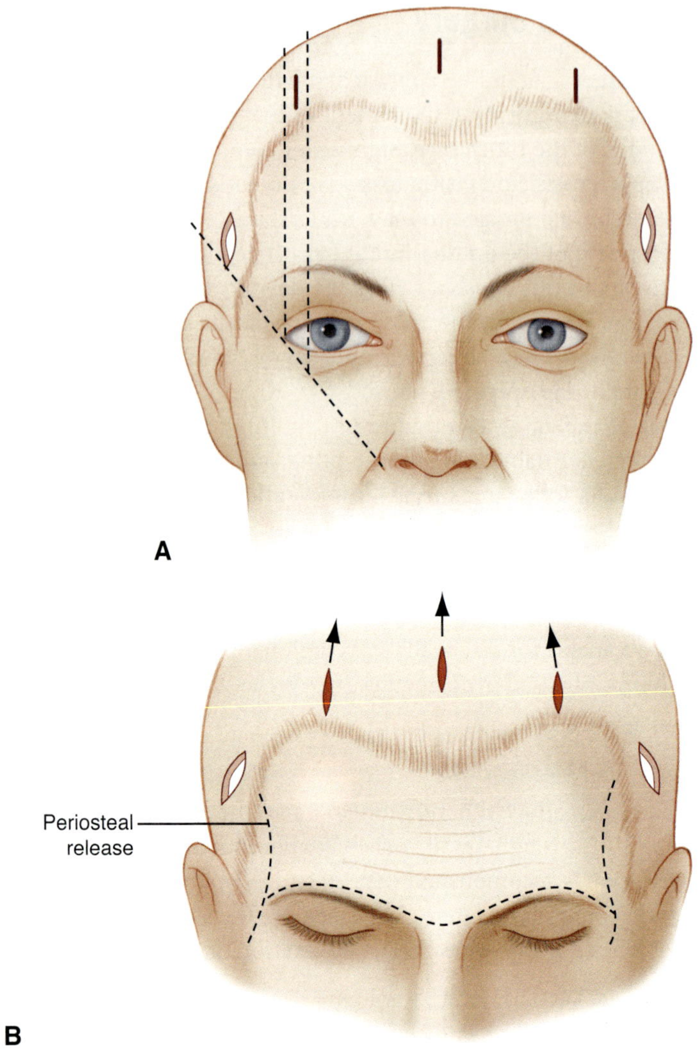


**Figure 11-27** **A,** Incisions for endoscopic forehead lift. **B,** After periosteal release, the scalp is retracted posteriorly and fixated in the 2 paracentral incisions with a fixation screw or drilled bone tunnel. *(Illustration by Christine Gralapp.)*

deformity. Attenuation of the orbitomalar, masseteric cutaneous, and zygomatic ligaments are the pathologic changes that occur with midfacial ptosis. Varying degrees of elevation of the suborbicularis oculi fat (SOOF) and midface, combined with conservative transconjunctival fat removal or redistribution, can restore youthful anterior projection of the midface, rendering a single smooth contour to the lower eyelid and midface region.

Midface elevation can be achieved through a preperiosteal (Fig 11-29) or subperiosteal approach. The preperiosteal plane can be accessed through the lower eyelid, with or without release of the lateral canthal tendon; or by using the temporal scalp incision

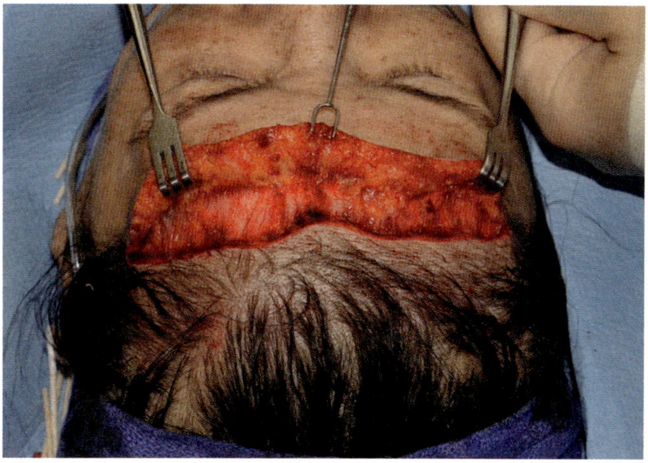

**Figure 11-28** Pretrichial incision used for forehead and brow elevation. The advantages of this incision are elevation of the brow without elevation of the hairline, a relatively well-hidden scar, and no need for endoscopic equipment. The disadvantage is a relatively high incidence of postoperative sensory paresthesias. *(Courtesy of Bobby S. Korn, MD, PhD.)*

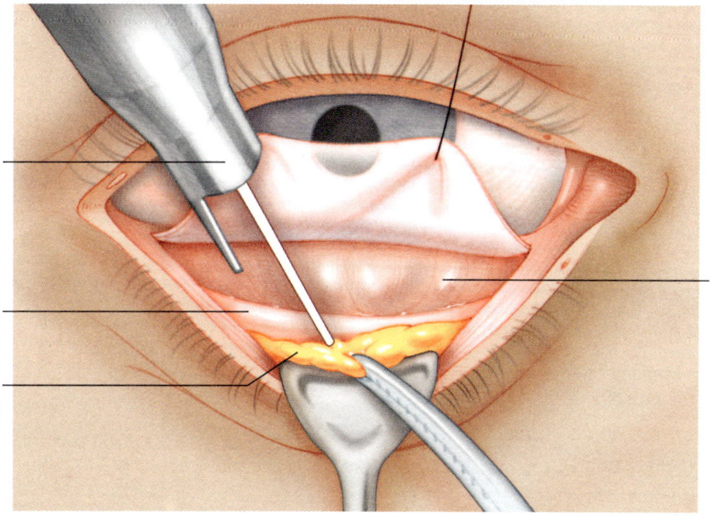


**Figure 11-29** Preperiosteal approach to suborbicularis oculi fat (SOOF) lift. *(Illustration by Christine Gralapp.)*

employed in an endoscopic brow-lift (endobrow). The subperiosteal midface can also be accessed through these incisions or, alternatively, through a superior gingival sulcus incision to elevate the periosteum (Fig 11-30). The goal of these procedures is to provide release of the midface tissues, followed by elevation and resuspension. Midface elevation is also commonly combined with a brow-lift or lower face-lift. Along with these techniques, a greater appreciation has developed regarding volume changes in the aging face. Such

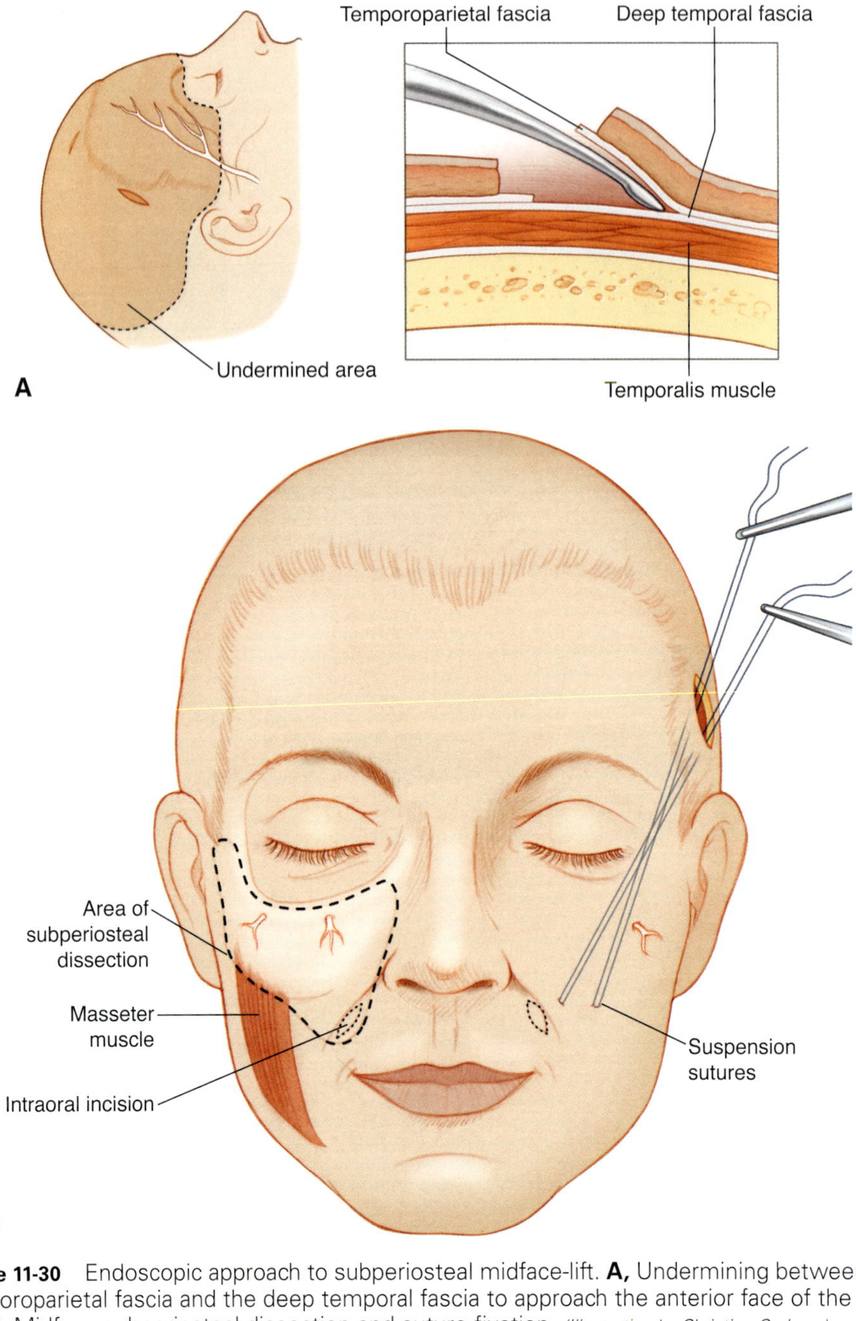


**Figure 11-30** Endoscopic approach to subperiosteal midface-lift. **A,** Undermining between the temporoparietal fascia and the deep temporal fascia to approach the anterior face of the maxilla. **B,** Midface subperiosteal dissection and suture fixation. *(Illustration by Christine Gralapp.)*

changes can also be addressed with liposculpture, in which autologous fat is strategically injected throughout the face.

Kikkawa DO, Lemke BN, Dortzbach RK. Relations of the superficial musculoaponeurotic system to the orbit and characterization of the orbitomalar ligament. *Ophthal Plast Reconstr Surg.* 1996; 12(2):77–88.

Lam SM, Glasgold MJ, Glasgold RA. *Complementary Fat Grafting.* Philadelphia: Lippincott William and Wilkins; 2007.
Lucarelli MJ, Khwarg SI, Lemke BN, Kozel JS, Dortzbach RK. The anatomy of midfacial ptosis. *Ophthal Plast Reconstr Surg.* 2000;16(1):7–22.
Williams EF III, Lam SM. Midfacial rejuvenation via an endoscopic browlift approach: a review of technique. *Facial Plast Surg.* 2003;19(2):147–156.

## Lower Face and Neck Rejuvenation

During preoperative evaluation, the face and neck should be considered as a single cosmetic unit. Correction of the cosmetic subunits of the upper face and midface without addressing the lower face and neck can create an unbalanced appearance. At the very least, these concerns must be discussed with the patient preoperatively along with surgical options.

### *Rhytidectomy*

The most commonly performed procedures include the vintage (subcutaneous) rhytidectomy, the rhytidectomy with superficial elevation and refixation of the superficial musculoaponeurotic system (SMAS) (Fig 11-31), and the deep-plane rhytidectomy. Rhytidectomies typically include surgical management of the jowls and neck, including liposuction with or without platysmaplasty. The 3 rhytidectomy procedures mentioned differ

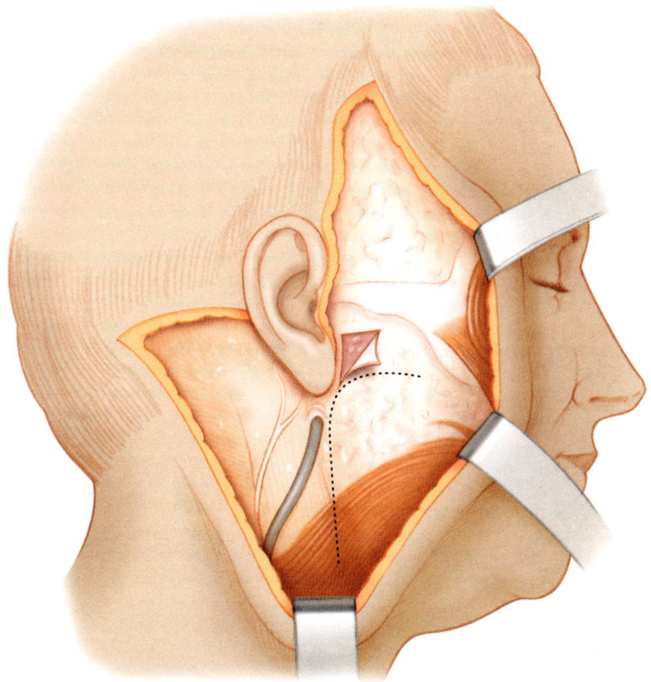

**Figure 11-31** The common goal of rhytidectomy procedures is modification of the superficial musculoaponeurotic system (SMAS) that translates to changes in the overlying anatomy. After release of the SMAS *(dotted line)*, the SMAS is pulled laterally and superiorly for elevation of the jowls and lower face. *(Illustration by Christine Gralapp.)*

mainly in the location and extent of dissection. Although the more superficial procedures are less likely to cause facial nerve damage, they may produce shorter-lasting results. The more extensive procedures have greater risks (eg, facial nerve injury), but the likelihood that they will produce dramatic, longer-lasting improvement is also greater.

Complications of rhytidectomy are directly related to the extent of subcutaneous undermining; they include hematoma, seroma, skin necrosis, hair loss, paresthesias, motor deficits, incisional scarring, asymmetry, earlobe distraction (pixie-ear deformity), and contour irregularities. Hematoma is the leading surgical face-lift complication, but patient dissatisfaction may be the most common problem for the surgeon postoperatively.

### Neck liposuction

Stab incisions, or *adits*, are made just posterior to the earlobe on each side and along the submental incision line, or they are made just anterior to the submental crease if liposuction is performed as a stand-alone procedure. Small liposuction cannulas are used for fat removal. A layer of fat is left on the dermis, and the liposuction cannula openings are always oriented away from the dermis to avoid injury to the vascular plexus deep to the dermis. In addition to abnormalities in skin quality, damage in this area can lead to unsightly scarring of the dermis of the underlying neck musculature. The adits are left open or sutured with prolene, and a compression bandage is worn for 1 week after the procedure.

### Platysmaplasty

Platysmaplasty is performed to correct platysmal bands and is typically done in conjunction with a lower face-lift. A subcutaneous dissection is carried out in the preplatysmal plane centrally under the chin to the level of the thyroid cartilage (Fig 11-32A). Lateral

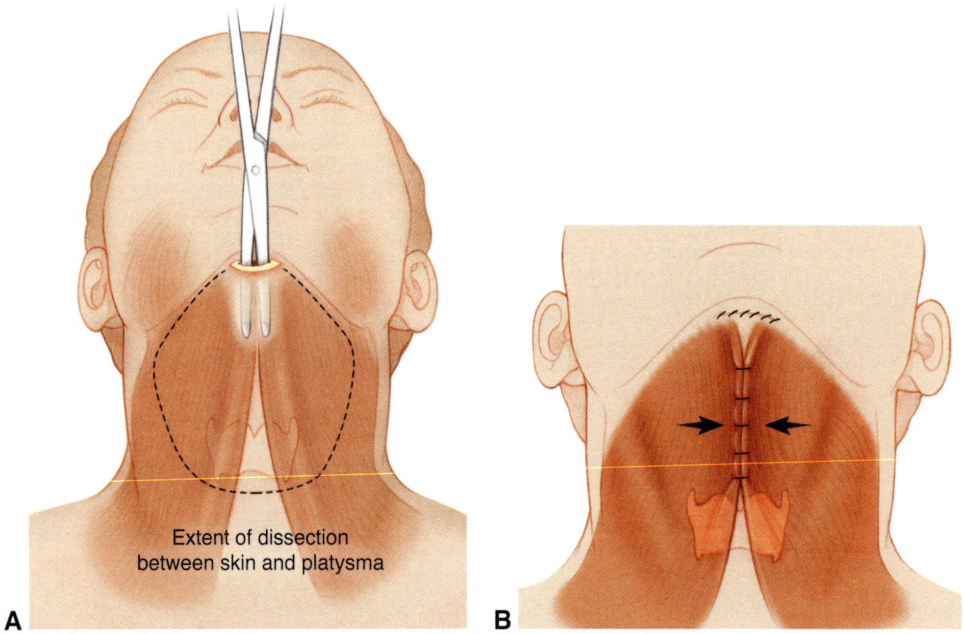


**Figure 11-32** Cervicoplasty. **A,** Undermining of the skin. **B,** Platysmaplasty. *(Illustrations by Christine Gralapp.)*

platysmal undermining and suspension may be performed as part of a rhytidectomy. Midline platysma resection and reconstruction (Fig 11-32B) are performed if midline neck support is needed. A drain and a light compression dressing are placed. Postoperatively, the cervicomental angle is more acute, yielding a more youthful look.

Baker DC. Minimal incision rhytidectomy (short scar face lift) with lateral SMASectomy: evolution and application. *Aesthet Surg J.* 2001;21(1):14–26.

Baylis HI, Goldberg RA, Shorr N. The deep plane facelift: a 20-year evolution of technique. *Ophthalmology.* 2000;107(3):490–495.

Dailey RA, Jones LT. Rejuvenation of the aging face. *Focal Points: Clinical Modules for Ophthalmologists.* San Francisco: American Academy of Ophthalmology; 2004, module 2.

Klein JA. *Tumescent Technique: Tumescent Anesthesia & Microcannular Liposuction.* St Louis: Mosby; 2000.

## Conclusion

The periocular area is part of the larger anatomical superstructure of the face, whose primary function is communication. Changes produced by aging, disease, or surgery can affect the messages transmitted by this entity. If a single subunit is altered without consideration of the other subunits, facial miscommunication and facial imbalance can result. It is therefore incumbent upon the oculofacial surgeon to understand the aging process, anatomy, and available surgical techniques before embarking on surgery that changes any portion of the face. Discussion of these issues with the patient preoperatively helps prevent patient dissatisfaction postoperatively.

# PART III

# Lacrimal System

CHAPTER 12

# Anatomy, Development, and Physiology of the Lacrimal Secretory and Drainage Systems

See Chapters 1 and 4 in BCSC Section 2, *Fundamentals and Principles of Ophthalmology,* for additional discussion, including illustrations, of some of the topics covered in this chapter.

## Normal Anatomy

### Secretory System

The lacrimal gland is an exocrine gland located in the superior lateral quadrant of the orbit within the lacrimal gland fossa. Embryologic development of the lateral horn of the levator aponeurosis indents the lacrimal gland, dividing it into orbital and palpebral lobes (see Chapter 1, Fig 1-7). The superior transverse ligament (Whitnall ligament) forms septa through the stroma of the gland, with some fibers also projecting onto the lateral orbital tubercle.

Some 8–12 major lacrimal ducts empty into the superior cul-de-sac approximately 5 mm above the lateral tarsal border after passing posterior to the levator aponeurosis, through the Müller muscle and conjunctiva. Because the lacrimal excretory ducts pass through the palpebral portion of the gland, removal of the palpebral lobe may reduce secretion from the entire gland. Therefore, biopsy of the lacrimal gland is preferentially performed on the orbital lobe.

Ocular surface irritation activates tear production from the lacrimal gland. The ophthalmic branch of the trigeminal nerve provides the sensory *(afferent)* pathway in this reflex tear arc. The *efferent* pathway is more complicated. Parasympathetic fibers, originating in the superior salivatory nucleus of the pons, exit the brainstem with the facial nerve, cranial nerve VII (CN VII) (Fig 12-1). Lacrimal fibers leave CN VII as the greater superficial petrosal nerve and pass to the sphenopalatine ganglion. From there, they are thought to enter the lacrimal gland via the superior branch of the zygomatic nerve, via an anastomosis between the zygomaticotemporal nerve and the lacrimal nerve. Whether

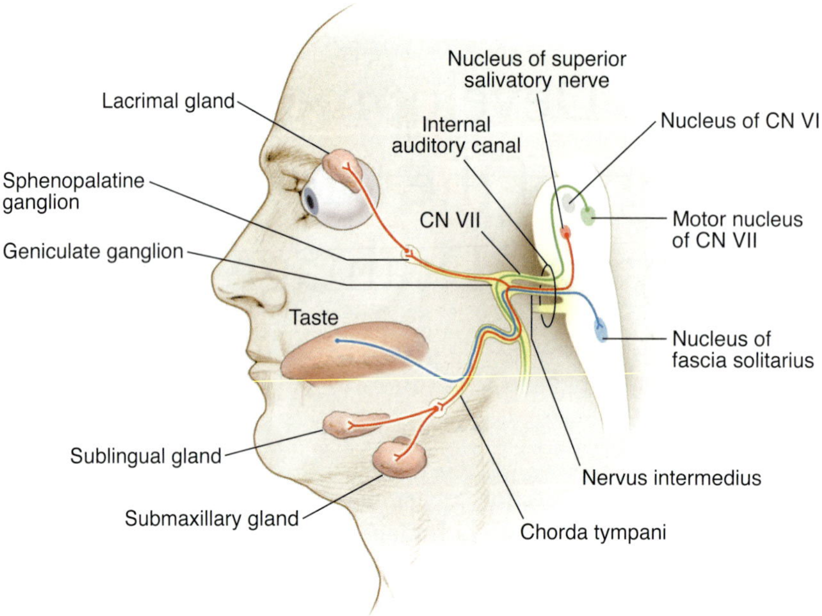


**Figure 12-1** Nonmotor pathways of the seventh cranial nerve (CN VII), including the efferent pathway to the lacrimal gland. *(Illustration by Christine Gralapp.)*

this anastomosis is uniformly present has been debated. What role, if any, the sympathetic nervous system plays in lacrimation is not well understood.

The *accessory glands of Krause* and *Wolfring* are exocrine glands located deep within the superior fornix and just above the superior border of the tarsus, respectively. Aqueous lacrimal secretion has traditionally been divided into basal secretion and reflex secretion. Previously it was thought that the accessory glands predominate in basal tear secretion; the lacrimal gland, in reflex tearing. It is now believed that all lacrimal glands respond as a unit.

The precorneal tear film covers the exposed surfaces of the cornea and globe and is composed of 3 layers:

- a deep mucin layer, secreted by goblet cells within the conjunctiva; it allows for even distribution of the tear film over the ocular surface
- a middle aqueous layer, secreted by the main and accessory lacrimal glands
- a superficial oily layer, produced by the meibomian glands; it reduces the evaporation of the aqueous layer

See BCSC Section 2, *Fundamentals and Principles of Ophthalmology,* for a more detailed discussion of the tear film.

## Drainage System

The entrance to the lacrimal drainage system is through puncta located medially on the margin of both the upper and the lower eyelids (Fig 12-2). The lower puncta lie slightly

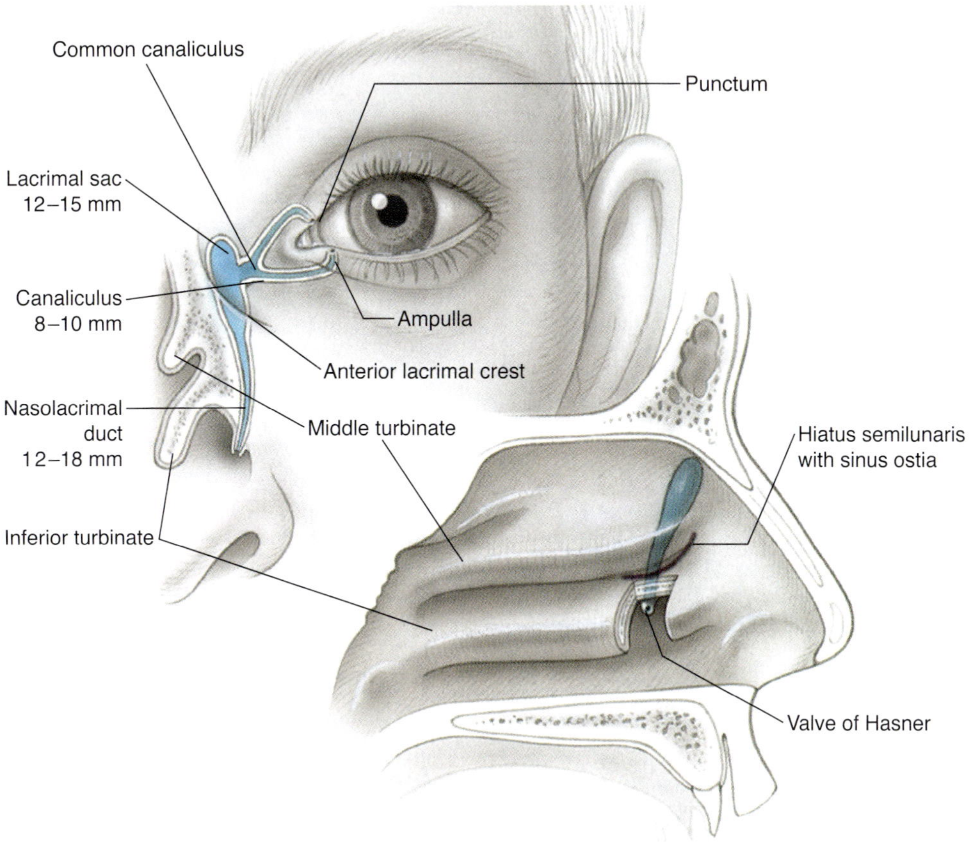


**Figure 12-2** Normal anatomy of the lacrimal drainage system. The measurements given are for adults. *(Illustration by Christine Gralapp.)*

farther lateral than the upper puncta. Normally, the puncta are slightly inverted and apposed to the globe, within the tear lake. Each punctum is surrounded by the ampulla, a fleshy elevation oriented perpendicular to the eyelid margin, and leads to a vertical segment of canaliculus. The *lacrimal canaliculi* are lined with nonkeratinized, non–mucin-producing stratified squamous epithelium. They run roughly 2 mm vertically from the punctum and then turn 90°, continuing 8–10 mm medially to join at the common canaliculus and connect with the *lacrimal sac* through the valve of Rosenmüller. In some individuals there is a unique configuration in which 2 independent canaliculi lead to the lacrimal sac.

The *valve of Rosenmüller* (Fig 12-3) has traditionally been described as the structure that prevents reflux of tears from the sac into the canaliculi. The presence of a mucosal fold was detected with electron microscopy. This fold (valve of Rosenmüller) presumably functions as a 1-way valve. Additional studies suggest that the common canaliculus consistently bends from posterior to anterior behind the medial canthal tendon before entering the lacrimal sac at an acute angle. This bend, in conjunction with the fold of mucosa, may play a role in blocking reflux.

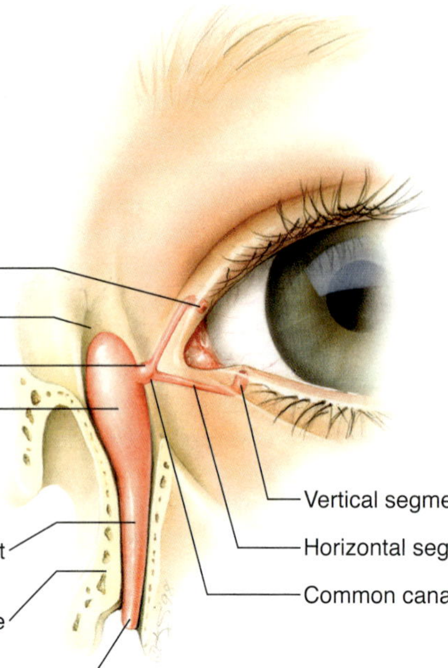


**Figure 12-3** The lacrimal drainage system. The valve of Rosenmüller has traditionally been described as the structure that prevents reflux of tears from the sac into the canaliculi. *(Reproduced with permission from Katowitz JA, ed.* Pediatric Oculoplastic Surgery. *Philadelphia: Springer-Verlag; 2002.)*

Located in the anterior medial orbit, the lacrimal sac lies within a bony fossa bordered by the anterior and posterior lacrimal crests. (See BCSC Section 2, *Fundamentals and Principles of Ophthalmology,* Figure 1-1 for a photo of this fossa.) Wrapping around the anterior and posterior aspects of the lacrimal sac, the medial canthal tendon is a complex structure composed of anterior and posterior crura. The superficial head attaches to the anterior lacrimal crest; the deep head (with the Horner muscle), to the posterior lacrimal crest. The medial wall of the fossa (the lamina papyracea) is composed of the lacrimal bone posteriorly and the frontal process of the maxilla anteriorly. Medial to the lamina papyracea is the middle meatus of the nose, sometimes with intervening ethmoid air cells. The dome of the sac extends several millimeters above the medial canthal tendon. Inferiorly, the lacrimal sac transitions into the *nasolacrimal duct (NLD).* When operating in the area of the lacrimal sac, the surgeon may encounter the angular artery and vein (see Chapter 1, Fig 1-9 in this volume), which lie 7–8 mm medial to the medial canthal angle and anastomose with the vascular systems of the face and orbit. If these vessels are cut during dacryocystorhinostomy, they may cause troublesome bleeding.

In adults, the NLD measures 12–18 mm in length. The interosseous portion of the duct is typically 12 mm in length, and the meatal soft tissue extends 5–6 mm inferior to the bony ostium. The NLD travels through bone within the nasolacrimal canal, which initially curves in an inferior and slightly lateral and posterior direction from the lacrimal sac. The NLD opens into the nose through an ostium under the inferior turbinate (the inferior meatus), which is usually partially covered by a mucosal fold (the valve of Hasner; see Fig 12-2). The mucosal ostium in adults is typically located 30–35 mm from the external nares.

## Development

### Secretory System

The lacrimal gland develops from multiple solid ectodermal buds in the anterior superolateral orbit. These buds branch, canalize, and form ducts and alveoli. The lacrimal glands are small and do not function fully until approximately 6 weeks after birth. Thus, newborn infants do not produce tears when crying.

### Drainage System

By the end of the fifth week of gestation, the nasolacrimal groove forms as a furrow lying between the nasal and maxillary prominence. In the floor of this groove, the NLD develops from a linear thickening of the ectoderm. A solid cord separates from adjacent ectoderm and sinks into the mesenchyme. The cord canalizes, forming the NLD and the lacrimal sac at its cranial end. The canalicular system is an outgrowth of the lacrimal sac. Caudally, the developing duct extends intranasally, exiting within the inferior meatus. The central tissue of this cord eventually breaks down, forming a lumen. Canalization of the NLD is usually complete around the time of birth. Failure of complete development and opening of the distal aspect of the duct is the most common cause of congenital NLD obstruction (NLDO). Obstruction at the valve of Hasner, at the distal end of the NLD, is symptomatic in approximately 5% of infants at birth. Patency usually occurs spontaneously within the first few months of life. As noted earlier, lacrimation does not function normally until around age 6 weeks; therefore, excessive tearing, which is often associated with this obstruction, may not be immediately obvious even if an obstruction exists.

## Physiology

Evaporation accounts for approximately 10% of tear elimination in the young and for 20% or more in elderly persons. Most of the tear flow is actively pumped from the tear lake by the actions of the orbicularis oculi muscle. Blinking pushes the tears from lateral to nasal on the eyelid margin, and then the action of the orbicularis muscle on the canaliculi and the lacrimal sac also promotes drainage (Fig 12-4). A weakened blink interferes with the normal pumping mechanism and contributes to epiphora in patients with eyelid laxity and seventh cranial nerve paresis.

Doane MG. Blinking and the mechanics of the lacrimal drainage system. *Ophthalmology.* 1981;88(8):844–851.

Rosengren B. On lacrimal drainage. *Ophthalmologica.* 1972;164(6):409–421.

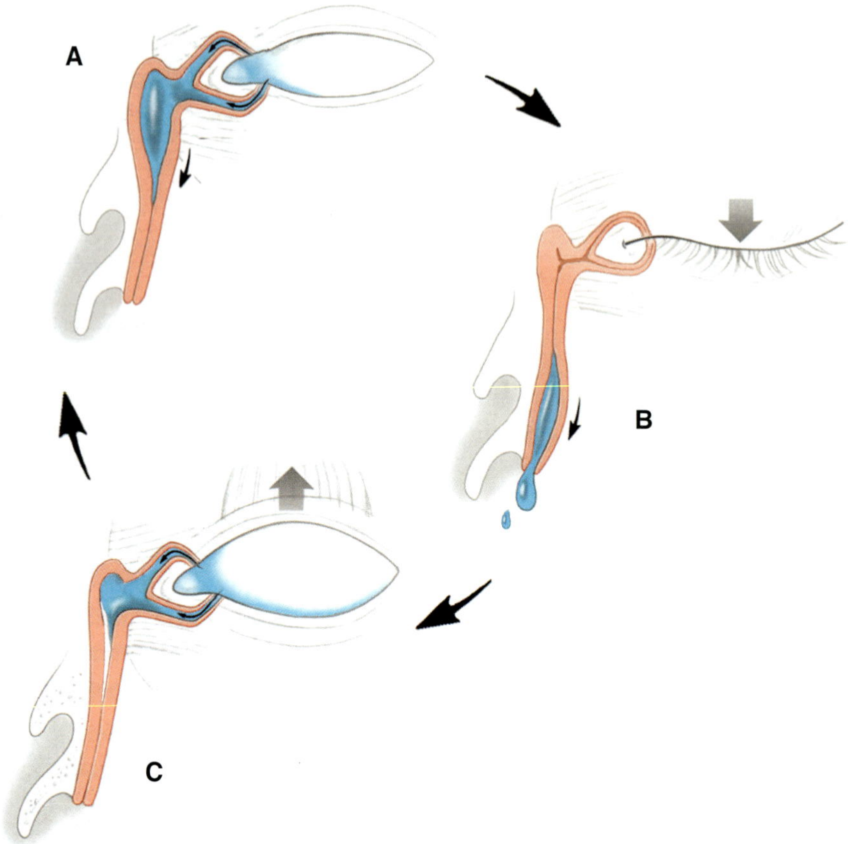


**Figure 12-4** Lacrimal pump mechanism. **A,** In the relaxed state, the puncta lie in the tear lake, and the lacrimal sac is filled with tears. **B,** With eyelid closure, contraction of the pretarsal orbicularis closes the puncta and canaliculi. The preseptal orbicularis fibers, which insert onto the sac, also compress the sac, creating positive pressure that propels tears through the duct. **C,** With eyelid opening, the orbicularis relaxes, and the puncta and sac open, creating negative pressure that draws tears into the canaliculi and lacrimal sac. As the eyelid closes, the cycle repeats. *(Original illustration by Christine Gralapp; revision based on an illustration by Cat N. Burkat, MD.)*

CHAPTER 13

# Abnormalities of the Lacrimal Secretory and Drainage Systems

## Developmental Abnormalities

### Lacrimal Secretory System

Congenital abnormalities of the lacrimal gland are relatively uncommon. Abnormalities include hypoplasia and agenesis of the lacrimal gland. Either can occur in isolation or, in some cases, in conjunction with congenital abnormalities of the salivary glands. Although they usually occur sporadically, both aplasia and hypoplasia have been reported to occur in an apparent autosomal dominant pattern. Lacrimal gland prolapse has been reported in association with craniosynostosis syndromes. Ectopic lacrimal gland tissue has also been found within the orbit and eyelids.

Occasionally, children are born with an aberrant ductule that exits externally through the eyelid overlying the lacrimal gland; this was previously referred to as a *lacrimal gland fistula.* These aberrant ductules exit laterally several millimeters above the eyelash line and are usually accompanied by an adjacent cluster of eyelashes. Tears produced from the aberrant ductules can mimic epiphora. These ductules can be successfully managed with simple excision.

### Lacrimal Drainage System

Most developmental abnormalities of the lacrimal drainage system relate to (1) errors in the genesis of the proximal system (multiple puncta or lacrimal–cutaneous fistula) or (2) incomplete patency, either at the eyelid (eg, punctal or canalicular hypoplasia or aplasia) or intranasally (eg, nasolacrimal duct [NLD] obstruction).

#### *Duplication*

Uncommonly, multiple puncta and additional canaliculi develop (Fig 13-1). When the extra opening is on the eyelid margin, it may be asymptomatic and requires no treatment. The term *congenital lacrimal–cutaneous fistula* has been used to describe uncommon fistulas that exit through the skin, typically infranasal to the medial canthus (Fig 13-2). These anlage ducts or fistulas from an otherwise normal canalicular system or lacrimal sac are sometimes asymptomatic, or they may be associated with tears that appear on the skin.

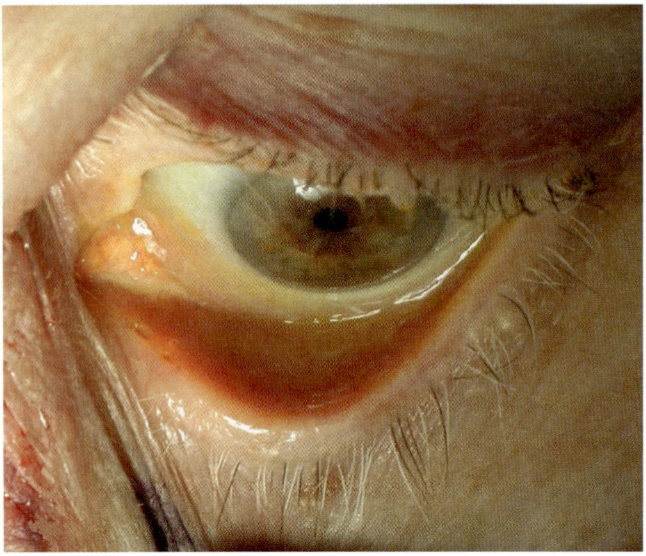

**Figure 13-1** Congenital accessory canaliculus of the lower eyelid. *(Courtesy of Jill Foster, MD.)*

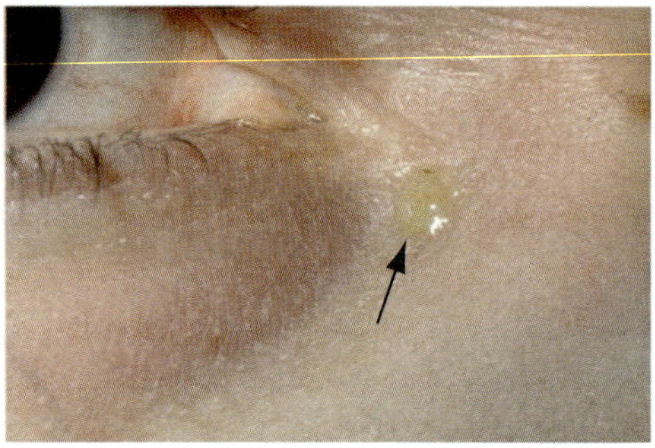

**Figure 13-2** Congenital lacrimal–cutaneous fistula draining to the skin surface *(arrow)*. *(Courtesy of Andrew Harrison, MD.)*

Approximately one-third of patients have an underlying NLD obstruction (NLDO); in these cases, chronic mucoid discharge from the affected nasolacrimal sac may be present.

In symptomatic patients, direct surgical excision of the epithelium-lined fistulous tract with direct suture closure is indicated. In patients with underlying NLDO and chronic dacryocystitis, silicone intubation or dacryocystorhinostomy may also be required. (See the management subsection under Acquired Nasolacrimal Duct Obstruction later in this chapter.)

Al-Salem K, Gibson A, Dolman PJ. Management of congenital lacrimal (anlage) fistula. *Br J Ophthalmol.* 2014;98(10):1435–1436.

### *Aplasia and hypoplasia*

Punctal hypoplasia or stenosis is encountered more frequently than true aplasia. Moreover, in many cases of presumed aplasia, close evaluation with magnification reveals an intact punctum with a thin overlying membrane. Management of punctal stenosis, membranes, and aplasia is discussed in the section addressing lacrimal drainage obstruction.

#### *Nasolacrimal duct obstruction*

In most cases, congenital NLDO is due to failure of the duct to fully canalize; however, associations with more severe abnormalities have been described. For example, major facial cleft deformities can pass through or be adjacent to the nasolacrimal drainage pathways and result in outflow disorders.

Treatment of lacrimal drainage obstruction differs according to the cause and location of the obstruction. Obstruction may involve the puncta, canaliculi, lacrimal sac, or NLD. Because the pathophysiology and management of congenital and acquired lacrimal drainage abnormalities differ, these disorders are addressed separately.

Sevel D. Development and congenital abnormalities of the nasolacrimal apparatus. *J Pediatr Ophthalmol Strabismus.* 1981;18(5):13–19.

## Congenital Lacrimal Drainage Obstruction

### Evaluation

The evaluation of congenital tearing is usually straightforward: the patient's parents report a history of tearing, mucopurulent discharge, or both beginning shortly after birth. In rare cases, visible distension of the lacrimal sac is present, suggesting a congenital dacryocystocele. Otherwise, distinction should be made among the following:

- constant tearing with minimal mucopurulence, suggesting blockage of the upper system (puncta, canaliculi, and common canaliculus) caused by punctal or canalicular dysgenesis
- constant tearing with frequent mucopurulence and matting of the eyelashes, suggesting complete obstruction of the NLD
- intermittent tearing with mucopurulence, suggesting intermittent obstruction of the NLD

Office examination includes inspection of the eyelid margins for patent puncta and evaluation for extrinsic causes of reflex hypersecretion, such as ocular surface irritation, infectious conjunctivitis, epiblepharon, trichiasis, and congenital glaucoma. Additional aspects of the examination include inspection of the medial canthal region to uncover a distended lacrimal sac (below the tendon), inflammation, or congenital defects such as an encephalocele (above the tendon). However, the single most important maneuver is application of digital pressure over the tear sac. If mucoid reflux is present, complete obstruction at the level of the NLD becomes the working diagnosis.

### Punctal and Canalicular Agenesis and Dysgenesis

The medial eyelid margin should be inspected for the presence of elevated lacrimal papillae and puncta. In patients who were initially thought to have complete punctal agenesis, close evaluation with magnification may reveal a punctum with a membranous occlusion. Such membranes can usually be opened with a sharp probe. Temporary intubation (discussed under Congenital Nasolacrimal Duct Obstruction) or placement of a silicone plug may help prevent recurrence. If the punctum is truly absent, the surgeon may cut down through the eyelid margin medial to the expected punctum location to try to identify the canaliculus. Alternatively, retrograde probing through an open lacrimal sac with direct visualization of the common canalicular opening (common internal punctum) may identify the canaliculi. Occasionally, these maneuvers reveal the presence of a relatively mature canalicular system with a patent nasolacrimal sac and duct, in which case intubation may be performed. Symptomatic patients with a single punctum may require surgery to relieve NLDO rather than canalicular obstruction. Symptomatic patients with complete absence of the puncta and the canalicular system require a conjunctivodacryocystorhinostomy (CDCR). This is performed when the patient is old enough to allow manipulation of, and to care for, the Jones tube. (CDCR is discussed later in this chapter in the section Canalicular Obstruction.)

Lyons CJ, Rosser PM, Welham RA. The management of punctal agenesis. *Ophthalmology.* 1993;100(12):1851–1855.

## Congenital Nasolacrimal Duct Obstruction

Congenital obstruction of the lacrimal drainage system is usually caused by a membrane blocking the valve of Hasner at the nasal end of the NLD. Many newborns are born with imperforate NLDs, but most obstructions open spontaneously within the first few months of life. Such an obstruction becomes clinically evident in only 2%–6% of full-term infants at 3–4 weeks of age. Of these, one-third have bilateral involvement. Approximately 90% of all symptomatic congenital NLD obstructions resolve in the first year of life.

Management options can be divided into conservative (nonsurgical) and surgical. Conservative options include observation, lacrimal sac massage, and topical or even oral antibiotics. The long-term use of topical antibiotics may be necessary to suppress chronic mucoid discharge with matting of the lashes.

When the obstruction fails to resolve with conservative measures, more invasive intervention may be required. Most often this consists of probing of the NLD to rupture the presumptive membrane occluding the NLD at the valve of Hasner (discussed in detail later in this chapter). In cases with airway obstruction secondary to nasal extension of an enlarged lacrimal sac or dacryocystitis, prompt treatment may be required. In uncomplicated cases, opinions differ regarding how long clinicians should continue with conservative management before probing.

Most cases of congenital NLDO—including infants with clinical symptoms at 6 months—resolve in the first year of life. Several reports have suggested that delaying probing past 13 months of age may be associated with a decreased success rate. Although the trend has been to perform probing with the patient under sedation if symptoms persist at 1 year of age, some advocate performing probing in the office earlier, usually at 6 months of age. In a younger child, probing in the office may sometimes be performed in selected patients with topical anesthesia and swaddling. Children aged 1 year or older usually require general anesthesia. Probing with topical anesthesia is inexpensive, avoids general anesthesia, and is relatively safe in well-trained hands, but it limits the acquisition of information about the nature of the obstruction and the physician's intervention choices at the time of the procedure.

In some instances of congenital NLDO, dacryocystitis manifests as an acutely inflamed lacrimal sac with cellulitis of the overlying skin. Treatment with systemic antibiotics should be started promptly. Management of the pediatric patient is similar to that of the adult patient (discussed in detail later). Following resolution of the infectious process, elective probing should be performed promptly to prevent recurrence of the dacryocystitis.

Casady DR, Meyer DR, Simon JW, Stasior GO, Zobal-Ratner JL. Stepwise treatment paradigm for congenital nasolacrimal duct obstruction. *Ophthal Plast Reconstr Surg.* 2006;22(4): 243–247.

Katowitz JA, Welsh MG. Timing of initial probing and irrigation in congenital nasolacrimal duct obstruction. *Ophthalmology.* 1987;94(6):698–705.

Miller AM, Chandler DL, Repka MX, et al; Pediatric Eye Disease Investigator Group. Office probing for treatment of nasolacrimal duct obstruction in infants. *J AAPOS.* 2014;18(1): 26–30.

### *Probing and irrigation*

Probing is a delicate surgical maneuver that is facilitated by immobilization of the patient and by contraction of the nasal mucosa with a topical vasoconstrictor, usually oxymetazoline hydrochloride. When probing, the physician should recall that the upper system begins at the punctum, with a 2-mm vertical segment followed by a horizontal segment of 8–10 mm (canaliculus; see Chapter 12, Fig 12-2). Punctal dilation is often needed to safely introduce a size 00 Bowman lacrimal probe (Fig 13-3). The probe is initially inserted into the punctum perpendicular to the eyelid margin and then turned parallel to the lid margin as it is advanced down the canalicular system, toward the medial canthal tendon. Manual lateral traction of the eyelid with the opposite hand straightens the canaliculus, decreasing the risk of damage to the canalicular mucosa and creation of a false passage.

Resistance to passage of the probe—along with medial movement of the eyelid soft tissue ("soft stop"), causing wrinkling of the overlying skin—may signify canalicular obstruction. More commonly, resistance is simply due to a kink in the canaliculus created by bunching of the soft tissues in front of the probe tip. If kinking is encountered, the probe is withdrawn and reinserted while lateral horizontal traction is maintained (Fig 13-4). If

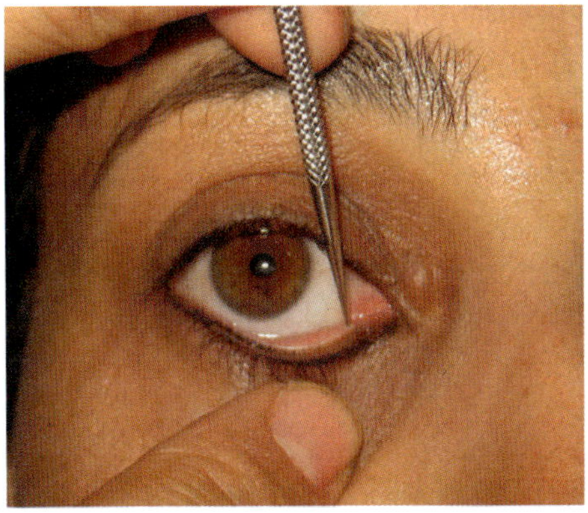
A

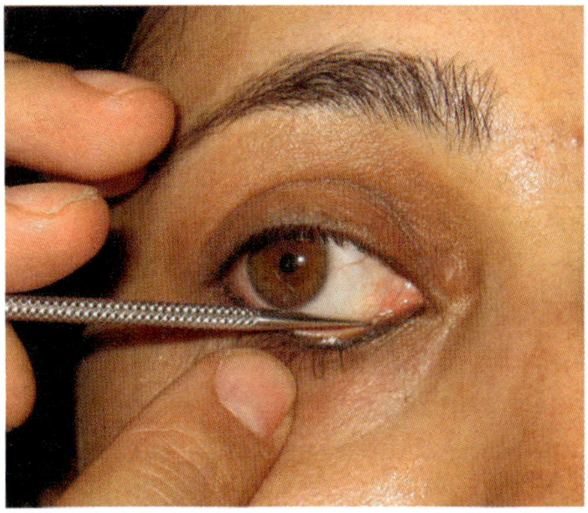
B

**Figure 13-3** **A,** Initial insertion of the dilator is perpendicular to the eyelid margin. **B,** While counter traction is applied, the dilator is advanced toward the nose. *(Courtesy of Morris E. Hartstein, MD.)*

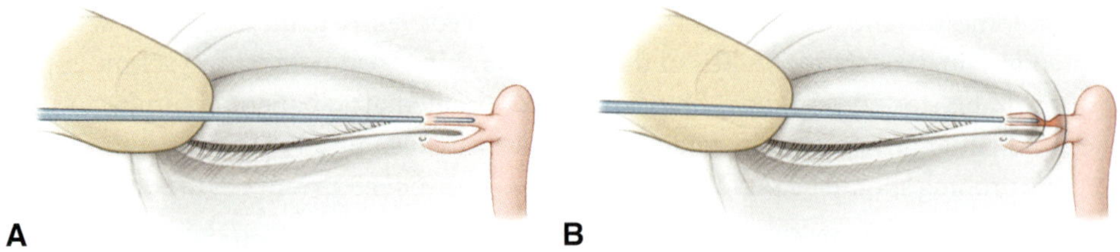


**Figure 13-4** **A,** Bowman probe in the right upper horizontal canaliculus. **B,** When canalicular obstruction is present or when the probe is not in the correct position, resistance to passage of the probe ("soft stop") with wrinkling of the overlying skin is encountered. *(Illustration by Christine Gralapp.)*

the probe advances successfully through the common canalicular system and across the lacrimal sac, the medial wall of the lacrimal sac and adjacent lacrimal bone will be encountered, resulting in a tactile "hard stop."

The probe is then rotated 90° superiorly toward the brow until it lies adjacent to the supraorbital notch. The probe is directed posteriorly and slightly laterally as it is advanced down the NLD. If significant resistance is encountered at any point during the probing procedure and the surgeon is uncertain whether the probe is in the natural pathway, the probe should be repositioned and passage attempted again. Creation of a false passage makes it difficult to redirect the probe back into the native lacrimal system. At some points of narrowing, particularly at the distal end of the NLD, gentle pressure may be necessary to push through the blockage. Direct visualization of the probe tip is sometimes possible with the use of a nasal speculum and a fiber-optic headlight or endoscope along the lateral wall of the nose under the inferior turbinate. In a child, the opening of the NLD is usually 20–22 mm back from the nostril. If the probe is not visualized, patency of the duct can be confirmed by metal-on-metal contact with another probe inserted through the naris or by irrigation with saline mixed with fluorescein (Fig 13-5). The fluorescein can be retrieved from the inferior meatus and visualized with a transparent suction catheter.

A single lacrimal probing successfully resolves congenital NLDO in 90% of patients who are 13 months or younger. In adults, irrigation and probing are limited to the canalicular system and are performed for diagnostic purposes only. Probing of the NLD in adults is potentially traumatic and rarely effective in permanently relieving an obstruction.

### *Intubation*

Intubation is usually performed with a silicone stent. It is indicated for children who have recurrent epiphora following nasolacrimal system probing and for older children in whom initial probing reveals significant stenosis or scarring. Intubation is also useful for the treatment of upper-system abnormalities such as canalicular stenosis, trauma, and agenesis of the puncta. Nasolacrimal intubation after failed probing has a reported success rate greater than 70%.

Many intubation techniques and types of intubation sets have been described. Figure 13-6 illustrates one of the more commonly utilized stents (Crawford stent). Keys to successful intubation include shrinkage of the nasal mucosa with a topical vasoconstrictor

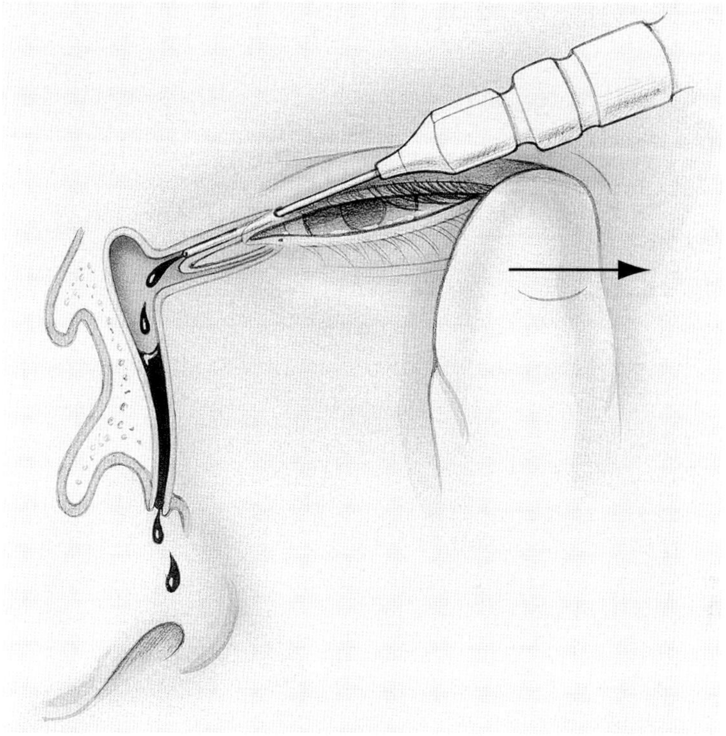

**Figure 13-5** Irrigation of the nasolacrimal system. Dye is injected from the syringe, and patency of the system is confirmed by suctioning the dye from the inferior meatus of the nose. *(Illustration by Christine Gralapp.)*

and adequate lighting with a fiber-optic headlight. In more difficult cases, an endoscope can be used, and medialization of the inferior turbinate is sometimes performed. The silicone tubing can be secured with a simple square knot, which allows removal of the tube through the canalicular system in a retrograde fashion. Alternatively, the silicone stent may be directly sutured to the lateral wall of the nose (without tension), or the limbs of the stent can be secured by passing them through either a silicone band or a sponge in the inferior meatus of the nose. These techniques allow the stent to be retrieved through the nose. Monocanalicular stents are also available (Fig 13-7). This type of stent is passed through a single punctum to the nasal cavity, where the end of the stent is simply cut and allowed to retract loosely into the nose. The proximal end has a punctal plug and is self-secured at the punctum. The monocanalicular stent is useful for patients with only one patent canaliculus.

### Balloon dacryoplasty

Balloon catheter dilation of the nasolacrimal canal has been used successfully in congenital nasolacrimal obstruction. A collapsed balloon catheter is placed in a manner similar to probing and inflated inside the duct at multiple levels. The role of this modality remains

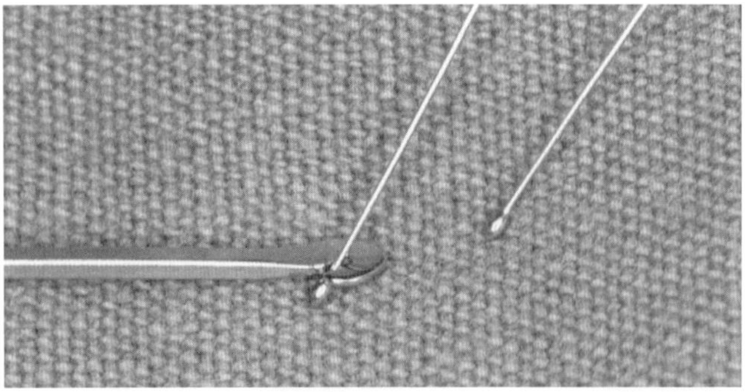

A

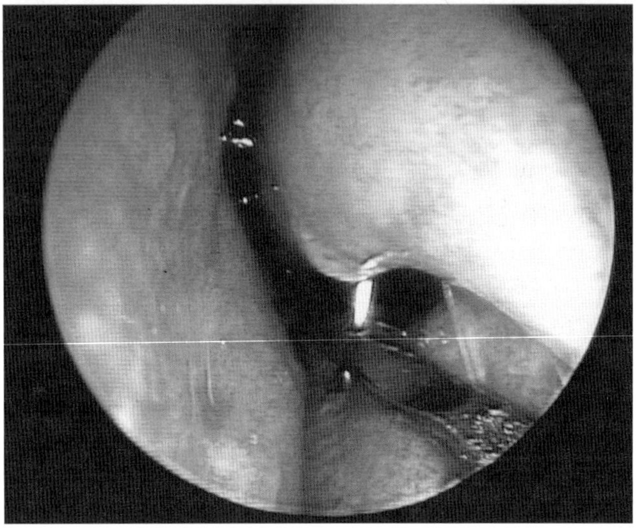

B

**Figure 13-6** Crawford stent and hook. **A,** Hook engaging the "olive tip" of the stent. **B,** Intranasal view of engaged hook retrieving the stent. *(Reproduced with permission from Nerad JA.* Oculoplastic Surgery: The Requisites in Ophthalmology. *Philadelphia: Mosby; 2001:233.)*

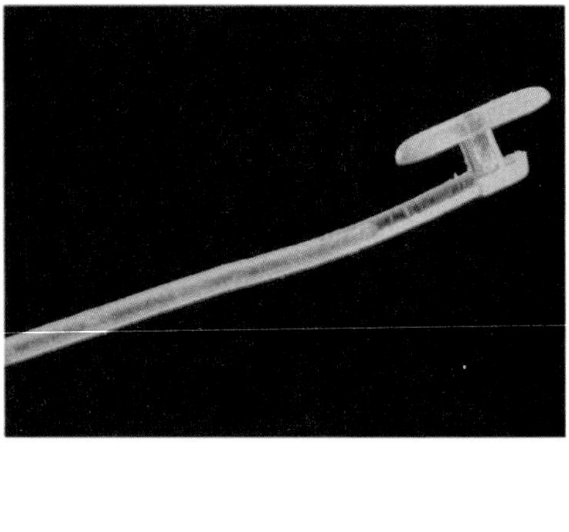

**Figure 13-7** Monocanalicular stent. At the proximal end are a soft barb and collarette, which secure the stent within the punctum. *(Courtesy of Roberta Gausas, MD.)*

undefined in part because the necessary catheter equipment is expensive and simple probing has a high success rate. Thus, balloon dacryoplasty is generally limited to complicated cases or to recurrence following standard probing techniques.

Repka MX, Chandler DL, Holmes JM, et al; Pediatric Eye Disease Investigator Group. Balloon catheter dilation and nasolacrimal duct intubation for treatment of nasolacrimal duct obstruction after failed probing. *Arch Ophthalmol.* 2009;127(5):633–639.

### *Turbinate infracture*

If the inferior turbinate appears to be lateralized against the NLD at the time of probing and irrigation, medial infracture of the inferior turbinate should be performed. This condition should be suspected in patients with recurrent intermittent obstruction and those whose symptoms appear primarily related to infections of the upper respiratory tract, in which swelling of the mucosa over the turbinate may cause intermittent obstruction of the inferior meatus. The blunt end of a periosteal elevator is placed within the inferior meatus along the lateral surface of the inferior turbinate. The inferior turbinate is then rotated medially toward the septum. Fracturing the turbinate at its base significantly enlarges the inferior meatus and permits direct visualization of the lacrimal probe tip.

Wesley RE. Inferior turbinate fracture in the treatment of congenital nasolacrimal duct obstruction and congenital nasolacrimal duct anomaly. *Ophthalmic Surg.* 1985;16(6): 368–371.

### *Dacryocystorhinostomy*

Dacryocystorhinostomy (DCR) is usually reserved for children who have persistent epiphora following intubation and/or balloon dacryoplasty, children who experience recurrent dacryocystitis, and patients with extensive developmental abnormalities of the nasolacrimal drainage system that prevent probing and intubation. The details of DCR are discussed later in this chapter under Acquired Nasolacrimal Duct Obstruction.

Dolmetsch AM, Gallon MA, Holds JB. Nonlaser endoscopic endonasal dacryocystorhinostomy with adjunctive mitomycin C in children. *Ophthal Plast Reconstr Surg.* 2008;24(5): 390–393.

## Dacryocystocele

Mucoceles may form within the lacrimal sac or within the nasal cavity as a consequence of congenital NLDO. The type of mucocele present in lacrimal sac distension has been termed a *dacryocystocele* (also called *amniotocele*) and may be present at birth or may develop within 1 to 4 weeks after birth (Fig 13-8). It occurs when the NLD is obstructed and amniotic fluid or mucus (secreted by lacrimal sac goblet cells) is trapped in the tear sac because of a functional block above the sac and a block or atresia at the lower end of the NLD. The dacryocystocele is initially sterile and may respond to conservative management with prophylactic topical antibiotics and massage. If there is no response in 1–2 weeks or if infection develops, probing of the lacrimal drainage system may be necessary to address the disorder. Distension of the nasal mucosa into the nasal cavity at the level of an occluded valve of Hasner may also occur. The intranasal portion often extends inferiorly under the inferior turbinate, where it

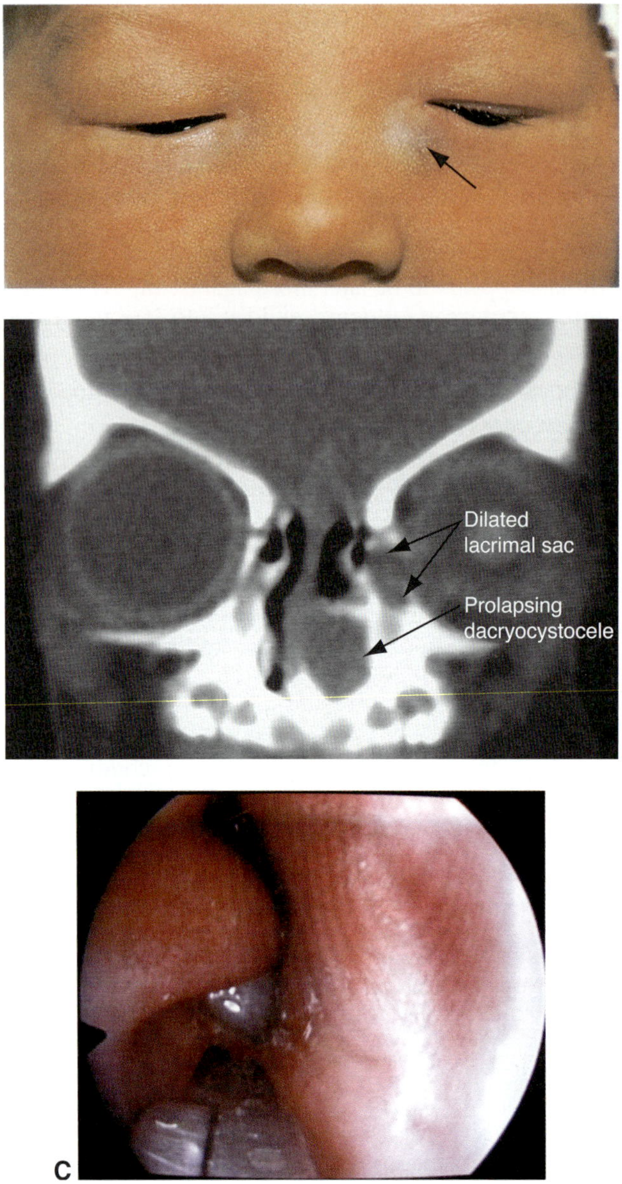


**Figure 13-8** **A,** Left congenital dacryocystocele *(arrow)* 1 week postpartum. **B,** Computed tomography scan of a congenital dacryocystocele. **C,** Endoscopic view of prolapsing dacryocystocele. *(Parts A and B courtesy of Pierre Arcand, MD; part C courtesy of Morris E. Hartstein, MD.)*

can be observed during nasal examination. Intranasal examination is recommended so that excision or marsupialization of the prolapsed duct can be performed if necessary. Urgent treatment may be needed if the condition is bilateral and causes airway obstruction.

In most patients, dacryocystoceles expand inferiorly to the medial canthal tendon. Congenital swelling above the medial canthal tendon, especially in the midline, should suggest alternate, often more serious, etiologies, such as a meningoencephalocele or dermoid cyst. Computed tomography (CT) or magnetic resonance imaging (MRI) is used to evaluate the patient for these more complex diagnoses.

## Acquired Lacrimal Drainage Obstruction

### Evaluation

#### *History*

Patients with acquired tearing can be loosely divided into 2 groups: those with hypersecretion of tears (lacrimation) and those with impairment of drainage (epiphora). The initial step in evaluating the tearing patient is differentiating between the 2 conditions. The following list aids in the assessment of the patient with acquired tearing:

- constant versus intermittent tearing
- periods of remission versus no remission
- unilateral versus bilateral condition
- subjective ocular surface discomfort
- history of allergies
- use of topical medications such as glaucoma drops
- history of probing during childhood
- prior ocular surface infections such as conjunctivitis or herpes simplex
- prior sinus disease or surgery, midfacial trauma, or nasal fracture
- previous episodes of lacrimal sac inflammation
- clear tears versus tears with discharge or blood (blood in the tear meniscus may indicate malignancy)

#### *Examination*

Systematic examination helps pinpoint the cause of acquired tearing. The initial step of the examination is to distinguish patients with obstruction of the lacrimal drainage system from those with secondary hypersecretion.

**Pseudoepiphora evaluation** *Epiphora* is defined as overflow tearing. Some patients feel like their eyes have too many tears but do not exhibit frank epiphora. These sensations are often caused by other ocular or eyelid abnormalities. For example, patients with dry eye may perceive foreign-body sensation or increased mucus production as excess tearing, but they do not exhibit true overflow of tears over the eyelid margin or down the cheek. In assessing pseudoepiphora, the ophthalmologist should consider the following:

- *Tear meniscus.* The size of the lacrimal lake as well as the presence of precipitated proteins and stringy mucus may indicate an abnormal tear film.
- *Tear breakup time.* This can be observed after fluorescein has been placed in the conjunctival cul-de-sac. The patient is asked to open his or her eyes and refrain from blinking. The ophthalmologist then examines the tear film using a broad beam of the slit lamp. The time before breakup should be at least 10 seconds. A more rapid tear film breakup time may indicate poor function of the mucin or meibomian layer despite a sufficient amount of tears. The mucin layer of the tear film

helps spread the other layers evenly over the corneal surface. The meibomian layer helps prevent tear evaporation.

- *Evaluation of corneal and conjunctival epithelium.* Topical rose bengal and lissamine green staining can detect subtle ocular surface abnormalities by staining devitalized conjunctival and corneal epithelium. Fluorescein staining indicates more severe tear film malfunction with epithelial loss.
- *Basal tear secretion.* In the basal tear secretion test, topical anesthetic is applied, and the inferior cul-de-sac is dried. The Schirmer strip is bent at the notch and placed with the short end resting on the conjunctiva and the fold crease on the eyelid margin at the lateral one-third of the lower eyelid. The strip is left in place for 5 minutes, and the amount of wetting is recorded. The normal amount is approximately 10–15 mm. Rapid saturation of the filter strip signifies hypersecretion. However, excess secretion may occur in response to irritation from the measuring strips themselves. Serial testing should be performed to confirm this assumption. Two classic but less often performed tests are the Schirmer I and Schirmer II tests. The Schirmer I test is performed like the basal tear secretion test, but no topical anesthetic is used. This allows the physician to evaluate both basic and reflex tearing. The Schirmer II test is used to distinguish between *fatigue block* (when reflex secretion is suppressed because of chronic irritation) and a lack of function of the reflex secretors. In this test, with the tear strip in place, a cotton-tipped applicator is placed in the nostril and moved back and forth for 2 minutes. Ocular surface fatigue block will be overcome, and wetting of the tear strip will occur. The classic Schirmer tests are reserved for special diagnostic circumstances. See also BCSC Section 8, *External Disease and Cornea,* for further discussion of tear film abnormalities.
- *Corneal irritation.* Patients should also be evaluated for mechanical irritation of the cornea. Corneal irritation from contact with eyelashes is a common cause of ocular irritation and secondary lacrimation. This can be seen with misdirected eyelashes (trichiasis) or eyelid malposition (entropion). Other ocular irritants include allergy; chronic infection, as seen, for example, with chlamydia or molluscum; and contact lens–related disease such as giant papillary conjunctivitis. Careful examination of the palpebral conjunctiva can aid in the identification of many such disorders.

#### *Lacrimal outflow examination*

Abnormal lacrimal outflow may result from problems in any number of structures. With eyelid malposition, tears might not reach the puncta. Thus, careful attention should be given to eyelid position and the position of the puncta. Slit-lamp examination during the blink cycle will help determine whether the punctum is properly positioned within the tear lake. Facial nerve dysfunction can result in a weakened or incomplete blink and poor lacrimal pump function. An enlarged caruncle or conjunctivochalasis can also mechanically block the aperture of the puncta and lead to tearing. Punctal stenosis, occlusion, or aplasia can be present.

Lacrimal sac evaluation is invaluable. Palpation with pressure on a distended lacrimal sac may cause reflux of mucoid or mucopurulent material through the canalicular system, confirming complete NLDO. No further diagnostic tests are needed if a lacrimal sac tumor is not suspected.

Nasal examination may uncover an unsuspected cause of the epiphora, such as an intranasal tumor, turbinate impaction, or chronic allergic rhinitis. These conditions may occlude the nasal end of the NLD.

### *Diagnostic tests*

The tear function tests routinely used in practice are the dye disappearance test, the basal tear secretion test (described earlier), and lacrimal irrigation. There are other tests of special diagnostic value or historical importance that should also be recognized. As originally outlined by Lester Jones, the clinical evaluation of the lacrimal drainage system historically comprised a dye disappearance test followed by the Jones I and Jones II tests.

The *dye disappearance test (DDT)* is useful for assessing the presence or absence of adequate lacrimal outflow, especially in unilateral cases. It is more heavily relied upon for children, in whom lacrimal irrigation is impossible without deep sedation. Using a drop of sterile 2% fluorescein solution or a moistened fluorescein strip, the examiner instills fluorescein into the conjunctival fornices of each eye and then observes the tear film with the cobalt blue filter of the slit lamp. Persistence of significant dye and, particularly, asymmetric clearance of the dye from the tear meniscus over a 5-minute period indicate an obstruction. Unilateral delayed dye disappearance is illustrated in Figure 13-9. If the DDT result is normal, severe lacrimal drainage dysfunction is highly unlikely. However, intermittent causes of tearing, such as allergy, dacryolith, or intranasal obstruction, cannot be ruled out.

The Jones I and Jones II tests have historically been used in the evaluation of epiphora. Like the DDT, the *Jones I test,* or *primary dye test,* investigates lacrimal outflow under normal physiologic conditions. The examiner instills fluorescein into the conjunctival fornices and recovers it in the inferior nasal meatus by passing a cotton-tipped applicator into the nose at 2 and 5 minutes. This test is no longer routinely performed.

The nonphysiologic *Jones II test* determines the presence or absence of fluorescein in the irrigating saline fluid retrieved from the nose. This test is performed as follows. The residual fluorescein is flushed from the conjunctival sac with clear saline lacrimal irrigation, following an unsuccessful Jones I test. The lacrimal system is then irrigated with clear saline using a cannula inserted into the canalicular system. Clear solution suggests that the tears never entered the lacrimal outflow system, and fluorescein-stained irrigant indicates partial obstruction. Although some clinicians continue to use and rely on formal Jones testing, most have found it technically difficult to retrieve the irrigating fluid from the nose and have abandoned the test. Instead, they employ a simplified approach, using only the DDT and lacrimal irrigation.

*Lacrimal drainage system irrigation* is most frequently performed immediately after the DDT to determine the level of lacrimal drainage system occlusion (Fig 13-10). After instillation of topical anesthesia, the lower eyelid punctum is dilated and any punctal

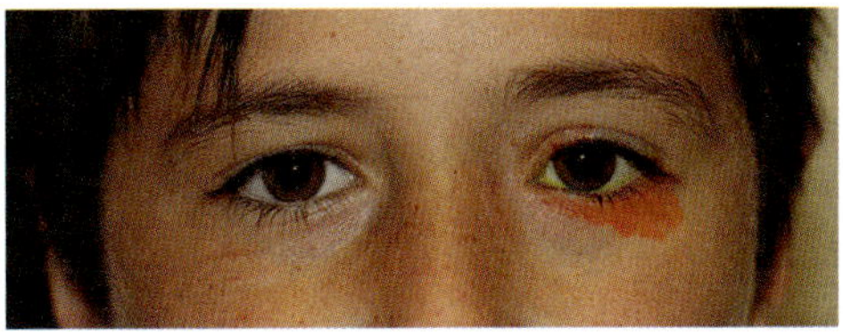

**Figure 13-9** Dye disappearance test. *(Courtesy of Jill Foster, MD.)*

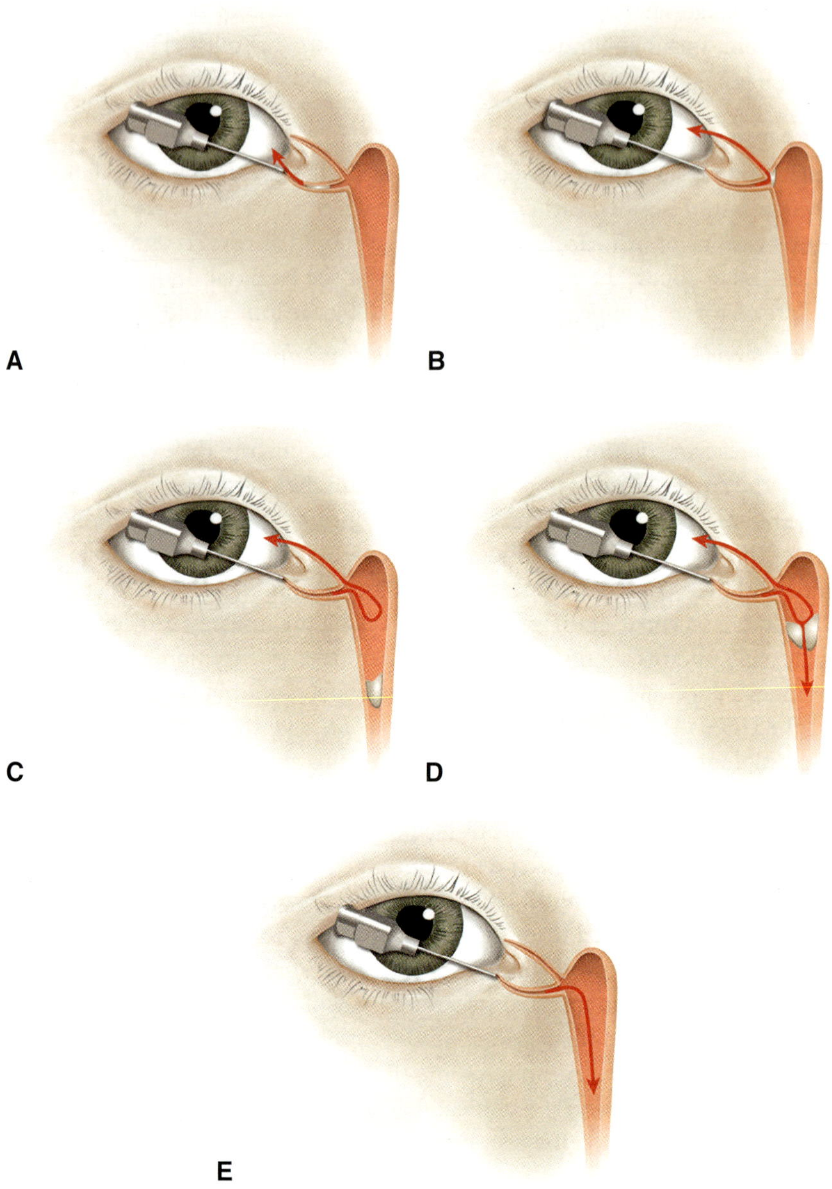


**Figure 13-10** Lacrimal drainage system irrigation. **A,** Complete canalicular obstruction. The cannula is advanced with difficulty, and irrigation fluid refluxes from the same canaliculus. **B,** Complete common canalicular obstruction. A "soft stop" is encountered at the level of the common canaliculus, and irrigated fluid refluxes through the opposite punctum and sometimes partially from the same canaliculus as well. **C,** Complete nasolacrimal duct obstruction (NLDO). The cannula is easily advanced to the medial wall of the lacrimal sac, then a "hard stop" is felt, and irrigation fluid refluxes through the opposite punctum. Often, the refluxed fluid contains mucus and/or pus. With a tight valve of Rosenmüller, lacrimal sac distension without reflux of irrigation fluid may occur. **D,** Partial NLDO. The cannula is easily placed, and irrigation fluid passes into the nose as well as refluxing through the opposite punctum. **E,** Patent lacrimal drainage system. The cannula is placed with ease, and most of the irrigation fluid passes into the nose. *(Illustration by Cyndie C. H. Wooley.)*

stenosis is noted. The irrigating cannula is placed in the canalicular system. To prevent canalicular kinking and difficulty in advancing the irrigating cannula, the clinician maintains lateral traction of the lower eyelid (see Fig 13-4). Canalicular stenosis or occlusion should be recorded and confirmed by subsequent diagnostic probing. Once the irrigating cannula has been advanced into the horizontal canaliculus, clear saline is injected and the results are noted. Careful observation and interpretation determine the area of obstruction without additional testing.

Difficulty advancing the irrigating cannula and an inability to irrigate fluid suggest *total canalicular obstruction.* If saline can be irrigated successfully but it refluxes through the upper canalicular system and no distension of the lacrimal sac is observed on palpation, *complete blockage of the common canaliculus* is probable (Fig 13-11). Subsequent probing determines whether the common canalicular stenosis is total or whether it can be dilated. If mucoid material or fluorescein refluxes through the opposite punctum and lacrimal sac distension is palpable, the diagnosis is *complete NLDO.* If saline irrigation is not associated with canalicular reflux or fluid passing down the NLD, the lacrimal sac will become distended, causing patient discomfort. This result confirms a complete NLDO with a functional valve of Rosenmüller, preventing reflux through the canalicular system. A combination of simultaneous saline reflux through the opposite canaliculus and saline irrigation through the NLD into the nose may indicate a *partial NLD stenosis.*

If saline irrigation passes freely into the nose with no reflux through the canalicular system, a *patent nasolacrimal drainage system* is present. However, it is important to note that even though this irrigation is successful under nonphysiologic conditions such as increased hydrostatic pressure due to the irrigating saline, a *functional obstruction* may still be present. A dacryolith may also impair tear flow without blocking irrigation.

*Diagnostic probing* of the upper system (puncta, canaliculi, and lacrimal sac) is useful in confirming the level of obstruction. In adults, this procedure can easily be performed with topical anesthesia. A small probe (size 00) should be used initially to detect any canalicular obstruction. If an obstruction is encountered, the probe is clamped at the punctum before withdrawal, thereby measuring the distance to the obstruction. A larger probe may be useful to determine the extent of a partial obstruction, but the probe should not be forced through any area of resistance.

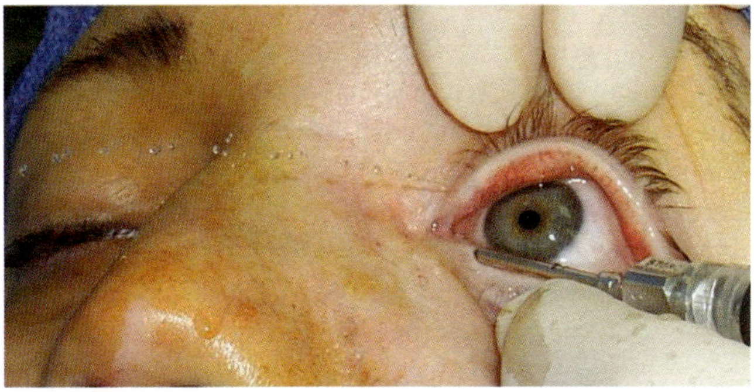

**Figure 13-11** Reflux from the opposite canaliculus caused by common canalicular obstruction or NLDO. *(Courtesy of Morris E. Hartstein, MD.)*

Diagnostic probing of the NLD has no place in adults because there are other means of diagnosing NLDO. Also, probing in adults has limited therapeutic value, rarely producing lasting patency. In contrast, probing in infants is a useful and largely successful procedure. This reflects the differing pathophysiologies of congenital and acquired NLDO: the former often results from occlusion of the NLD by a thin membrane and the latter from more extensive fibrosis of the duct itself.

Intranasal examination is performed with a nasal speculum and light source. When available, diagnostic nasal endoscopy is helpful in the evaluation of the nasal anatomy and in the identification of disease processes.

*Contrast dacryocystography* and *dacryoscintigraphy* aid in evaluation of the anatomy and function of the lacrimal drainage system. However, they are now used infrequently, primarily because alternate methods of evaluation, such as simple irrigation and modern imaging techniques (CT and MRI), are available. Contrast dacryocystography, which involves dye injection into the lacrimal system followed by computerized digital subtraction imaging, provides anatomical information. Dacryoscintigraphy provides a physiologic picture of lacrimal outflow by using radionucleotide eyedrops to follow tear flow on a scintigram.

*CT* and *MRI* are useful after craniofacial injury, in congenital craniofacial deformities, or for suspected neoplasia. CT is superior for the evaluation of suspected bony abnormalities, such as fractures. MRI is superior for the evaluation of suspected soft-tissue disease, such as malignancy. Either CT or MRI may be helpful in evaluating concomitant sinus or nasal disease that may contribute to excess tearing.

Guzek JP, Ching AS, Hoang TA, et al. Clinical and radiologic lacrimal testing in patients with epiphora. *Ophthalmology.* 1997;104(11):1875–1881.

Kashkouli MB, Mirzajani H, Jamshidian-Tehrani M, Pakdel F, Nojomi M, Aghaei GH. Reliability of fluorescein dye disappearance test in assessment of adults with nasolacrimal duct obstruction. *Ophthal Plast Reconstr Surg.* 2013;29(3):167–169.

Wright MM, Bersani TA, Frueh BR, Musch DC. Efficacy of the primary dye test. *Ophthalmology.* 1989;96(4):481–483.

## Punctal Disorders

Several punctal abnormalities can result in epiphora. Puncta may be stenotic, occluded, or too big (usually due to iatrogenic causes); or they may be malpositioned or occluded by adjacent structures.

Punctal stenosis and occlusion can occur due to numerous causes, including those that are congenital, inflammatory (eg Stevens-Johnson syndrome, mucous membrane pemphigoid [ocular cicatricial pemphigoid]), infectious (eg, herpes), or iatrogenic (eg, glaucoma medications, deliberate occlusion in the treatment of dry eye disease) in nature. Punctal stenosis may be associated with punctal ectropion, perhaps from atrophy in the absence of tear flow. Punctal stenosis may be treated with dilation, punctoplasty, or stenting. Most often, the benefits of dilation are short-lived and punctoplasty is required. This is usually accomplished with a snip procedure, in which a small portion of the ampulla is excised. If stenosis recurs, stenting may be required during healing to prevent contraction. Treatment of complete occlusion consists of surgical canalization and, in most cases, stenting.

Abnormally large puncta can also cause epiphora, although this is counterintuitive. In such cases, epiphora is thought to be the result of disruption of the lacrimal pump. The expanded opening prevents formation of an adequate seal when the eyes are closed. This in turn prevents development of negative pressure such that suctioning of the tears does not occur. Punctal enlargement is almost exclusively the result of iatrogenic injury. Stenting of the lacrimal drainage system can result in "cheese-wiring" of the puncta and adjacent canaliculi; therefore, patients with stents require periodic monitoring. Stents should be removed if punctal deformation is detected. Punctal enlargement can also result from overly aggressive punctoplasty and, occasionally, from excision of adjacent neoplasms. Damage to the puncta should be avoided because no consistently effective treatment is available. Attempts at reconstruction usually fail, leaving a CDCR as the only reasonable alternative. Fortunately, symptoms are rarely severe enough to require this procedure.

In order to drain, tears must have access to the puncta. This access can be disrupted by a punctum that is malpositioned and no longer lies within the tear lake. In cases of epiphora secondary to punctal malposition, the anatomical abnormality must be corrected. Medial ectropion repair by resection of a horizontal ellipse of conjunctival and subconjunctival connective tissue below the punctum, with reapposition of the edges, rotates the punctum inward into the tear lake. This procedure may be combined with horizontal eyelid tightening if laxity is present. Frequently, punctal stenosis is also present and may require a punctoplasty.

Puncta may also become obstructed or malpositioned by adjacent structures, such as a hypertrophied caruncle or conjunctivochalasis. In most cases, this is easily corrected with excision of the abnormal caruncle or conjunctiva.

## Canalicular Obstruction

### *Evaluation*

Obstruction can occur within the common, upper, or lower canaliculus. Diagnostic canalicular probing may reveal a canalicular obstruction proximal to the common canaliculus. *Partial obstruction* may be discovered during lacrimal system irrigation if there is partial fluid flow into the nose and partial reflux. *Total common canalicular obstruction* is characterized by flow from the lower to the upper canaliculus with no flow into the lacrimal sac during lacrimal system irrigation. After insertion, the lacrimal probe advances only about 8 mm from the punctum before encountering a tactile soft stop: the probe cannot be advanced beyond a total common canalicular obstruction. In normal conditions, a hard stop would be reached when the probe successfully passes through the open canalicular system into the lumen of the lacrimal sac and then encounters the medial lacrimal sac and lacrimal bone. When common canalicular obstruction is present, lacrimal system irrigation results in a high-velocity reflux from the opposite canaliculus (see Fig 13-11).

The clinician should keep in mind that what appears to be a partial obstruction may sometimes be a *total functional occlusion.* This can be seen with weakness of the lacrimal pump or inability of tears to pass through the partial obstruction under normal physiologic conditions. Some functional obstructions may be overcome with irrigation due to creation of exceptionally high hydrostatic pressure.

### *Etiology*

**Lacrimal plugs** Punctal and canalicular plugs, which are designed to obstruct lacrimal outflow in the treatment of dry eye disease, come in various shapes and sizes. Although any type of plug can result in obstruction, this is most commonly seen with intracanalicular plugs. The permanent intracanalicular plug is a poorly conceived device that leads to partial canalicular obstruction and infection. Punctal plugs that are too small may migrate within the canaliculi and also result in obstruction. Even temporary or absorbable plugs have been known to cause a local inflammatory response and canalicular constriction. Canalicular probing is diagnostic. High-frequency ultrasound has also been used to identify silicone plugs causing obstructions within canaliculi. Once identified, the problematic plug is surgically excised. Often, excision of a short segment of scarred canaliculus is required. The canaliculus is then repaired with reanastomosis over a stent. This technique is similar to reconstruction following trauma or after injury of the canaliculus during excision of a neoplasm.

White WL, Bartley GB, Hawes MJ, Linberg JV, Leventer DB. Iatrogenic complications related to the use of Herrick Lacrimal Plugs. *Ophthalmology.* 2001;108(10):1835–1837.

**Medication** Medications occasionally cause canalicular obstruction. This is often encountered with idoxuridine and chemotherapeutic agents such as 5-fluorouracil and docetaxel. These drugs are secreted in the tears, leading to inflammation and scarring of the canaliculi. Use of topical steroid drops and artificial tears during chemotherapy may prevent the scarring. If this condition is identified early—before the obstruction is complete—stents can be placed to prevent progression while the patient completes the course of chemotherapy. A special canalicular-only stent is available for these cases. Less commonly, canalicular obstruction has also been reported to follow the use of topical medication (eg, phospholine iodide, eserine).

**Infection** Numerous infections can cause canalicular obstruction. Most frequently, obstruction occurs in the setting of more diffuse conjunctival infection (eg, vaccinia virus, herpes simplex virus). Isolated canalicular infection (canaliculitis; discussed in the section titled Infection) can also result in obstruction.

**Inflammatory disease** Inflammatory conditions such as mucous membrane pemphigoid (ocular cicatricial pemphigoid), Stevens-Johnson syndrome, and graft-vs-host disease often cause loss of the puncta and/or canaliculi. However, because of concurrent loss of tear secretion, patients often do not experience epiphora.

**Trauma** Traumatic injury to the canaliculi can result in permanent damage if the injury is not managed in a timely, appropriate manner. This is discussed in greater detail later in this chapter in the section titled Trauma.

**Neoplasm** When a neoplasm is present in the medial canthal area, complete resection may include removal of the puncta and canaliculi. Complete tumor excision must be confirmed by histologic examination of excised tissue before connection of the lacrimal drainage system with the middle meatus is considered. When the distal lacrimal drainage system remains intact, the remaining portion of the canaliculi may be marsupialized to the conjunctival surface with or without intubation.

### *Management*

**Canalicular stenting** *Intubation* or *stenting* of the lacrimal drainage system should be considered as a first-line therapy whenever possible. Intubation of the nasolacrimal drainage system can usually be performed successfully when the patient has symptomatic canalicular constriction but not complete occlusion. For canalicular scarring, the use of a balloon catheter alone is usually not sufficient to correct this condition.

**Reconstruction** Reconstruction of an obstructed canaliculus is often successful when only a few millimeters are involved. If a limited area of total occlusion is discovered near the punctum, the occluded canaliculus can be resected and the cut ends of the canaliculus anastomosed over a stent. When a focal obstruction is found distally or within the common canaliculus, trephination of the scarred segment establishes a patent lumen. Stenting is then required to prevent contracture and to provide a scaffold for proper epithelialization. Also, during removal of a punctal or canalicular plug, a small segment of scarred canaliculus is often excised, then the canaliculus is reconstructed over a stent. Laser canaliculoplasty with a holmium laser followed by stenting has had some success in recanalizing a scarred canaliculus.

**Canaliculodacryocystorhinostomy** If the common canaliculus is totally obstructed, or if the lacrimal sac is sclerotic, a canaliculodacryocystorhinostomy or canaliculorhinostomy may be performed. In these procedures, the area of total common canalicular obstruction is removed, and the remaining patent canalicular system is directly anastomosed to the lacrimal sac mucosa or the lateral nasal wall mucosa. Use of a silicone stent for the reconstructed canalicular system is an important part of these types of reconstruction. Because the failure rate of canalicular resection surgery for total obstruction is significant, Jones tube placement is a surgical alternative.

**Conjunctivodacryocystorhinostomy** When one or both canaliculi are severely obstructed, a CDCR may be required. This procedure creates a complete bypass of the lacrimal drainage system. A CDCR is indicated when the canalicular abnormality is so severe that the canalicular system cannot be used or reconstructed. After creating a rhinostomy opening into the nose, a Jones tube is placed through an opening created at the inferior half of the caruncle and then through the osteotomy site into the middle nasal meatus (Fig 13-12). Gold dilators may be used to enlarge the mucosal opening prior to insertion of the Jones tube. Before the tube is inserted, the desired tube length can be determined with a sizer. A partial carunculectomy may be needed to prevent obstruction of the tube. The ocular end of the tube must be situated in the tear lake, whereas the nasal end must clear the anterior end of the middle turbinate. Subtotal resections of the anterior middle turbinate may be necessary. The surgeon should have tubes of different lengths available at the time of surgery, to ensure implantation of a tube that emerges clearly in the nose without abutting the nasal septum.

Postoperative care and complications, including obstruction of the tube with mucus and migration of the tube, can be troublesome. Forced inspiration, with the mouth and nose manually closed, creates significant airflow through the tube into the nasal airway and usually clears mucous debris and prevents obstruction. Patients should be instructed to perform this maneuver daily. They should also be informed that loss of the tube, even

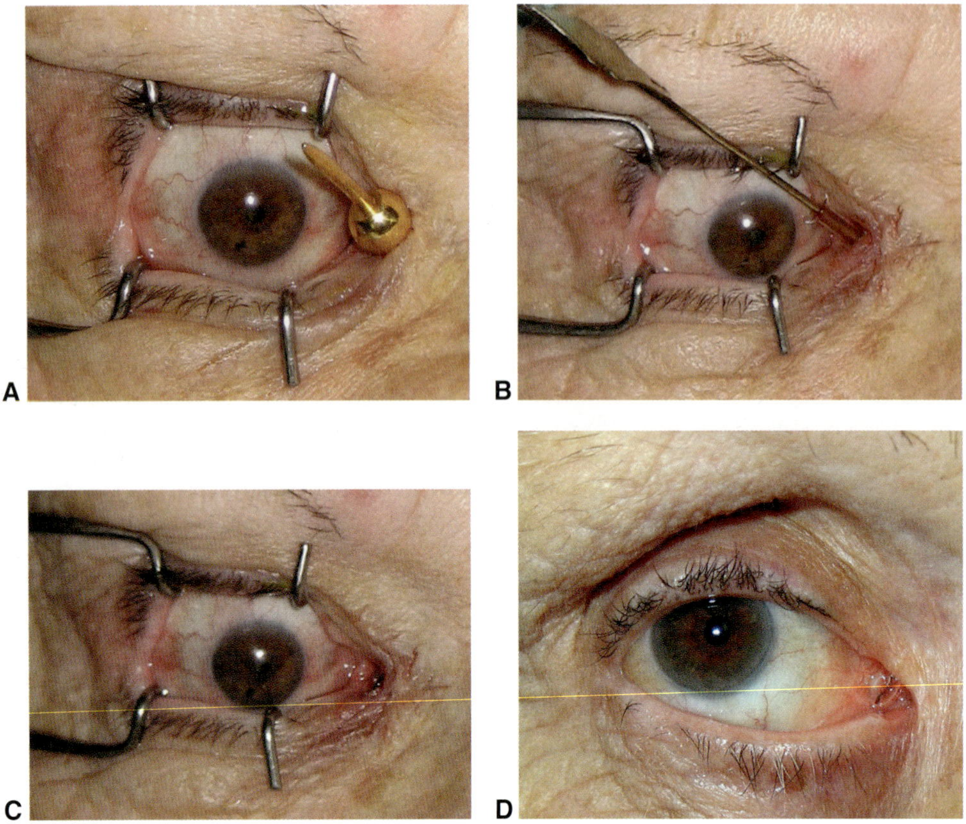

**Figure 13-12** Steps in conjunctivodacryocystorhinostomy. **A,** The tract through the caruncle is enlarged using a dilator. **B,** The Jones tube is advanced over the probe to determine the proper length of the tube. **C,** Jones tube in place at the conclusion of the procedure. **D,** Well-positioned Jones tube postoperatively. *(Courtesy of Morris E. Hartstein, MD.)*

if only for a few days, may lead to closure of the soft-tissue tract for the Jones tube. Periodic removal, cleaning, and replacement of the Jones tube in the office may be necessary. Jones tubes may cause chronic foreign-body sensation and mucus production and can incite pyogenic granuloma formation. Despite these drawbacks, the procedure helps many patients with otherwise intractable epiphora. Patients who have problems with recurrent migration or loss of the tube may benefit from placement of a frosted, angled, or modified Jones tube. Another alternative is the porous polyethylene-coated tube, which allows ingrowth of fibrous tissue into its outer covering to better secure the tube.

Rosen N, Ashkenazi I, Rosner M. Patient dissatisfaction after functionally successful conjunctivodacryocystorhinostomy with Jones tube. *Am J Ophthalmol.* 1994;117(5): 636–642.

## Acquired Nasolacrimal Duct Obstruction

Nasolacrimal duct obstruction can usually be diagnosed with irrigation. Clinicians tend to assume that NLDO is a relatively benign condition and proceed directly to a discussion of surgery. Although this is true in most cases, the alternate causes of NLDO merit consideration.

Bartley GB. Acquired lacrimal drainage obstruction: an etiologic classification system, case reports, and a review of the literature. Part 1. *Ophthal Plast Reconstr Surg.* 1992;8(4): 237–242.

Bartley GB. Acquired lacrimal drainage obstruction: an etiologic classification system, case reports, and a review of the literature. Part 3. *Ophthal Plast Reconstr Surg.* 1993;9(1):11–26.

### *Etiology*

**Involutional stenosis** Involutional stenosis is probably the most common cause of NLDO in older persons. It affects women twice as frequently as men. Although the inciting event in this process is unknown, clinicopathologic study suggests that inflammatory infiltrates and edema cause compression of the lumen of the NLD. This may be the result of anatomical predisposition, unidentified infection, or possibly autoimmune disease. Management almost always consists of DCR.

**Dacryolith** Dacryoliths, or concretions formed within the lacrimal sac (Fig 13-13), can also obstruct the NLD. Dacryoliths consist of shed epithelial cells, lipids, and amorphous debris with or without calcium. In most cases, no inciting event or abnormality is identified. Occasionally, infection with *Actinomyces israelii* or *Candida* species or long-term administration of topical medications such as epinephrine can lead to the formation of a concretion.

Dacryoliths can form in patients with otherwise normal lacrimal drainage systems. When this occurs, patients often experience intermittent symptoms, depending on the location of the dacryolith. Dacryoliths also tend to form following a preexisting obstruction; in this situation, symptoms are unremitting. Acute impaction of a dacryolith in the NLD can produce lacrimal sac distension and substantial pain. Dacryoliths can be removed during external DCR.

Repp DJ, Burkat CN, Lucarelli MJ. Lacrimal excretory system concretions: canalicular and lacrimal sac. *Ophthalmology.* 2009;116(11):2230–2235.

**Sinus disease** Sinus disease often occurs in conjunction with, and may contribute to, the development of NLDO. Clinicians should inquire about previous sinus surgery, as the NLD is sometimes inadvertently damaged during sinus procedures.

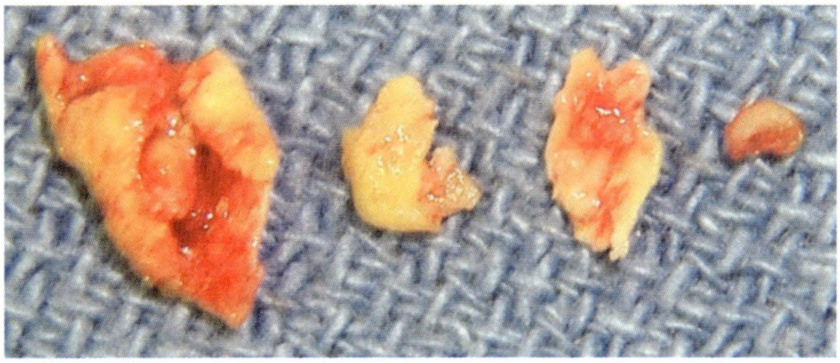

**Figure 13-13** Dacryoliths removed from the lacrimal sac. *(Courtesy of Morris E. Hartstein, MD.)*

**Trauma** Naso-orbital fractures may involve the NLD. Early treatment with fracture reduction and stenting of the entire lacrimal drainage system should be considered. However, such injuries are often not recognized or are initially neglected as more serious injuries are managed. In such cases, late treatment of persistent epiphora usually requires DCR. Injuries may also occur during rhinoplasty or endoscopic sinus surgery; the management of these injuries is similar to the treatment of injuries occurring with fractures.

**Inflammatory disease** Granulomatous disease, including sarcoidosis, granulomatosis with polyangiitis (formerly, Wegener granulomatosis), and lethal midline granuloma, may also lead to NLDO. When systemic disease is suspected, a biopsy of the lacrimal sac or the NLD performed at the time of DCR may provide additional diagnostic input.

**Lacrimal plugs** As with similar cases of canalicular obstruction, dislodged punctal and canalicular plugs can migrate to and occlude the NLD. As with most forms of NLDO, treatment consists of DCR. Remaining segments of a partially removed silicone stent have also been known to cause NLDO.

**Radioactive iodine** Therapeutic radioactive iodine for the treatment of thyroid cancer may also lead to closure of the lacrimal apparatus, specifically the sac and duct. This is not seen with the lower dosages used for treatment of the thyroid gland in patients with Graves hyperthyroidism.

**Neoplasm** Neoplasm should be considered as a possible etiology in any patient presenting with NLDO. In patients with an atypical presentation, including younger age and male sex, further workup is appropriate. Bloody punctal discharge or lacrimal sac distension above the medial canthal tendon is also suggestive of neoplasm. A history of malignancy, especially of sinus or nasopharyngeal origin, warrants further investigation. When malignancy is suspected, appropriate imaging studies (CT or MRI) should be obtained. Preoperative endoscopy is performed to evaluate for intranasal neoplasm. In addition, if an unexpected mass or other suggestive abnormality is encountered during surgery, a biopsy specimen should be obtained.

When a neoplasm is found to contribute to NLDO, initial treatment should focus on the neoplasm. In patients with benign tumors, a DCR or CDCR can then be performed. In patients with malignant tumors, surgical correction of the nasolacrimal drainage system should be postponed until there is certainty of clear margins or freedom from recurrence, after which a DCR or CDCR may be undertaken. Tumors of the lacrimal sac and NLD are discussed in further detail later in this chapter, in the section titled Neoplasm.

### *Management*

**Intubation and stenting** Some clinicians have reported that partial stenosis of the NLD with symptomatic epiphora may respond to surgical intubation of the entire lacrimal drainage system. This procedure should be performed only if the tubes can be passed easily. In some cases of partial NLDO, the balloon catheter has proved to be a helpful adjuvant. In complete NLDO, intubation alone is not effective and a DCR should be considered.

**Dacryocystorhinostomy** A DCR is the treatment of choice for most patients with acquired NLDO. Surgical indications include recurrent dacryocystitis, chronic mucoid reflux, painful distension of the lacrimal sac, and bothersome epiphora. For patients with dacryocystitis, active infection should be treated, if possible, before DCR is performed.

Although there are many minor variations in surgical technique, all share the feature of creating an anastomosis between the lacrimal sac and the nasal cavity through a bony ostium. One distinction between techniques is whether the surgeon uses an internal (intranasal) approach or the more traditional external (transcutaneous) approach.

The advantages of an *internal (endonasal) DCR* include lack of a visible scar, a shorter recovery period, and less discomfort. Recent data have demonstrated higher success rates for internal DCR than were previously reported. When selecting a surgical technique, the surgeon should remember that second attempts following failed DCR—no matter which approach was used—have a higher failure rate. Therefore, patients should be informed that if an internal DCR fails, the likelihood of a successful external DCR is somewhat decreased. An external DCR allows better exposure for management of canalicular stenosis, unexpected neoplasm, or dacryoliths.

DCR can be performed under general anesthesia, but in most adults, local anesthesia with intravenous sedation can be used. Whether DCR is performed under general anesthesia or monitored anesthesia care, intraoperative hemostasis can be enhanced by preoperative injection of lidocaine with epinephrine into the medial canthal soft tissues and by the use of intranasally injected anesthetic and nasal packing with vasoconstrictive agents (oxymetazoline hydrochloride or phenylephrine. In *external DCR* (Fig 13-14), the skin incision should be made so as to avoid the angular blood vessels and prevent wound contractures leading to epicanthal folds. The osteotomy adjacent to the medial wall of the lacrimal sac can be created with a hemostat, rongeur, trephine, or drill. A large osteotomy site facilitates the formation of posterior and anterior mucosal flaps from both the lacrimal sac and the nasal mucosa. Suturing of the corresponding posterior flaps and anterior flaps is common, but sometimes only anterior flaps are anastomosed. Simultaneous stenting of the canaliculi with silicone tubes may be needed, especially in patients who have common canalicular stenosis.

A biopsy with frozen section examination should be considered if abnormal tissue is found. Some surgeons routinely perform a biopsy of the excised lacrimal sac. However, evidence suggests that in the absence of a grossly visible abnormality or an indicative history, lacrimal sac biopsies are unlikely to reveal occult disease. *Endonasal DCR* usually consists of removal of a nasal mucosal flap or en bloc resection over the area corresponding to the nasolacrimal sac and duct (Fig 13-15). An osteotomy is performed to remove the frontal process of the maxilla and the lacrimal bone covering the lacrimal sac. Often, the surgeon also has to remove the uncinate process to allow proper exposure of the superior aspect of the lacrimal passage. The lacrimal sac is then opened, and the medial wall of the sac is removed, marsupializing the sac into the nose. Bicanalicular intubation is usually performed at the end of the procedure. Preservation of the lacrimal and nasal mucosa may result in less scarring and a higher success rate, and techniques to preserve these structures have been proposed. Careful selection of patients with an adequate normal nasal cavity is crucial for success. The surgeon should be prepared to modify the nasal anatomy for better exposure and access, such as by performing nasal septoplasty. Several variations of endonasal DCR are available. Some surgeons use a fiber-optic probe passed through a canaliculus to transilluminate the lacrimal sac (as shown in Figure 13-15). This

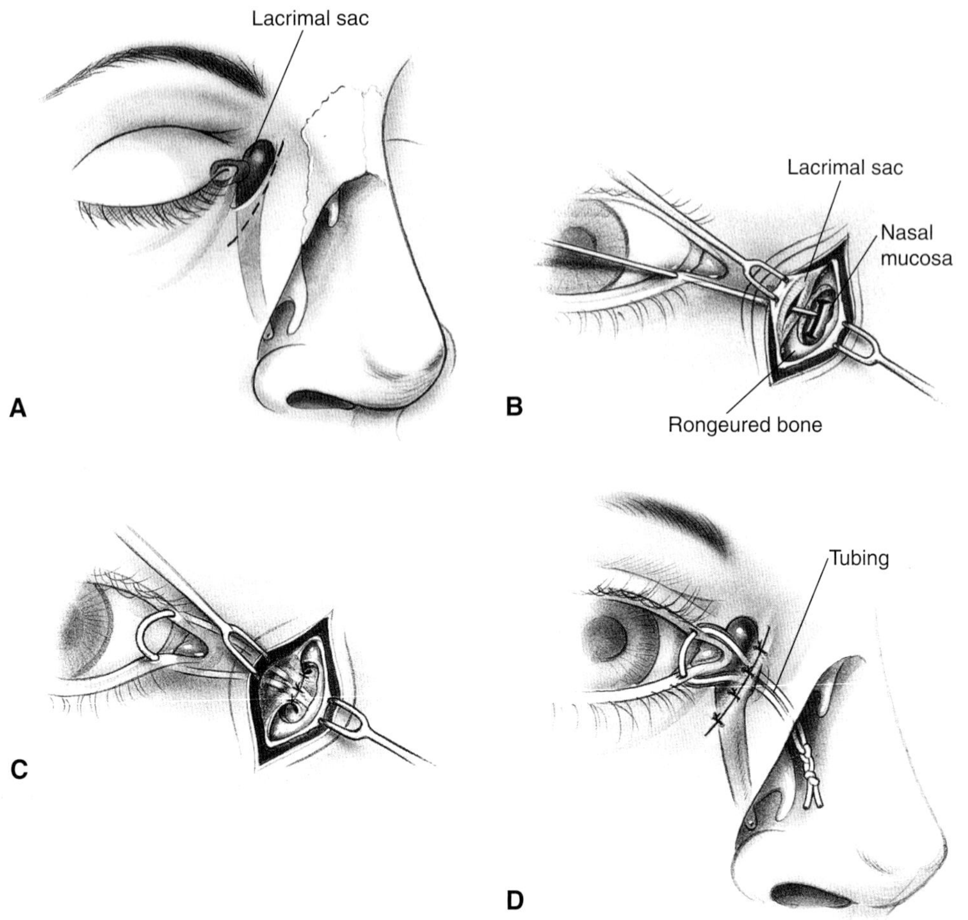


**Figure 13-14** External dacryocystorhinostomy (DCR). **A,** The incision is marked 10 mm from the medial canthus, starting just above the medial canthal tendon and extending inferiorly. **B,** Bone from the lacrimal fossa and anterior lacrimal crest has been resected. Flaps have been fashioned in the nasal mucosa. A lacrimal probe extends through an incision in the lacrimal sac. **C,** The anterior lacrimal sac flap is sutured to the anterior nasal mucosal flap after a silicone tube is placed. **D,** Final position of the silicone tube following closure of the skin incision. *(Illustration by Christine Gralapp.)*

probe helps identify the thin lacrimal bone. Internal DCR can be performed endoscopically *(endoscopic DCR).* Internal DCRs through the nostril may also be performed under direct visualization.

Although DCRs are successful in most patients, failures do occur. DCR failures may be caused by fibrosis and occlusion of the osteotomy, common canalicular obstruction, or inappropriate placement or size of the bony ostium. The outcome of the DCR is also influenced by other factors, including the patient's history of trauma, coexisting autoimmune inflammatory disease, the presence of active dacryocystitis, the development of postoperative infection, or hypersensitivity or foreign-body reactions to the stent. When an initial DCR fails, most surgeons attempt a second DCR before resorting to CDCR. In

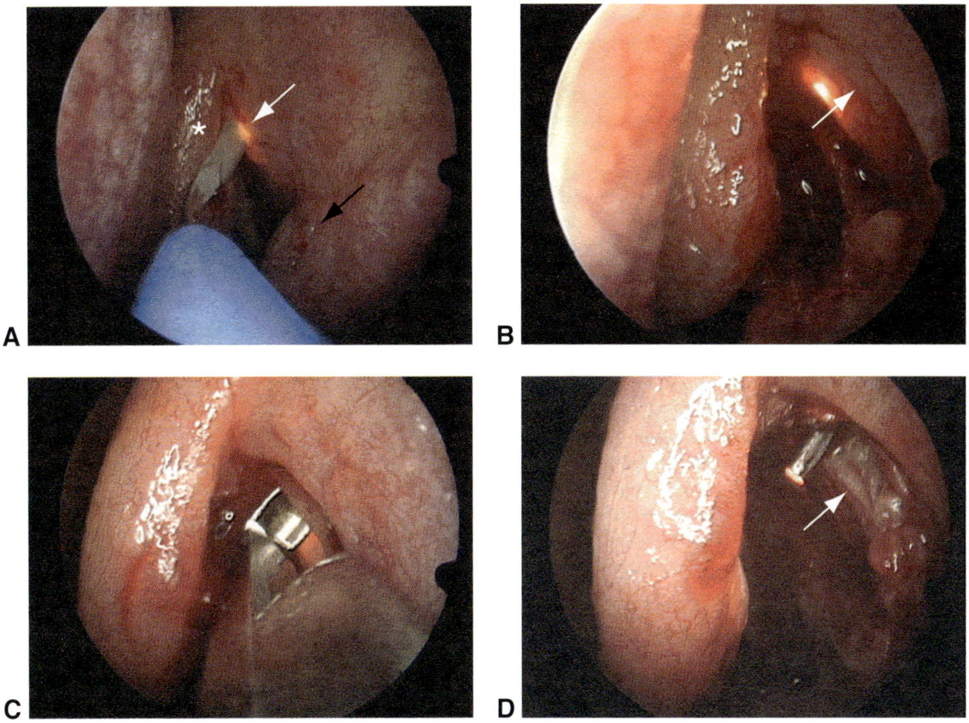


**Figure 13-15** Endonasal DCR. **A,** Posterior incision behind the intracanalicular transilluminator *(white arrow)*, above the inferior turbinate *(black arrow)*, and just anterior to the insertion of the middle turbinate *(*)*. **B,** Frontal process of the maxilla after removal of nasal mucosa *(white arrow)*. **C,** Removal of the frontal process of the maxilla with rongeurs. **D,** The lacrimal sac has been opened *(white arrow)*, and the transilluminator can be seen in the nose. *(Courtesy of François Codère, MD.)*

an attempt to increase the likelihood of success, some surgeons apply topical mitomycin C, a potent antiproliferative alkylating agent, to the surgical site. This is thought to prevent fibrosis at the osteotomy site. The appropriate role of mitomycin C in a secondary DCR performed after initial failure continues to evolve.

Dolman PJ. Comparison of external dacryocystorhinostomy with nonlaser endonasal dacryocystorhinostomy. *Ophthalmology.* 2003;110(1):78–84.

Huang J, Malek J, Chin D, et al. Systematic review and meta-analysis on outcomes for endoscopic versus external dacryocystorhinostomy. *Orbit.* 2014;33(2):81–90.

## Therapeutic Closure of the Lacrimal Drainage System

In cases of severe dry eye disease, occlusion of the lacrimal drainage system may be helpful. Dissolvable collagen plugs may be used on a trial basis. More commonly, permanent plugs made of silicone are used. The advantages of permanent plugs are that placement is fairly straightforward and that, in most cases, they can be removed, if necessary. Although permanent plugs are usually well tolerated, complications are occasionally encountered.

Minor problems include ocular surface irritation and a foreign-body reaction. Pyogenic granulomas may develop, requiring removal of the plug. In most cases, the pyogenic granuloma regresses once the plug is removed, but surgical excision is needed on occasion. More serious complications usually relate to plug displacement.

*Plug extrusion* or *migration* is not uncommon. The ophthalmologist can best avoid these complications by using a plug that is the appropriate size. An instrument that measures punctal diameter is available. When appropriately fitted, punctal plugs usually stay in place. In most cases, a plug that is too small will simply be extruded. However, if the plug migrates within the lacrimal drainage system, obstruction of either the canaliculus or the NLD may result. Most instances of canalicular obstruction have been caused by plugs that were designed to be placed within the canaliculus. Use of these plugs is not recommended. *Canaliculitis* may also result from canalicular plugs or from punctal plugs that have migrated to the canaliculus.

When occlusion with plugs is not successful, the clinician may consider surgical occlusion. Surgery should be reserved for severe cases and must be performed with caution. Surgical closure is almost always permanent. If a patient suffers from subsequent epiphora, no simple solution is available; most cases require a CDCR. To avoid this complication, all patients should undergo a trial of temporary closure before permanent closure.

Once the decision has been made to proceed with surgical occlusion, the puncta should be closed in a stepwise fashion, one punctum at a time. The upper and lower puncta of the same eye should never be closed simultaneously. Complete loss of lacrimal outflow can result in epiphora even in patients with fairly severe dry eye disease.

Numerous surgical techniques for occluding the lacrimal drainage system have been described. *Thermal obliteration* of the puncta and adjacent canaliculi can be performed with a handheld cautery unit or a needle-tip unipolar cautery unit. Although an argon laser can be used for thermal punctal occlusion, it offers no advantage over conventional techniques. *Ampullectomy* can be performed with either direct closure or placement of an overlying conjunctival graft. Often, despite fairly aggressive attempts, the puncta persist or reform. In these recalcitrant cases, the punctal and adjacent canalicular epithelium can be completely excised.

Kim BM, Osmanovic SS, Edward DP. Pyogenic granulomas after silicone punctal plugs: a clinical and histopathologic study. *Am J Ophthalmol.* 2005;139(4):678–684.

Mazow ML, McCall T, Prager TC. Lodged intracanalicular plugs as a cause of lacrimal obstruction. *Ophthal Plast Reconstr Surg.* 2007;23(2):138–142.

## Trauma

### Canaliculus

Most traumatic injuries to the canaliculi occur in one of 2 ways: by direct laceration, such as from a stab wound, or by traction, which occurs when sudden lateral displacement of the eyelid tears the medial canthal tendon and associated canaliculus. Because it lacks tarsal support, the canaliculus lies within the weakest part of the eyelid and is often the first structure to yield. Whenever blunt trauma, such as from a fist or an airbag, results in a full-thickness eyelid laceration, the clinician should suspect and evaluate for an associated medial injury. The avulsion injury often appears trivial on superficial inspection, its full extent revealed only on detailed examination of the area. When possible, diagnostic canalicular probing and irrigation should be performed.

Because patients who have only one functioning canaliculus may be asymptomatic, some clinicians consider the repair of an isolated canalicular laceration to be optional. However, some patients with only one functioning canaliculus may experience symptomatic epiphora, especially with ocular irritation. Moreover, the success rate of primary repair is much higher than that of secondary reconstruction. Therefore, given the common occurrence of epiphora and the difficulties associated with delayed reconstruction, most surgeons recommend repair of all canalicular lacerations.

Repair of injured canaliculi should be performed as soon as possible, preferably within 48 hours of injury. The first step of the repair is locating the severed ends of the canalicular system. This can be frustrating, but the controlled conditions of an operating room, including the use of general anesthesia and magnification with optimal illumination, facilitate the search. A thorough understanding of the medial canthal anatomy guides the surgeon to the appropriate area to begin exploration for the medial end of the severed canaliculus. Laterally, the canaliculus is located near the eyelid margin, but for lacerations close to the lacrimal sac, the canaliculus is deep to the anterior limb of the medial canthal tendon. Irrigation using air, fluorescein, or yellow viscoelastic material through an intact adjacent canaliculus may be helpful. Methylene blue should be avoided, as it tends to stain the entire operative field. In difficult cases, the careful use of a smooth-tipped pigtail probe may help identify the medial cut end. The probe is introduced through the opposite, uninvolved punctum; passed through the common canaliculus; and finally passed through the medial cut end.

Stenting of the injured canaliculus is usually performed to help prevent postoperative canalicular strictures. By putting the stent on traction, the surgeon draws together the severed canalicular ends and other soft-tissue structures, putting them back in their normal anatomical positions. Direct anastomosis of the cut canaliculus over the silicone tube can be accomplished with closure of the pericanalicular tissues. Direct suturing of the canaliculi is probably not necessary. Lacrimal intubation also facilitates the soft-tissue reconstruction of the medial canthal tendon and eyelid margin.

Traditionally, bicanalicular stents have been used, but monocanalicular stents are also available (see Fig 13-7). One type of monocanalicular stent is attached distally to a metal guiding probe. This probe is retrieved intranasally. A type of silicone monocanalicular stent without the metallic probe is inserted into the punctum and threaded directly into the lacerated canaliculus to bridge the laceration but does not extend into the nose. This also allows the procedure to be performed under local anesthesia in the office or the emergency department.

Stents are usually left in place for 2 months or longer. However, cheese-wiring, ocular irritation, infection, local inflammation, or pyogenic granuloma formation may necessitate early removal. Bicanalicular stents are usually cut at the medial canthus and retrieved from the nose. Monocanalicular stents are simply pulled through the punctum.

Jordan DR, Gilberg S, Mawn LA. The round-tipped, eyed pigtail probe for canalicular intubation: a review of 228 patients. *Ophthal Plast Reconstr Surg.* 2008;24(3):176–180.

Kersten RC, Kulwin DR. "One-stitch" canalicular repair. A simplified approach for repair of canalicular laceration. *Ophthalmology.* 1996;103(5):785–789.

### Lacrimal Sac and Nasolacrimal Duct

The lacrimal sac and NLD may be injured by direct laceration or by fracture of surrounding bones. Injuries of the lacrimal sac or NLD may also occur during rhinoplasty or endoscopic sinus surgery when the physiologic maxillary sinus ostium is being enlarged anteriorly. Early treatment of the lacrimal sac and NLD is appropriate and consists of fracture reduction, soft-tissue repair, and silicone intubation of the entire lacrimal drainage system. Late treatment of persistent epiphora may require DCR.

## Infection

### Dacryoadenitis

Acute inflammation of the lacrimal gland *(dacryoadenitis)* is most often seen in inflammatory disease and occasionally is the consequence of malignancy, such as lymphoproliferative disease. Noninfectious disease of the lacrimal gland is covered in Chapter 4. Dacryoadenitis is unusual, and gross purulence and abscess formation are uncommon. However, with the emergence of community-acquired methicillin-resistant *Staphylococcus aureus (MRSA),* this condition is seen more frequently. Most cases are the result of bacterial infection, which may develop secondary to an adjacent infection, after trauma, or hematogenously. Alternatively, MRSA infection may appear without preexisting risk factors. Given the rare occurrence of these infections, large case series are lacking, as are a precise breakdown of causative organisms and suggestions on management. Presumably, most cases are due to gram-positive bacteria, but cases due to gram-negative bacteria have been documented. There are case reports of dacryoadenitis related to tuberculosis, involving the formation of discrete tuberculomas in several cases. Epstein-Barr virus is the most frequently reported viral pathogen. Many nonsuppurative cases are treated empirically, without isolation of the alleged pathogen; coverage for MRSA infection should be considered.

Mathias MT, Horsley MB, Mawn LA, et al. Atypical presentations of orbital cellulitis caused by methicillin-resistant *Staphylococcus aureus. Ophthalmology.* 2012;119(6):1238–1243.

### Canaliculitis

Canaliculitis can be a challenge for patients and clinicians. A variety of bacteria, viruses, and mycotic organisms can cause infection within the canaliculus. The most common pathogen is a filamentous gram-positive rod, *Actinomyces israelii.* The patient presents with persistent weeping and discharge, sometimes accompanied by a follicular conjunctivitis centered in the medial canthus. The punctum is often erythematous and dilated, or "pouting." A cotton-tipped applicator can be used to apply pressure to the canaliculus ("milking"). The expression of purulent discharge confirms the diagnosis (Fig 13-16).

Canaliculitis can be somewhat difficult to eradicate; the clinician should warn the patient that treatment may require several stages. Culture of the discharge may be useful in identifying the cause of the infection. Conservative management consists of warm

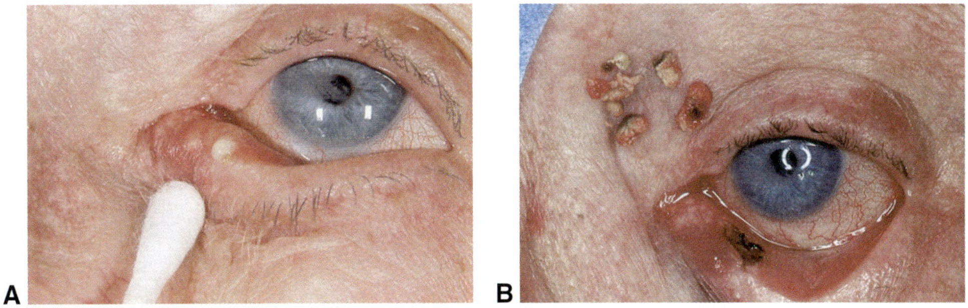


**Figure 13-16** Canaliculitis. **A,** "Pouting" punctum expressing purulent material. **B,** Several small stones curetted from the infected canaliculus. *(Courtesy of Jeffrey A. Nerad, MD.)*

compresses, digital massage, and topical and sometimes oral antibiotic therapy. Many patients require more aggressive treatment, particularly those with *A israelii* infection, which has a tendency to form concretions, or "stones." Within these stones, organisms are protected from lethal antibiotic concentrations. Curettage through the punctum is sometimes successful at removing multiple stones. However, in some cases a canaliculotomy is required to completely remove all particulate matter.

The canaliculotomy should be limited to the horizontal canaliculus and approached from the conjunctival surface. The incision is left open to heal by second intention and does not require stenting. Some surgeons irrigate or paint the canaliculus with povidone-iodine or irrigate with specially formulated penicillin-fortified drops perioperatively. If the infection is the consequence of an obstruction, such as plug placement, the surgeon may need to correct the obstruction to prevent recurrence.

## Dacryocystitis

Inflammation of the lacrimal sac *(acute dacryocystitis)* has various causes. However, in most cases the common factor is complete NLDO, which prevents normal drainage from the lacrimal sac into the nose. Chronic tear retention and stasis lead to secondary infection. Clinical findings include edema and erythema with distension of the lacrimal sac (Fig 13-17). The degree of discomfort ranges from none to severe pain. Complications include dacryocystocele formation, chronic conjunctivitis, and spread to adjacent structures (orbital or facial cellulitis).

The following steps may be used in the treatment of acute dacryocystitis:

- Irrigation or probing of the canalicular system should be avoided until the infection subsides. In most cases, irrigation is not needed to establish the diagnosis, and it is extremely painful for patients with active infection.
- Similarly, diagnostic or therapeutic probing of the NLD is not indicated in adults with acute dacryocystitis.
- Topical antibiotics are of limited value. They do not reach the site of the infection because of stasis within the lacrimal drainage system. They also do not penetrate sufficiently within the adjacent soft tissue.

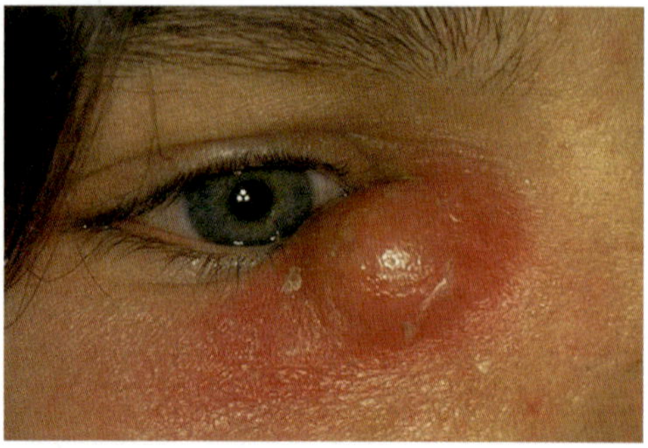

**Figure 13-17** Acute dacryocystitis with cellulitis. *(Courtesy of Morris E. Hartstein, MD.)*

- Oral antibiotics are effective for most infections. Gram-positive bacteria are the most common cause of acute dacryocystitis. However, the clinician should suspect gram-negative organisms in patients who are diabetic or immunocompromised and in those who have been exposed to atypical pathogens (eg, individuals residing in nursing homes).
- Parenteral antibiotics are necessary for the treatment of severe cases, especially if cellulitis or orbital extension is present.
- Aspiration of the lacrimal sac may be performed if a pyocele or mucocele is localized and approaching the skin. Smears and cultures of the aspirate may inform the selection of systemic antibiotic therapy.
- A localized abscess involving the lacrimal sac and adjacent soft tissues may require incision and drainage. The incised abscess is allowed to heal by second intention and may be packed open. This treatment should be reserved for cases that do not respond to more conservative measures or for patients in severe discomfort. A chronically draining epithelialized fistula that communicates with the lacrimal sac can form, but this is rare.

Dacryocystitis indicating total NLDO requires a DCR in most cases because of inevitable persistent epiphora and recurrence. In general, such surgery is deferred until the acute inflammation is resolved. Some patients, however, continue to have a subacute infection until definitive drainage surgery is performed.

*Chronic dacryocystitis,* a smoldering low-grade infection, may develop in some individuals. It usually results in distension of the lacrimal sac. Massage may reflux mucoid material through the canalicular system onto the surface of the eye. If a tumor is not suspected, no further diagnostic evaluation is indicated to confirm the diagnosis of total NLDO. Chronic dacryocystitis is treated before elective intraocular surgery.

## Neoplasm

### Lacrimal Gland

Neoplasms of the lacrimal gland are discussed in Chapter 5.

## Lacrimal Drainage System

Neoplastic causes of acquired obstruction of the lacrimal drainage system may be classified into the following groups:

- primary lacrimal drainage system tumors (most commonly papilloma and squamous cell carcinoma)
- primary tumors of tissues surrounding the lacrimal drainage system that secondarily invade or compromise lacrimal system structures (most commonly basal and squamous cell carcinoma of the eyelid skin; others include adenoid cystic carcinoma, infantile [capillary] hemangioma, inverted papilloma, epidermoid carcinoma, osteoma, and lymphoma)
- tumors metastatic to the nasolacrimal region

*Primary lacrimal sac tumors* are rare and may present clinically as a mass located above the medial canthal tendon. They may be associated with epiphora or chronic dacryocystitis. Dacryocystitis associated with tumor may differ from simple NLDO in that the irrigation fluid may pass into the nose. Also, blood may reflux from the punctum on irrigation, and more ominously, some patients report spontaneous bleeding. Tumors that invade the skin may produce ulceration with telangiectasia over the lacrimal sac. Metastasis to regional lymph nodes may also occur. Dacryocystography is useful for outlining uneven, mottled densities in the dilated lacrimal sac. However, CT or MRI is far superior in identifying neoplasms and determining disease extent. CT also has the advantage of clearly revealing bone erosion.

Histologically, approximately 45% of lacrimal sac tumors are benign and 55% are malignant. Squamous cell papillomas and carcinomas are the most common tumors of the sac. Many papillomas initially grow in an inverted pattern and into the lacrimal sac wall; consequently, their excision is often incomplete. With recurrence, malignant degeneration may occur.

Treatment of benign lacrimal sac tumors commonly requires a *dacryocystectomy.* Malignant tumors may require a dacryocystectomy combined with a lateral rhinotomy and medial maxillectomy sometimes performed in concert with an otolaryngologist. *Exenteration,* including bone removal in the medial canthal area, is necessary if a malignant epithelial tumor has involved bone and the soft tissues of the orbit (see Chapter 8). *Radiation* is useful for treatment of lymphomatous lesions, as an adjuvant after removal of malignant lesions, or as a palliative measure for unresectable lesions. The recurrence rate for invasive squamous and transitional cell carcinoma of the lacrimal sac is approximately 50%, with 50% of these cases being fatal. See Chapter 5 for further discussion.

Parmar DN, Rose GE. Management of lacrimal sac tumours. *Eye (Lond).* 2003;17(5):599–606.

# Basic Texts

## Orbit, Eyelids, and Lacrimal System


Albert DM, Lucarelli MJ, eds. *Clinical Atlas of Procedures in Ophthalmic and Oculofacial Surgery*. 2nd ed. New York: Oxford University Press; 2012.

Baker SR. *Local Flaps in Facial Reconstruction*. 3rd ed. Philadelphia: Mosby; 2014.

Black EH, Nesi FA, Calvano CJ, Gladstone GJ, Levine MR, eds. *Smith and Nesi's Ophthalmic Plastic and Reconstructive Surgery*. 3rd ed. New York: Springer; 2012.

Bron AJ, Tripathi RC, Tripathi BJ. *Wolff's Anatomy of the Eye and Orbit*. 8th ed. Philadelphia: A Hodder Arnold Publication; 1997.

Chen WP. *Asian Blepharoplasty and the Eyelid Crease*. 2nd ed. Philadelphia: Butterworth-Heinemann; 2006.

Codner MA, McCord CD Jr, eds. *Eyelid and Periorbital Surgery*. St Louis: Quality Medical Pub; 2008.

Dutton JJ. *Atlas of Clinical and Surgical Orbital Anatomy*. 2nd ed. Philadelphia: Elsevier/Saunders; 2011.

Dutton JJ. *Atlas of Oculoplastic and Orbital Surgery*. Philadelphia: Wolters Kluwer/Lippincott Williams & Wilkins; 2013.

Dutton JJ, Byrne SF, Proia AD. *Diagnostic Atlas of Orbital Diseases*. Philadelphia: Saunders; 2000.

Ellis E, Zide MF. *Surgical Approaches to the Facial Skeleton*. 2nd ed. Philadelphia: Lippincott Williams & Wilkins; 2006.

Fagien S. *Putterman's Cosmetic Oculoplastic Surgery*. 4th ed. Philadelphia: Saunders; 2007.

Holck D. *Evaluation and Treatment of Orbital Fractures: A Multidisciplinary Approach*. Philadelphia: Saunders; 2005.

Hurwitz JJ, ed. *The Lacrimal System*. Philadelphia: Lippincott-Raven; 1996.

Katowitz JA. *Pediatric Oculoplastic Surgery*. New York: Springer-Verlag; 2002.

Korn BS, Kikkawa DO, eds. *Video Atlas of Oculofacial Plastic and Reconstructive Surgery*. Philadelphia: Elsevier/Saunders; 2011.

Lemke BN, Della Rocca RC, eds. *Surgery of the Eyelids and Orbit: An Anatomical Approach*. East Norwalk, CT: Appleton & Lange; 1992.

Levine MR. *Manual of Oculoplastic Surgery*. 4th ed. Thorofare, NJ: SLACK Incorporated; 2010.

Massry GG, Murphy MR, Azizzadeh B. *Master Techniques in Blepharoplasty and Periorbital Rejuvenation*. New York: Springer; 2011.

McCord CD, Tanenbaum M, Nunery WR, eds. *Oculoplastic Surgery*. 3rd ed. New York: Raven Press; 1995.

Nerad JA. *Oculoplastic Surgery*. St Louis: Mosby; 2001.

Nerad J. *Techniques in Ophthalmic Plastic Surgery: A Personal Tutorial*. Philadelphia: Saunders; 2009.

Rootman J, ed. *Diseases of the Orbit: A Multidisciplinary Approach.* 2nd ed. Philadelphia: Lippincott Williams & Wilkins; 2002.

Shields JA, Shields CL. *Eyelid, Conjunctival, and Orbital Tumors: An Atlas and Textbook.* 2nd ed. Philadelphia: Lippincott Williams & Wilkins; 2007.

Spencer WH, ed. *Ophthalmic Pathology: An Atlas and Textbook.* 4th ed. Philadelphia: WB Saunders; 1996.

Tse DT. *Color Atlas of Oculoplastic Surgery.* 2nd ed. Philadelphia: Wolters Kluwer/Lippincott Williams & Wilkins; 2011.

Tyers AG, Collin JRO. *Colour Atlas of Ophthalmic Plastic Surgery.* 3rd ed. Oxford: Butterworth-Heinemann; 2007.

Yen MT, ed. *Surgery of the Eyelids, Lacrimal System, and Orbit.* 2nd ed. New York: Oxford University Press; 2012.

Zide BM. *Surgical Anatomy Around the Orbit: The System of Zones.* Philadelphia: Lippincott Williams & Wilkins; 2005.

# Related Academy Materials

The American Academy of Ophthalmology is dedicated to providing a wealth of high-quality clinical education resources for ophthalmologists.

### Print Publications and Electronic Products

For a complete listing of Academy products related to topics covered in this BCSC Section, visit our online store at http://store.aao.org/clinical-education/topic/oculoplastics-orbit.html. Or call Customer Service at 866.561.8558 (toll free, US only) or +1 415.561.8540, Monday through Friday, between 8:00 AM and 5:00 PM (PST).

### Online Resources

Visit the Ophthalmic News and Education (ONE®) Network at aao.org/onenetwork to find relevant videos, online courses, journal articles, practice guidelines, self-assessment quizzes, images and more. The ONE Network is a free Academy-member benefit.

Access free, trusted articles and content with the Academy's collaborative online encyclopedia, EyeWiki, at aao.org/eyewiki.

## Requesting Continuing Medical Education Credit

The American Academy of Ophthalmology is accredited by the Accreditation Council for Continuing Medical Education (ACCME) to provide continuing medical education for physicians.

The American Academy of Ophthalmology designates this enduring material for a maximum of 10 *AMA PRA Category 1 Credits*™. Physicians should claim only the credit commensurate with the extent of their participation in the activity.

The American Medical Association requires that all learners participating in activities involving enduring materials complete a formal assessment before claiming continuing medical education (CME) credit. To assess your achievement in this activity and ensure that a specified level of knowledge has been reached, a posttest for this Section of the Basic and Clinical Science Course is provided online. A minimum score of 80% must be obtained to pass the test and claim CME credit.

**To take the posttest and request CME credit online:**

1. Go to www.aao.org/cme-central and log in.
2. Click on "Claim CME Credit and View My CME Transcript" and then "Report AAO Credits."
3. Select the appropriate media type and then the Academy activity. You will be directed to the posttest.
4. Once you have passed the test with a score of 80% or higher, you will be directed to your transcript. *If you are not an Academy member, you will be able to print out a certificate of participation once you have passed the test.*

CME expiration date: June 1, 2018. *AMA PRA Category 1 Credits*™ may be claimed only once between June 1, 2015, and the expiration date.

For assistance, contact the Academy's Customer Service department at 866-561-8558 (US only) or +1 415-561-8540 between 8:00 AM and 5:00 PM (PST), Monday through Friday, or send an e-mail to customer_service@aao.org.

# Study Questions

Please note that these questions are not part of your CME reporting process. They are provided here for your own educational use and identification of any professional practice gaps. The required CME posttest is available online (see "Requesting CME Credit"). Following the questions are a blank answer sheet and answers with discussions. Although a concerted effort has been made to avoid ambiguity and redundancy in these questions, the authors recognize that differences of opinion may occur regarding the "best" answer. The discussions are provided to demonstrate the rationale used to derive the answer. They may also be helpful in confirming that your approach to the problem was correct or, if necessary, in fixing the principle in your memory. The Section 7 faculty thanks the Self-Assessment Committee for reviewing these self-assessment questions.

1. The nasolacrimal duct opens into what anatomical structure?
   a. sphenoethmoidal recess
   b. middle meatus
   c. inferior meatus
   d. superior meatus

2. What is the largest paranasal sinus?
   a. maxillary sinus
   b. sphenoid sinus
   c. frontal sinus
   d. ethmoid sinus

3. In what anatomical layer is the temporal (frontal) branch of cranial nerve VII found?
   a. deep temporal fascia
   b. temporoparietal fascia
   c. temporal fat pad
   d. subcutaneous tissue

4. What term is used to describe a wider-than-normal separation between the medial orbital walls?
   a. exorbitism
   b. hypertelorism
   c. telecanthus
   d. exophthalmos

5. Failure of what embryonal developmental process results in microphthalmia with orbital cyst?
   a. neural crest cell migration
   b. choroidal fissure closure
   c. primary optic vesicle growth
   d. secondary optic vesicle degeneration

6. A 60-year-old man presents with a 10-day history of left periorbital and facial erythema and edema but no orbital signs. Visual acuity is 20/20 OU, and extraocular motility is full. There is no relative afferent pupillary defect. The history is negative for previous trauma, recent insect bite, and other inciting event. What is the most appropriate next step of action?
   a. steroids
   b. orbital ultrasonography
   c. computed tomography (CT)
   d. topical antibiotics

7. A 4-year-old child presents with lytic bony changes on CT and a superotemporal orbital mass. Histologic examination of the tissue shows fibrous connective tissue and an infiltrate of eosinophils and histiocytes. What systemic condition is most likely to be associated with these findings?
   a. diabetes mellitus
   b. growth hormone deficiency
   c. absence of the septum pellucidum
   d. diabetes insipidus

8. What is the best method to diagnose pleomorphic adenoma?
   a. incisional biopsy
   b. biopsy of pseudocapsule
   c. complete excision
   d. CT

9. Le Fort fractures always involve what structure?
   a. maxilla
   b. nasal bone
   c. ethmoid bone
   d. pterygoid plates

10. Which answer best represents the current standard of care for treatment of traumatic optic neuropathy?
    a. high-dose corticosteroids
    b. surgical decompression of the optic canal
    c. calcium channel blocker
    d. It is controversial; observation alone is acceptable.

11. A tumor is suspected in the lacrimal gland region. What is the best initial surgical approach for a mass in this area?
    a. eyelid crease incision
    b. vertical eyelid-splitting orbitotomy
    c. sub-brow incision
    d. "swinging lower eyelid" approach

12. A mass is found within the medial subperiosteal space. What is the best surgical approach to reach the lesion and create the least-visible scar?
    a. lateral orbitotomy
    b. eyelid crease incision
    c. transcaruncular incision
    d. direct skin incision over the medial canthus

13. What typically does not contribute to socket contraction?
    a. radiation
    b. multiple socket operations
    c. persistent wearing of a conformer or prosthesis
    d. extrusion of an orbital implant

14. In non-Asian persons, where does the orbital septum of the upper eyelid fuse with the levator aponeurosis?
    a. 2–5 mm above the superior tarsal border
    b. inferior third of the tarsus
    c. arcus marginalis
    d. Whitnall ligament

15. What congenital eyelid condition is more common in Asian children and may contribute to mechanical entropion of the lower eyelid margin?
    a. epiblepharon
    b. euryblepharon
    c. ankyloblepharon
    d. congenital ectropion

16. Which characteristic is consistent with infantile (capillary) hemangioma of the eyelid?
    a. It is most often present at birth.
    b. It can be associated with Muir-Torre syndrome.
    c. It tends to show progressive growth into adulthood.
    d. It can be associated with amblyopia.

17. If a basal cell carcinoma involves the lacrimal area and tumor removal leads to destruction of the lacrimal sac or nasolacrimal duct, when should reconstruction of the lacrimal outflow system be performed?
   a. in 4–6 weeks to allow healing
   b. in 3–4 months to see whether tearing will be symptomatic
   c. in 5 years to minimize tumor spread
   d. Reconstruction should never be performed.

18. What histopathologic evaluation is necessary when an eyelid specimen suspicious for sebaceous cell carcinoma is being evaluated?
   a. Congo red stain
   b. S-100 protein stain
   c. lipid stains (oil red O)
   d. immunofluorescence studies

19. What technique is usually needed to repair a large lower eyelid defect involving more than 50% of the eyelid?
   a. primary closure
   b. spontaneous granulation
   c. Cutler-Beard procedure
   d. modified Hughes procedure

20. What is a characteristic finding in blepharophimosis–ptosis–epicanthus inversus syndrome (BPES)?
   a. telecanthus
   b. epicanthus tarsalis
   c. dermatochalasis
   d. epiblepharon

21. What is a typical feature of cicatricial ectropion of the lower eyelid?
   a. anterior lamellar deficiency
   b. lateral canthal tendon laxity
   c. lower eyelid retractor disinsertion
   d. medial canthal tendon laxity

22. What finding is often associated with cicatricial entropion of the lower eyelid?
   a. horizontal eyelid laxity
   b. overriding preseptal orbicularis oculi muscle
   c. lower eyelid retractor disinsertion
   d. posterior lamellar shortening

23. What finding is typically seen in involutional ptosis?
    a. elevated eyelid crease
    b. lagophthalmos
    c. levator function of <10 mm
    d. ipsilateral eyebrow depression

24. What lesion is the most common eyelid malignancy?
    a. squamous cell carcinoma
    b. basal cell carcinoma
    c. sebaceous cell carcinoma
    d. Merkel cell carcinoma

25. What is a characteristic sign of hemifacial spasm?
    a. abatement of symptoms during sleep
    b. unilateral involvement of eyelid protractor muscles
    c. involvement of the procerus and corrugator superciliaris muscles
    d. bilateral lower facial involvement consistent with Meige syndrome

26. Which statement correctly describes the anatomy of the lacrimal sac?
    a. The lacrimal sac lies between the anterior and posterior crura of the medial canthal tendon.
    b. The superficial head of the medial canthal tendon is known as the Horner muscle.
    c. The lacrimal sac contains a distensible superior portion.
    d. The lacrimal sac is located anterior to the angular artery and vein.

27. Which statement best describes the valve of Rosenmüller?
    a. It is located at the distal portion of the nasolacrimal duct.
    b. It prevents reflux of tears from the lacrimal sac into the canaliculi.
    c. It contains no mucosal folds.
    d. It functions as a 2-way valve.

28. Which statement is the most accurate regarding congenital nasolacrimal duct obstruction?
    a. It is caused by a blockage at the valve of Hasner.
    b. It resolves by 2 months of age in most cases.
    c. It is bilateral in 75% of cases.
    d. It should be managed conservatively in all cases.

29. Which is a correct helpful tip for probing of the lacrimal drainage system?
    a. Visualization of the properly placed probe is facilitated by contraction of the nasal mucosa with a topical vasoconstrictor.
    b. Wrinkling of the skin is normal and not an indication to stop probing.
    c. Puncturing scar tissue can help relieve the obstruction.
    d. Once the probe cannot be advanced further, it can be assumed to have exited beneath the inferior turbinate.

30. What is the first diagnostic test for a patient who reports constant epiphora?
    a. Jones I
    b. Jones II
    c. probing and irrigation
    d. dye disappearance test

31. Which treatment has the highest success rate in eliminating epiphora in patients with total obstruction at the common canaliculus?
    a. dacryocystorhinostomy (DCR)
    b. conjunctivodacryocystorhinostomy (CDCR)
    c. canaliculorhinostomy
    d. trephine and silicone intubation

32. What is the most crucial step in successful external DCR?
    a. use of general anesthesia
    b. biopsy of the lacrimal sac
    c. osteotomy through the lacrimal sac fossa and into the nose
    d. suturing of posterior mucosal flaps

33. What is the first line of treatment for an adult with an acute erythematous, tender medial canthal mass inferior to the medial canthal tendon?
    a. incision and drainage
    b. external DCR
    c. oral antibiotics
    d. CT scan of the orbit

# Answer Sheet for Section 7
# Study Questions

| Question | Answer | Question | Answer |
|---|---|---|---|
| 1 | a b c d | 18 | a b c d |
| 2 | a b c d | 19 | a b c d |
| 3 | a b c d | 20 | a b c d |
| 4 | a b c d | 21 | a b c d |
| 5 | a b c d | 22 | a b c d |
| 6 | a b c d | 23 | a b c d |
| 7 | a b c d | 24 | a b c d |
| 8 | a b c d | 25 | a b c d |
| 9 | a b c d | 26 | a b c d |
| 10 | a b c d | 27 | a b c d |
| 11 | a b c d | 28 | a b c d |
| 12 | a b c d | 29 | a b c d |
| 13 | a b c d | 30 | a b c d |
| 14 | a b c d | 31 | a b c d |
| 15 | a b c d | 32 | a b c d |
| 16 | a b c d | 33 | a b c d |
| 17 | a b c d | | |

# Answers

1. **c.** The nasolacrimal duct opens into the inferior meatus. The sphenoid sinus drains just cephalad to the superior concha in the sphenoethmoidal recess. The frontal sinus, maxillary sinus, and anterior and middle ethmoid air cells drain into the middle meatus. The posterior ethmoidal cells open into the superior meatus under the superior turbinate.
2. **a.** The maxillary sinuses are the largest of the paranasal sinuses. The roof of each maxillary sinus forms the floor of each orbit. The maxillary sinus extends posteriorly to the inferior orbital fissure.
3. **b.** In the temporal area, the temporal (frontal) branch of cranial nerve VII crosses the zygomatic arch and courses superomedially in the deep layers of the temporoparietal fascia (also called the superficial temporalis fascia), often near branches of the temporal artery.
4. **b.** Hypertelorism is a wider-than-normal separation between the medial orbital walls. Exorbitism refers to an angle between the lateral orbital walls that is greater than 90°, which may also be associated with shallow orbital depth. Telecanthus refers to a wide intercanthal distance. Exophthalmos refers specifically to proptosis of the eye associated with thyroid eye disease.
5. **b.** Microphthalmia with orbital cyst results from failure of the choroidal fissure to close in the embryo. Craniofacial clefts occur as a result of a developmental arrest or mechanical disruption of development. Etiologic theories include a failure of neural crest cell migration and a failure of fusion or movement of facial processes. Anophthalmia occurs when the primary optic vesicle fails to grow out from the cerebral vesicle at the 2-mm stage of embryonic development. Consecutive anophthalmia is thought to result from a secondary degeneration of the optic vesicle.
6. **c.** In a patient with preseptal cellulitis of unknown etiology, an imaging scan is used to evaluate for possible neoplasm or to obtain other diagnostic information. In preseptal cellulitis, there would typically have been an inciting event such as trauma, insect bite, or brow-hair removal. Sinus neoplasms may present with orbital and/or facial swelling, which can be confused with preseptal cellulitis. Nonspecific orbital inflammation (NSOI; also known as idiopathic orbital inflammatory disease) or sinusitis may also be considered in the differential diagnosis of this patient.
7. **d.** The findings are consistent with a diagnosis of eosinophilic granuloma. In this disease, the orbital lesion is usually located in the superotemporal quadrant of the orbit and most commonly results in lytic bony lesions of the orbital roof. Patients may be unsuccessfully treated for allergy or infection until the proper diagnosis is made by biopsy. Diabetes insipidus is a possible systemic manifestation.
8. **c.** Treatment is complete removal of the tumor with its pseudocapsule intact. When a pleomorphic adenoma (benign mixed cell tumor) is suspected, no preliminary biopsy should be performed. Although the lesion is benign, partial excision is more likely to result in residual orbital disease and recurrence. Residual tumor may also show malignant transformation.
9. **d.** By definition, Le Fort fractures must extend posteriorly through the pterygoid plates. They can have orbital and nasal involvement.

10. **d.** The treatment of optic neuropathy remains controversial, and currently there is no standard of care. Observation alone is an acceptable treatment option. A recent multicenter, prospective nonrandomized trial failed to show benefit from corticosteroid or surgical treatment of optic neuropathy. Calcium channel blockers have been shown to have neuroprotective properties, but their use in traumatic optic neuropathy has not been established.
11. **a.** For a tumor in the lacrimal gland region, an eyelid crease incision provides excellent exposure and good cosmesis. The vertical eyelid-splitting incision would disrupt the eyelid anatomy more than is necessary to reach the lacrimal gland. A sub-brow incision will result in a scar. The "swinging eyelid" approach is better suited for inferior masses.
12. **c.** A transcaruncular incision provides the most direct access to the medial subperiosteal space and excellent cosmesis. As stated in the previous discussion, an eyelid crease incision provides good access to the superior orbital rim and periosteum. A direct skin incision provides exposure but may produce scarring.
13. **c.** Wearing a prosthesis or conformer 24 hours a day does not cause socket contraction. The other choices are associated with socket contraction.
14. **a.** In non-Asian persons, the orbital septum fuses with the levator aponeurosis 2–5 mm above the superior tarsal border. The levator aponeurosis attaches to the tarsus at the inferior third of the tarsus. The fusion of the periosteum of the facial bones, the periorbita, and the orbital septum is the arcus marginalis. Whitnall ligament acts as a pulley for the force of the levator muscle and provides suspensory support for the upper eyelid and the superior orbital tissues.
15. **a.** In epiblepharon, the lower eyelid pretarsal muscle and skin ride above the lower eyelid margin to form a horizontal fold of tissue that causes the cilia to assume a vertical position. The condition is most common in Asian children. With maturation of the facial bones, the epiblepharon may become less pronounced and the eyelash position may improve without surgical intervention.
16. **d.** Infantile (capillary) hemangiomas can cause amblyopia by inducing astigmatism or anisometropia or by occluding the visual axis. They are not typically present at birth but appear thereafter. Hemangiomas tend to enlarge until age one, after which they decrease in size over the next several years. Sebaceous hyperplasia can be associated with Muir-Torre syndrome and visceral malignancies; it is thus important to recognize this entity.
17. **c.** Lacrimal outflow reconstruction is best deferred for 5 years to minimize the likelihood of tumor spread. If there are unsuspected residual tumor cells, early lacrimal intervention with dacryocystorhinostomy (DCR) or conjunctivodacryocystorhinostomy (CDCR) could potentially lead to tumor spread into the nasolacrimal passages. Lacrimal reconstruction can be performed if the patient has symptomatic tearing 5 years after surgery and there is no sign of recurrence at that point.
18. **c.** Lipid stains are important for accurate diagnosis of sebaceous cell carcinoma of the eyelid. The other pathologic studies have relevance in ophthalmology but are not necessary for this particular eyelid malignancy.
19. **d.** The eyelid-sharing technique of a Hughes flap combined with skin grafting of the anterior lamella would be the best repair technique for a large defect of the lower eyelid. Note that repair of a large full-thickness eyelid defect requires reconstruction of the mucosa-

lined posterior lamella and the cutaneous anterior lamella. At least one of the lamellae should be a vascularized flap; free grafts of both lamellae will not survive. Thus, another option in this case would be a free tarsoconjunctival graft from the contralateral upper eyelid with vascular supply from a pedicled skin–muscle flap.

The Cutler-Beard procedure is an eyelid-sharing technique in which a full-thickness lower eyelid flap is moved into the defect of the upper eyelid by advancement of the flap behind the remaining lower eyelid margin. Primary closure of a large defect involving more than 50% of the lower lid is unlikely to be possible, and granulation alone would lead to a poor functional and cosmetic result.

20. **a.** The most typical features of blepharophimosis–ptosis–epicanthus inversus syndrome (BPES), also known as *blepharophimosis syndrome,* are telecanthus, epicanthus inversus, and severe ptosis, usually with limited levator function. Hypertelorism, ectropion, and hypoplasia of the superior orbital rims may also occur. Dermatochalasis is not a typical finding in BPES.
21. **a.** Anterior lamellar deficiency is a hallmark of cicatricial ectropion. Lower eyelid laxity is a common pathologic change seen in patients with involutional ectropion. This can involve the medial or lateral canthal tendon or both. Lower eyelid retractor disinsertion may also be a component of involutional ectropion and is typically manifested by tarsal ectropion, in which the palpebral conjunctival surface is outwardly rotated.
22. **d.** Posterior lamellar shortening is characteristic of cicatricial entropion, and treatment is directed toward supplementing this defect. Lower eyelid retractor disinsertion, lower eyelid laxity, and overriding preseptal orbicularis muscle are characteristics of involutional entropion.
23. **a.** Involutional ptosis is characterized by a higher than normal eyelid crease, normally functioning levator muscle (>15 mm), and, often, ipsilateral compensatory eyebrow elevation. The eyelid crease is often found at a higher level than normal secondary to levator attenuation or frank disinsertion. Aponeurotic disinsertion also results in superior migration of the orbital septum and underlying preaponeurotic fat, which in turn results in hollowing of the upper eyelid ("deep superior sulcus"). An absent or poorly formed eyelid crease is a characteristic finding in congenital ptosis.
24. **b.** Basal cell carcinoma is the most common malignant lesion of the eyelid, accounting for 90%–95% of eyelid malignancies.
25. **b.** Unilateral symptoms that persist at night are typical for hemifacial spasm. Bilateral involvement of eyelid protractors is seen in patients with benign essential blepharospasm (BEB). The symptoms of BEB abate at night, and all of the eyelid protractors can be involved. Patients with BEB may present with or progress to Meige syndrome.
26. **a.** The Horner muscle is defined as the extension of orbicularis in the deep head of the medial canthal tendon. Both the angular artery and vein lie anterior to the lacrimal sac. The superior portion of the sac is fibrous; thus, in dacryocystitis, the sac is more likely to be distended inferiorly.
27. **b.** The "valve" of Rosenmüller is actually a mucosal fold. Located at the junction of the common canaliculus and the lacrimal sac, it functions as a 1-way valve to prevent the reflux of tears into the common canaliculus during the lacrimal pump cycle. The valve of Hasner is located in the inferior meatus at the distal end of the nasolacrimal duct.

28. **a.** Most cases of symptomatic congenital nasolacrimal duct obstruction resolve by 12 months of age. Bilateral obstruction occurs in about one-third of cases. Many cases may respond to conservative treatment or resolve spontaneously; however, surgical intervention may be needed, especially if dacryocystitis is present.

29. **a.** Wrinkling of overlying skin may indicate canalicular kinking, in which case the probe should be withdrawn and reinserted. Scar tissue will recur with simple puncturing. Furthermore, attempted puncturing of scar tissue may result in formation of a false passage. The probe's location intranasally should always be confirmed by metal-on-metal contact or direct visualization.

30. **d.** The dye disappearance test helps distinguish between true epiphora resulting from lacrimal drainage obstruction and other conditions causing excessive tearing. The Jones I and II tests are used to determine tear flow under normal physiologic and nonphysiologic conditions, respectively. Probing and irrigation play a role in the workup, but they are not used as the initial test.

31. **b.** A DCR will not address the problem at the canaliculus. In a canaliculorhinostomy, the scarred canalicular segment is removed and the remaining patent canalicular system is anastomosed to the lacrimal sac mucosa or the lateral nasal wall mucosa. When successful, a canaliculorhinostomy results in the most natural anatomy. Unfortunately, the success rate for this procedure is lower with common canalicular obstruction. While it is preferable to use the native anatomy when possible, a CDCR has the highest likelihood of creating an intact lacrimal drainage system. Silicone intubation will be insufficient to relieve the obstruction.

32. **c.** An osteotomy from the lacrimal sac, through the lacrimal sac fossa, and into the nose must be performed for successful rerouting of the lacrimal drainage. DCR may be performed under local anesthesia or local anesthesia with intravenous sedation. General anesthesia is not mandatory. Unless an obvious abnormality is noted intraoperatively, routine biopsy of the sac usually does not reveal any pathology. Anterior mucosal flaps alone are typically adequate in successful DCR.

33. **c.** If there is no improvement with antibiotics or if relief of acute pain is necessary, incision and drainage can be performed. External DCR is generally performed after the acute infection resolves. CT scan is not indicated in acute dacryocystitis unless atypical features are present.

# Index

( *f* = figure; *t* = table)

A-scan ultrasonography/echography, orbital, 31
AAPOX. *See* Adult-onset asthma with periocular xanthogranuloma
Abducens nerve. *See* Cranial nerve VI
Aberrant nerve regeneration, synkinesis and, 211, 229
AbobotulinumtoxinA, 238. *See also* Botulinum toxin
Abscesses
  in dacryocystitis, 286
  orbital, 47, 47*f*
Accessory lacrimal glands
  of Krause, 146*f*, 152, 252
  of Wolfring, 146*f*, 152, 252
ACE. *See* Angiotensin-converting enzyme
Acetylcholine receptor antibody tests, for myasthenia gravis, 217
Acrocephalosyndactyly (Apert syndrome), 37, 38*f*
Acrochordon (skin tag), 166, 166*f*
Acrolentiginous melanoma, 185
Acropachy, in thyroid eye disease, 56
Actinic keratosis, 175–176, 176*f*
  squamous cell carcinoma and, 182
*Actinomyces israelii*
  canaliculitis caused by, 284–285, 285*f*
  dacryolith formation and, 277
Acute lymphoblastic leukemia, orbital involvement and, 98
Acute spastic entropion, 205–206
Adenocarcinoma
  secondary, of orbit, 96–97
  sebaceous, of eyelid 183–184, 183*f*
Adenoid cystic carcinoma (cylindroma)
  of eyelid, 171
  of lacrimal gland, 91, 93
Adenoma
  pleomorphic (benign mixed tumor)
    of eyelid, 170
    of lacrimal gland, 91, 92–93, 92*f*
  sebaceous, of eyelid, 170
Adits, for neck liposuction, 246
Adnexa. *See* Ocular adnexa
Adult-onset asthma with periocular xanthogranuloma (AAPOX), 90, 91
Adult-onset xanthogranuloma (AOX), 90, 91
Advancement flaps
  for canthal repair, 195
  for eyelid repair, 191, 192, 193*f*, 194
Afferent pupillary defects
  in meningioma, 81
  in optic nerve glioma, 74
  in traumatic optic neuropathy, 113
Age/aging
  ectropion and (involutional ectropion), 198*f*, 199–201, 200*f*
  entropion and (involutional entropion), 202–204, 203*f*, 204*f*, 205*f*
  eyelid changes associated with
    orbital septum changes and, 149
    retro-orbicularis oculi fat (ROOF) and, 153
    suborbicularis oculi fat (SOOF) and, 152
  facial changes associated with
    communication and, 235–236
    facial rejuvenation surgery and, 241–247, 242*f*, 243*f*, 244*f*, 245*f*, 246*f*. *See also specific procedure*
    pathogenesis of, 236
    physical examination of, 197, 236–237
    skin changes and, 236–237
  periorbital changes associated with, 229–230, 229*f*
Air cells, ethmoid (ethmoid sinuses), 8, 8*f*, 18, 19, 19*f*
Albright syndrome, 84
Allergic aspergillosis sinusitis, 51
Alveolar nerves
  anterior superior, 17*f*
  posterior superior, 17*f*
Alveolar rhabdomyosarcoma, 83
Amblyopia
  in congenital ptosis, 211–212
  eyelid-sharing techniques in children and, 161, 195
  in infantile (capillary) hemangioma, 68, 161
  in traumatic ptosis, 190
American Society of Ocularists, 132
Amniotic membrane graft
  for contracted socket, 134
  for eyelid repair, in burn injury, 190
  for symblepharon, 208
Amniotocele (dacryocystocele), 265–267, 266*f*
  in dacryocystitis, 285
Ampulla, 253
Ampullectomy, 282
ANCA (antineutrophil cytoplasmic autoantibody), in granulomatosis with polyangiitis (Wegener granulomatosis), 33–34, 61–62
Anesthesia (anesthetics)
  for dacryocystorhinostomy, 279
  for lacrimal probing, 260
Angiography/arteriography
  in carotid-cavernous fistulas, 73
  in orbital evaluation, 32
Angiotensin-converting enzyme (ACE), serum levels of, in sarcoidosis, 34, 63
Angular artery, 16*f*, 254
  eyelids supplied by, 16*f*, 154
Angular vein, 254
  eyelids drained by, 154
Animal bites, eyelid injuries caused by, 190
Anisometropia, in infantile (capillary) hemangioma, 68, 161
Ankyloblepharon, 157*f*, 158
Ankyloblepharon filiforme adnatum, 158
Annulus of Zinn, 11, 12–13, 13*f*, 14*f*, 15*f*, 16
Anophthalmia, 35, 127. *See also* Anophthalmic socket
  surgical, 127–137
  treatment of, 36
Anophthalmic ectropion, 135
Anophthalmic ptosis, 135

Anophthalmic socket, 127–137. *See also specific aspect*
complications and treatment of, 132–136, 133*f*, 134*f*, 135*f*
contracted, 134–135, 135*f*
enucleation and, 128–129, 130
evisceration and, 129–130, 130
exenteration and, 136–137, 137*f*
goals for surgery of, 129
implants and, 131–132, 131*f*
in children, 129
Anophthalmic surgery, 127–137. *See also* Anophthalmic socket
Anterior ciliary artery, 14*f*, 15*f*
Anterior clinoid process, 7*f*
Anterior cranial fossa, 7*f*
Anterior lamellar deficiency, surgery for eyelid retraction and, 224
Anterior orbitotomy. *See also* Orbitotomy
incisions for, 116*f*
Anterior superior alveolar nerve, 17*f*
Antimicrosomal antibody, in thyroid eye disease, 53
Antineutrophil cytoplasmic autoantibody (ANCA), in granulomatosis with polyangiitis (Wegener granulomatosis), 33–34, 61–62
Antithyroid antibodies, in thyroid eye disease, 53
Antithyroid drugs, for hyperthyroidism, 58
Antiviral agents, laser skin resurfacing and, 238
Antoni A pattern/Antoni B pattern, in schwannomas, 82
AOX. *See* Adult-onset xanthogranuloma
Apert syndrome (acrocephalosyndactyly), 37, 38*f*
Apocrine glands, of eyelid, 170. *See also* Glands of Moll
tumors originating in, 171, 171*f*
Apocrine hidrocystoma, 171, 171*f*
Aponeurotic ptosis, 214, 214*f*, 214*t*
Aqueous layer, of tear film, 252
Arcus marginalis, 11
Argon laser therapy, for trichiasis, 208
Arteriography. *See* Angiography/arteriography
Arteriovenous fistulas, 72–74, 72*f*, 73*f*
Arteriovenous malformations (AVMs), 72
Arteritis, giant cell (GCA/temporal), 61
Artificial tears, for paralytic ectropion, 224–225
Asian eyelid, 147, 147*f*
epicanthus tarsalis and, 158, 159
*Aspergillus* (aspergillosis), 50–51
Astrocytoma, pilocytic. *See* Optic nerve (optic pathway/chiasm) glioma
Auricular nerves, 144*f*, 145*f*
Auriculotemporal nerve, 145*f*
Auscultation, in orbital disorders, 26
Autoantibodies
in granulomatosis with polyangiitis (Wegener granulomatosis), 33–34, 61–62
in thyroid eye disease, 53, 55
Autogenous fascia lata, for frontalis suspension, 221
AVMs. *See* Arteriovenous malformations
Axial displacement of globe, in orbital disorders, 24

B-cell lymphomas, orbital, 86
B-scan ultrasonography/echography, orbital, 31
Bacteria, orbital infection caused by
cellulitis, 44
necrotizing fasciitis, 48–49
"Balanced" orbital decompression, 122, 123*f*
Balloon dacryoplasty (balloon catheter dilation)
for acquired nasolacrimal duct obstruction, 278
for canalicular obstruction, 275
for congenital nasolacrimal duct obstruction, 263–265
Bandage contact lenses, for involutional entropion, 203
Banked fascia lata, for frontalis suspension, 221
Basal cell carcinoma, of eyelid, 177–182, 178*f*, 179*f*
Basal cell nevus syndrome (Gorlin syndrome), 178
Basal tear secretion test, 268
BEB. *See* Benign essential blepharospasm
Bell phenomenon, in ptosis evaluation, 211
Benign essential blepharospasm (BEB), 226–228, 227*f*
Benign mixed tumor (pleomorphic adenoma)
of eyelid, 170
of lacrimal gland, 91, 92–93, 92*f*
Beta (β)-blockers, for infantile (capillary) hemangioma, 68
Beta (β)-hemolytic group A streptococci, orbital necrotizing fasciitis caused by, 48
Bicanalicular stents
for canalicular trauma, 283
after dacryocystorhinostomy, 279
Bick procedure, 199
Bites, eyelid injuries caused by, 190
Blepharochalasis, 230
Blepharophimosis–ptosis–epicanthus inversus syndrome (BPES/blepharophimosis syndrome), 155–156, 156*f*, 158, 212
with congenital ectropion, 155, 156
with euryblepharon, 155, 156
Blepharophimosis syndrome. *See* Blepharophimosis–ptosis–epicanthus inversus syndrome
Blepharoplasty, 230–234, 232*f*
complications of, 233–234
eyelid retraction, 223, 234
cosmetic/functional indications and, 230–231
infraciliary incision for, orbitotomy and, 118
laser resurfacing as adjunct to, 237
preoperative evaluation for, 231
techniques for, 232–233, 232*f*
Blepharoptosis. *See* Ptosis
Blepharospasm
botulinum toxin for, 227–228, 227*f*
essential/benign essential (BEB), 226–228, 227*f*
reflex, 227
Blindness. *See also* Vision loss
after blepharoplasty, 233–234
functional, in benign essential blepharospasm, 226
Blinking (blink reflex), tear secretion and, 255, 256*f*
Blowout (indirect) fractures
of medial orbital wall, 8, 108
orbital cellulitis following, 47
of orbital floor, 108–112, 110*f*
diplopia after, 108
infraorbital nerve and, 19
surgery for, 111–112
indications for, 110–111
of orbital roof, 106
Blue nevus, 175
Blunt trauma
canalicular injury and, 282–283
eyelid, 187
optic canal fracture caused by, 10

Bone, eosinophilic granuloma of, 90
Botryoid rhabdomyosarcoma, 83
Botulinum toxin, 227–228, 227*f*
for acute spastic entropion, 206
for blepharospasm, 227–228, 227*f*
cosmetic uses of, 238–239
for hemifacial spasm, 229
for paralytic ectropion, 225
ptosis caused by, 216
for thyroid eye disease, 59
Bowen disease, 176
Bowman probe, 261, 261*f*, 262*f*
BPES. *See* Blepharophimosis–ptosis–epicanthus inversus syndrome
Breast cancer, eye involvement and, 100, 100*f*
Bronchogenic carcinoma, eye involvement and, 100
Brow- and forehead-lift, 241, 242*f*, 243*f*
Brow ptosis, 234–235, 235*f*
dermatochalasis and, 229, 234, 235
Browpexy, 235
Bruits, in orbital disorders, 26, 73
Buccal fat pad, 142*f*
Buccal mucous membrane graft
for contracted socket, 134
for eyelid repair, 190
for symblepharon, 208
Buccal nerve, 142*f*, 143, 144*f*, 145*f*
Buccinator muscle, 141, 143*f*
Budge-Waller, ciliospinal center/nucleus of, 16
Burns, eyelid, 190

C-reactive protein, in giant cell arteritis, 61
CA-MRSA. *See* Community-acquired methicillin-resistant *Staphylococcus aureus*
Caldwell-Luc procedure, for orbital decompression, 121
Canal. *See specific type*
Canalicular plugs, for dry eye, 281–282
canalicular obstruction and, 274, 282
nasolacrimal duct obstruction and, 278, 282
Canalicular stenting
for canalicular obstruction, 274, 275
for canalicular trauma, 283
for congenital lacrimal drainage obstruction, 262–263, 264*f*
Canaliculi, lacrimal, 253, 253*f*, 254*f*
agenesis/dysgenesis of, 259–260
development of, 255
duplication of, 257, 258*f*
infection of, 284–286, 285*f*. *See also* Canaliculitis
obstruction and, 274
obstruction of, 273–276, 276*f*
functional occlusion, 273
irrigation/probing in evaluation of, 270*f*, 271–272, 271*f*, 273
reconstruction/repair of, 275, 283
stenosis of, 271
trauma to, 282–284
obstruction caused by, 274
Canaliculitis, 284–285, 285*f*
lacrimal plug migration causing, 282
obstruction and, 274
Canaliculodacryocystorhinostomy, for canalicular obstruction, 275
Canaliculoplasty, laser, for canalicular reconstruction, 275
Canaliculorhinostomy, for canalicular obstruction, 275
Canaliculotomy, for canaliculitis, 285
*Candida* (candidiasis), dacryolith formation and, 277
Canthal reconstruction, 189, 195–196. *See also* Eyelids, surgery/reconstruction of
Canthal soft tissues, trauma involving, 189
Canthal tendons, 152*f*, 153
lateral, 7, 14*f*, 152*f*, 153
laxity in, in involutional ectropion, 199
medial, 152*f*, 153, 254
trauma involving, 189
Cantholysis
lateral
for orbital decompression, 122, 122*f*
for orbitotomy, 116*f*, 118, 119*f*
for orbital hemorrhage, 112
for traumatic vision loss, 113
Canthotomy, lateral
for orbital decompression, 122, 122*f*
for orbital hemorrhage, 112
for orbitotomy, 116*f*, 118, 119*f*
for traumatic vision loss, 113
Capillary hemangioma. *See* Infantile (capillary) hemangioma
Capsulopalpebral fascia, 151
Capsulopalpebral head, 146*f*, 151
Capsulopalpebral orbital septum complex, 149
Carbon dioxide laser
for infantile (capillary) hemangioma, 162
for skin resurfacing, 237
Carcinoma
adenoid cystic (cylindroma)
of eyelid, 171
of lacrimal gland, 91, 93
basal cell, of eyelid, 177–182, 178*f*, 179*f*
sebaceous, of eyelid, 183–184, 183*f*
squamous cell
of eyelid, 182, 182*f*
actinic keratosis and, 176, 182
in situ (Bowen disease), 176
of orbit, secondary, 96–97, 96*f*
Carcinoma in situ, of eyelid
keratoacanthoma, 176–177, 177*f*
squamous cell (Bowen disease), 176
Carotid arteries
external, 13, 154
eyelids supplied by, 154
internal, 13, 14*f*, 15*f*, 154
orbit supplied by, 13
Carotid-cavernous sinus fistula, 72–74, 72*f*, 73*f*
direct, 72, 72–73
dural (indirect), 72, 73
Caruncle
edema of, in thyroid eye disease, 54
hypertrophied, punctal obstruction/malposition and, 273
incision through. *See* Transcaruncular incision
Carunculectomy, conjunctivodacryocystorhinostomy for canalicular obstruction and, 275
CAS (Clinical Activity Score), for thyroid eye disease, 57
Cautery, thermal, for punctal occlusion, 282

Cavernous hemangioma, of orbit, 68–69, 69*f*
Cavernous sinus, 14*f*, 15*f*
  carotid artery fistulas and, 72–74, 72*f*, 73*f*
    direct, 72, 72–73
    dural (indirect), 72, 73
Cavernous sinus thrombosis, orbital infection/cellulitis and, 48
CD20 receptor blockers, for thyroid eye disease, 58
CD40, orbital fibroblast, thyroid eye disease and, 55
CD154, orbital fibroblast, thyroid eye disease and, 55
CDCR. *See* Conjunctivodacryocystorhinostomy
Cell-marker studies, in orbital tumor evaluation, 33
Cellulitis, 44–48, 46*f*, 46*t*, 47*f*
  dacryocystitis and, 44, 285, 286*f*
  orbital, 46–48, 46*f*, 46*t*, 47*f*
  preseptal, 44, 44–46
Central orbital fat pad, 149
Central retinal artery occlusion (CRAO), hyaluronic filler injection causing, 239, 240*f*
Central surgical space (intraconal fat/surgical space), 11, 115*f*, 116
Cervical fascia, deep and superficial, 143
Cervical nerve, 143, 144*f*
Chalazion (chalazia), 162–163, 163*f*
  sebaceous carcinoma misdiagnosed as, 183–184
Check ligament of lateral rectus muscle, 7
Cheek advancement/rotation flap (Mustardé flap/procedure), for eyelid repair, 194*f*, 195
Cheek elevation, in eyelid repair, 193
Chemosis
  in nonspecific orbital inflammation, 64
  in thyroid eye disease, 52, 52*f*, 54
Chemotherapy (cancer)
  canalicular obstruction caused by, 274
  for lacrimal gland tumors, 93
  for optic nerve glioma, 77
  for rhabdomyosarcoma, 83
Chiasm (optic), gliomas involving, 74–77, 75*f*
Children
  enucleation in, 129
  eyelid anomalies in, 155–162, 157*f*
  infantile (capillary) hemangiomas in
    of eyelid, 161–162
    of orbit, 67–68, 67*f*
  lateral orbitotomy in, 120
  optic nerve gliomas in, 74, 75, 75*f*, 77
  orbital cellulitis in, 47
  orbital fractures in, 106
  orbital inflammation in, nonspecific, 65
  orbital metastatic disease in, 98–99, 98*f*
  orbital tuberculosis in, 49, 49*f*
  preseptal cellulitis in, 44, 45
Chloasma, 173
Chloroma (granulocytic sarcoma), 98–99
Chondrosarcoma, of orbit, 84
Choristomas, orbital, 39–41, 39*f*, 41*f*
Choroid, melanoma of, enucleation for, 128
Chronic lymphocytic lymphoma (CLL), of orbit, 86
Cicatricial ectropion, 198*f*
  after blepharoplasty, 234
Cicatricial entropion, 198*f*, 201, 202*f*, 206–207, 206*f*, 207*f*
  trichiasis in, 208
Cigarette smoking
  basal cell carcinoma and, 177
  thyroid disease and, 52, 56, 58
Cilia (eyelashes), 153
  entropion/ptosis of. *See also* Trichiasis
    in anophthalmic socket, 136
  in epiblepharon, 157*f*, 159, 159*f*
  follicles of, 154*f*
    tumors arising in, 172, 172*f*, 173*f*
  misdirection of. *See* Trichiasis
  in trichotillomania, 165
Ciliary arteries, anterior/posterior, 14*f*, 15*f*
Ciliary ganglion, 14*f*, 15*f*, 16, 17*f*
Ciliary margin, 153
Ciliary nerves
  long, 14*f*, 15*f*, 16
  short, 12*f*, 14*f*, 15*f*, 16, 17*f*
Ciliospinal center/nucleus of Budge-Waller, 16
Cleft syndromes, 36–38, 37*f*, 38*f*
  nasolacrimal duct obstruction and, 259
Clinical Activity Score (CAS), for thyroid eye disease, 57
Clinoid process, anterior, 7*f*
CLL. *See* Chronic lymphocytic lymphoma
Clobetasol, for infantile (capillary) hemangioma, 162
Clonality, in orbital lymphoma, 88
Clonazepam, for benign essential blepharospasm, 228
$CO_2$ laser. *See* Carbon dioxide laser
Collagen, as dermal filler for facial rejuvenation, 239
Collagen plugs, for dry eye, 281. *See also* Lacrimal plugs
Colobomas, eyelid, 160–161, 160*f*
Community-acquired methicillin-resistant *Staphylococcus aureus* (CA-MRSA)
  dacryoadenitis caused by, 284
  preseptal cellulitis caused by, 45
Compartment syndrome, 125
  vision loss after orbital trauma and, 109, 113
Compound nevi, 173
Compressive optic neuropathy
  orbital varices and, 71
  in thyroid eye disease, 52, 54, 56, 59
Computed tomography (CT scan)
  helical (spiral), in orbital evaluation, 27
  in lacrimal drainage evaluation, 272
  in orbital cellulitis, 47, 47*f*
  in orbital evaluation, 26–27, 26*f*, 27*f*, 30*f*
    dermoid cysts and, 39–40, 39*f*
    MRI compared with, 29–31, 29*t*, 30*f*
  in preseptal cellulitis, 44–45
Computed tomography angiography (CTA), in orbital evaluation, 32
Concave (minus) lenses, anophthalmic socket camouflage and, 136
Conchae (turbinates), nasal, 18, 253*f*, 254*f*
  infracture of, for congenital nasolacrimal duct obstruction, 265
Conformer
  after anophthalmic surgery, 132
    contracture of fornices and, 133
  in congenital anophthalmia/microphthalmia management, 36
Congenital anomalies. *See also specific type*
  of eyelid, 155–162, 157*f*
  of orbit, 35–41, 37*f*, 38*f*, 39*f*, 41*f*

Congenital infantile hemangioma
of eyelid, 161–162
of orbit, 67
Congenital lacrimal–cutaneous fistula, 257, 258*f*
Congenital nasolacrimal duct obstruction. *See* Nasolacrimal duct (NLD), obstruction of
Congenital ptosis. *See* Ptosis
Conjunctiva, 146*f*, 152, 154*f*
epithelium of, evaluation of, in pseudoepiphora, 268
incision through. *See* Transconjunctival incision
infection/inflammation of, canalicular obstruction and, 274
Conjunctival erythema, in thyroid eye disease, 52, 53*f*
Conjunctival flaps, for symblepharon, 208
Conjunctivochalasis, punctal obstruction/malposition and, 273
Conjunctivodacryocystorhinostomy (CDCR)
for canalicular obstruction, 275–276, 276*f*
after canthal repair, 195
for punctal/canalicular agenesis/dysgenesis, 260
Connective tissue, eyelid, 152–153
Consecutive anophthalmia, 35
Consent, informed, for facial rejuvenation surgery, 241
Contact lenses, bandage, for involutional entropion, 203
Contracted fornices, anophthalmic socket and, 133
socket contracture and, 135
Contracted socket, 134–135, 135*f*
Contrast dacryocystography, for lacrimal drainage evaluation, 272
Convex (plus) lenses, anophthalmic socket camouflage and, 136
Cornea
epithelium of, evaluation of, in pseudoepiphora, 268
irritation of, pseudoepiphora and, 268
Corneal light reflex, eyelid margin distance to (margin-reflex distance), in ptosis, 209–210, 210*f*, 214*t*
Coronal incision, for orbitotomy, 117
Corrugator superciliaris muscle, 16
Corrugator supercilii muscle, 141, 143*f*
Corticosteroids (steroids)
for infantile (capillary) hemangioma, 68, 161, 161–162
for nonspecific orbital inflammation, 63, 64–65, 65
for orbital floor/blowout fracture, 109
for thyroid eye disease, 58, 59
for traumatic vision loss, 114
Cosmetic facial surgery. *See specific procedure and* Facial surgery
Cosmetic optics, for anophthalmic socket, 136
Cranial fossae, anterior, 7*f*
Cranial nerve II. *See* Optic nerve
Cranial nerve III (oculomotor nerve), 10*f*, 12, 12*f*, 13*f*, 14*f*, 15*f*
aberrant regeneration of, synkinesis in, 211
extraocular muscles innervated by, 12, 12*f*
levator muscle innervated by, 151
palsy of, ptosis caused by, 215, 215–216
Cranial nerve IV (trochlear nerve), 10*f*, 12, 13*f*, 14*f*, 15*f*
extraocular muscles innervated by, 12
Cranial nerve V (trigeminal nerve), 12, 17*f*, 144, 145*f*
facial innervation and, 144, 145*f*
$V_1$ (ophthalmic nerve), 14*f*, 15*f*, 16, 17*f*, 144, 145*f*
in reflex tear arc, 251
$V_2$ (maxillary nerve), 14*f*, 15*f*, 16, 17*f*, 144, 145*f*
$V_3$ (mandibular nerve), 14*f*, 15*f*, 17*f*, 144, 145*f*
Cranial nerve VI (abducens nerve), 10*f*, 12, 13*f*, 14*f*, 15*f*
extraocular muscles innervated by, 12
Cranial nerve VII (facial nerve), 16, 142*f*, 143, 144*f*
aberrant regeneration of, synkinesis in, 211, 229
buccal branch of, 142*f*, 143, 144*f*
cervical branch of, 143, 144*f*
marginal mandibular branch of, 142*f*, 143, 144*f*
palsy/paralysis/weakness of. *See* Facial paralysis/weakness
in reflex tear arc, 251, 252*f*
surgical ablation of, for essential blepharospasm, 228
surgical decompression of, for hemifacial spasm, 229
temporal (frontal) branch of, 142*f*, 143, 144, 144*f*
zygomatic branch of, 142*f*, 143, 144*f*
Cranial nerves
extraocular muscles supplied by, 11, 14, 15*f*
orbit supplied by, 16–18, 17*f*
Cranial sutures, premature closure of, in craniosynostosis, 37
Craniofacial clefts, 36–38, 37*f*, 38*f*. *See also specific type and* Craniofacial malformations
nasolacrimal duct obstruction and, 259
Craniofacial dysostosis (Crouzon syndrome), 37, 38*f*
Craniofacial malformations, 36–38, 37*f*, 38*f*. *See also specific type*
Apert syndrome (acrocephalosyndactyly), 37, 38*f*
craniosynostosis/syndromic craniosynostosis, 37–38, 38*f*
Crouzon syndrome, 37, 38*f*
Goldenhar syndrome/oculoauricular dysplasia, 37
Treacher Collins–Franceschetti syndrome (mandibulofacial dysostosis), 37, 37*f*
Craniosynostosis, 37–38, 38*f*
Craniotomy, frontal, for orbital surgery, 124
CRAO. *See* Central retinal artery occlusion
Crawford stent, for nasolacrimal intubation, 262, 264*f*
Creases, eyelid. *See* Eyelids, creases of
Crouzon syndrome (craniofacial dysostosis), 37, 38*f*
Cryotherapy
for basal cell carcinoma of eyelid, 181
for trichiasis/distichiasis, 160, 208
Cryptophthalmos, 161, 161*f*
CT scan. *See* Computed tomography
Cutaneous horn (exuberant hyperkeratosis), 168
Cutler-Beard procedure, 192, 193*f*
Cylindroma (adenoid cystic carcinoma)
of eyelid, 171
of lacrimal gland, 91, 93
Cystic carcinoma, adenoid (cylindroma)
of eyelid, 171
of lacrimal gland, 91, 93
Cysticercosis, orbital involvement and, 51

Dacryoadenitis, 284
lacrimal gland masses and, 91
nonspecific orbital inflammation and, 64
Dacryocystectomy, for lacrimal sac tumors, 287
Dacryocystitis, 285–286, 286*f*
acute, 285–286, 286*f*
cellulitis and, 44, 285, 286*f*
chronic, 286
dacryocystocele and, 285

in nasolacrimal duct obstruction, 260, 285, 286
tumor associated with, 287
Dacryocystocele, 265–267, 266*f*
in dacryocystitis, 285
Dacryocystography
for lacrimal drainage evaluation, 272
for lacrimal sac tumor evaluation, 287
Dacryocystorhinostomy (DCR), 265, 278–281, 280*f*, 281
for acquired nasolacrimal duct obstruction, 278–281, 280*f*, 281
for congenital nasolacrimal duct obstruction, 265
for dacryocystitis, 286
Dacryoliths, 277, 277*f*
Dacryoplasty, balloon (balloon catheter dilation)
for acquired nasolacrimal duct obstruction, 278
for canalicular obstruction, 275
for congenital nasolacrimal duct obstruction, 263–265
Dacryoscintigraphy, for lacrimal drainage evaluation, 272
DCR. *See* Dacryocystorhinostomy
DDT. *See* Dye disappearance test
Decompression
optic canal, for traumatic vision loss, 114
orbital, 121–123, 122*f*, 123*f*
complications of, 125
for orbital hemorrhage, 112
for thyroid eye disease, 52, 58, 59, 121
for traumatic vision loss, 113
for vision loss after blepharoplasty, 233
Deep cervical fascia, 143
Deep facial fascia, 141
Deep mimetic muscles, 141
Deep-plane rhytidectomy, 245
Deep superior sulcus deformity, anophthalmic socket and, 132–133, 133*f*
Deep temporal fascia, 141, 142*f*, 144
Depression of eye (downgaze)
disorders/limitation of, in orbital floor/blowout fracture, 108
surgery and, 110
ptosis exacerbation in, 209
ptotic eyelid position in, 211, 214*t*
Depressor anguli oris muscle, 143, 143*f*
Depressor labii inferioris muscle, 143, 143*f*
Depressor septi muscle, 143*f*
Dermal fillers, in facial rejuvenation, 239–240, 239*f*, 240*f*
Dermal nevus, 173
Dermal/oculodermal melanocytosis (nevus of Ota), 175, 175*f*
Dermatochalasis, 218, 218*f*, 229–230, 229*f*
brow ptosis and, 229, 234, 235
pseudoptosis and, 218, 218*f*
ptosis and, 229, 229*f*
Dermis-fat grafts, 132
in children, 129
in congenital anophthalmia/microphthalmia management, 36
for exposure and extrusion of orbital implant, 134
for superior sulcus deformity, 132–133
Dermoids (dermoid cysts/tumors), orbital, 39–40, 39*f*
Dermolipomas, of orbit, 40, 41*f*
Developmental defects. *See also specific type and* Congenital anomalies
of orbit, 35–41, 37*f*, 38*f*, 39*f*, 41*f*
Dexamethasone, for nonspecific orbital inflammation, 65
Diffuse soft-tissue histiocytosis, 90
Digital eversion test, for cicatricial entropion, 206
Diplopia
after blepharoplasty, 234
in orbital floor/blowout fracture, 108
surgery and, 110, 111
in orbital roof fractures, 106
in thyroid eye disease, 56, 58, 59
Direct carotid-cavernous fistula, 72, 72–73
Distichiasis
acquired, 154*f*
congenital, 154*f*, 160, 160*f*
Distraction test, 199, 203
Dog bites, eyelid injuries caused by, 190
Dog tapeworm *(Echinococcus granulosus)*, orbital infection caused by, 51
Doppler imaging, in orbital evaluation, 31
Dorsal nasal nerve, 17*f*
Double-convexity deformity, 236, 241–242
Double-elevator palsy (monocular elevation deficiency), 213
Double freeze–thaw technique, for trichiasis, 208
Down syndrome, congenital ectropion and, 156
Downgaze
disorders/limitation of, in orbital floor/blowout fracture, 108
surgery and, 110
ptosis exacerbation in, 209
ptotic eyelid position in, 211, 214*t*
Drugs, canalicular obstruction caused by, 274
Dry eye
blepharoplasty and, 232
in blepharospasm, 227
lacrimal lymphoepithelial lesions and, 94
lacrimal plugs for, 281–282
canalicular obstruction and, 274, 282
extrusion/migration of, 282
nasolacrimal duct obstruction and, 278, 282
Duane retraction syndrome, synkinesis in, 211, 215
Dumbbell dermoid cyst, 39–40
Dural (indirect) carotid-cavernous fistula, 72, 73
Dye disappearance test (DDT), 269, 269*f*
Dystonia, facial, 226–229, 227*f*

Ear cartilage graft
for cicatricial entropion, 207
for eyelid retraction, 224
for paralytic ectropion, 226
Ecchymoses, periorbital, 22, 22*f*
in neuroblastoma, 98, 98*f*
in orbital floor/blowout fracture, 108
in orbital roof fracture, 106
Eccrine hidrocystoma, 170
Eccrine sweat glands, of eyelid, 170
tumors originating in, 170, 171*f*
ECD. *See* Erdheim-Chester disease
*Echinococcus granulosus* (echinococcosis), orbital infection caused by, 51
Ectropion, 197–201, 198*f*, 200*f*
anophthalmic, 135
cicatricial, 198*f*, 201, 202*f*
after blepharoplasty, 234

congenital, 156, 157*f*
in blepharophimosis–ptosis–epicanthus inversus syndrome, 155, 156
involutional, 198*f*, 199–201, 200*f*
mechanical, 198*f*, 201
paralytic, 198*f*, 224–226, 225*f*
tarsal, 200
Edema, eyelid, 164
in blepharochalasis, 230
in orbital floor/blowout fracture, 108
in rhabdomyosarcoma, 82
Edrophonium chloride, in myasthenia gravis diagnosis, 217
EGFR inhibitors. *See* Epidermal growth factor receptor (EGFR) inhibitors
Elderly patients. *See* Age/aging
Electrolysis, for trichiasis/distichiasis, 160, 208
Electromyography/electromyogram, in myasthenia gravis, 217
Electron microscopy, in orbital tumor evaluation, 33
Elevated intraocular pressure, in traumatic optic neuropathy, 113
Elevation of eye (upgaze), disorders/limitation of
in monocular elevation deficiency (double-elevator palsy), 213
in orbital floor/blowout fracture, 108
surgery and, 110
Embryonal rhabdomyosarcoma, 83
Emphysema (ocular), of orbit and eyelids, in orbital floor/blowout fracture, 109
Encephaloceles, 37
Endobrow incision, 243
Endonasal (internal) dacryocystorhinostomy (DCR), 279, 280, 281*f*
endoscopic, 280
Endophthalmitis, evisceration for, 130
Endoscopic brow- and forehead-lift, 241, 242*f*
Endoscopic dacryocystorhinostomy (DCR), 280
Endoscopic subperiosteal midface lift, 243, 244*f*
Endoscopy, nasal
for lacrimal drainage evaluation/obstruction, 272
for orbital decompression, 122
Enophthalmos, 23–24
breast carcinoma metastasis to orbit and, 100, 100*f*
in medial orbital wall/blowout fracture, 108
in orbital floor/blowout fracture, 109
surgery and, 110–111, 111
orbital varices and, 71
Entropion, 202–207, 203*f*, 204*f*, 205*f*, 206*f*, 207*f*
cicatricial, 198*f*, 201, 202*f*, 206–207, 206*f*, 207*f*
congenital, 159–160, 160*f*
involutional, 202–204, 203*f*, 204*f*, 205*f*
lash margin
in anophthalmic socket, 136
tarsal fracture operation for, 207, 207*f*
trichiasis in, 208
spastic/acute spastic, 203, 204*f*
Enucleation, 127, 128–129
in childhood, 129
congenital anophthalmia/microphthalmia treatment and, 36
goals of, 129
intraoperative complications of, 130
ocular prostheses after, 132
orbital implants after, 129
ptosis/extraocular muscle damage and, 130
for sympathetic ophthalmia prevention, 128
wrong eye removal and, 130
Eosinophilic granuloma of bone, orbital, 90
Ephelis, of eyelid, 174
Epiblepharon, 157*f*, 159, 159*f*
Epicanthus, 157*f*, 158–159, 158*f*
inversus, 158, 159
in blepharophimosis–ptosis–epicanthus inversus syndrome, 155, 158
palpebralis, 158
supraciliaris, 158
tarsalis, 158, 159
Epidermal/epidermoid cysts
of eyelid, 168–169, 168*f*, 169*f*
of orbit, 39
Epidermal growth factor receptor (EGFR) inhibitors, for squamous cell carcinoma, 182
Epidermal inclusion cysts, of eyelid, 168, 168*f*
Epidermis, eyelid, neoplasms of, 155, 168–169, 168*f*, 169*f*, 175–176, 176*f*. *See also* Eyelids, tumors of
benign, 168–169, 168*f*, 169*f*
premalignant, 175–176, 176*f*
Epidermoid/epidermal cysts
of eyelid, 168–169, 168*f*, 169*f*
of orbit, 39
Epilation, for trichiasis/distichiasis, 160, 208
Epimyoepithelial islands, 94
Epinephrine, with local anesthetic, for dacryocystorhinostomy, 279
Epiphora, 267. *See also* Tearing
Episcleral (sub-Tenon) surgical space, 115, 115*f*
Epithelial cysts, of eyelids, benign, 168–169, 168*f*, 169*f*
Epithelial hyperplasias, of eyelids, 166–168, 166*f*, 167*f*
Epithelial tumors
of eyelids
benign lesions, 168–169, 168*f*, 169*f*
hyperplasias, 166–168, 166*f*, 167*f*
in situ carcinoma, 176–177, 177*f*
of lacrimal gland, 91–94, 92*f*
exenteration for, 93, 136
Epithelium
conjunctival, in pseudoepiphora, 268
corneal, in pseudoepiphora, 268
eyelid
benign lesions of, 168–169, 168*f*, 169*f*
hyperplasia of, 166–168, 166*f*, 167*f*
in situ carcinoma of, 176–177, 177*f*
Epstein-Barr virus, dacryoadenitis caused by, 284
Erbium:YAG laser, for skin resurfacing, 237
Erdheim-Chester disease (ECD), 90, 91
Erythema
in nonspecific orbital inflammation, 64
in thyroid eye disease, 52, 53*f*, 54
Essential blepharospasm/benign essential blepharospasm (BEB), 226–228, 227*f*
Ethanol, retrobulbar injection of, for pain control, 128
Ethmoid air cells/sinuses, 8, 8*f*, 18, 19, 19*f*
Ethmoid arteries, anterior/posterior, 14*f*, 15*f*
Ethmoid bone, 6*f*, 7*f*, 8, 8*f*
Ethmoid nerves, anterior/posterior, 14*f*, 15*f*, 17*f*

Ethmoidal foramina, anterior/posterior, 6*f*, 7*f*, 9
Euryblepharon, 156–158, 157*f*, 158*f*
Evisceration, 127, 129–130
goals of, 129
intraoperative complications of, 130
ocular prostheses after, 132
sympathetic ophthalmia and, 130
wrong eye removal and, 130
Examination
periocular malpositions/involutional changes and, 197
in ptosis evaluation, 209–212, 210*f*, 211*f*, 212
Excisional biopsy, 179*f*, 180
Excretory lacrimal system, 252–255, 253*f*, 254*f*. *See also* Lacrimal drainage system
anatomy of, 252–255, 253*f*, 254*f*
development of, 255
abnormalities of, 257–259, 258*f*
disorders of
acquired, 267–281
congenital, 259–267
therapeutic closure of, 281–282
tumors of, 287
Exenteration, 127, 136–137, 137*f*
for basal cell carcinoma, 180
for lacrimal gland tumors, 93, 136
for lacrimal sac tumors, 287
ocular prosthesis after, 137
for sebaceous adenocarcinoma, 184
for squamous cell carcinoma, 182
for teratoma, 41
Exophthalmometry, 24, 24*f*
Exophthalmos, 23. *See also* Proptosis
in orbital roof fractures, 106
in thyroid eye disease, 56. *See also* Thyroid eye disease
Exorbitism, 23. *See also* Proptosis
External carotid artery, 13, 154
External dacryocystorhinostomy (DCR), 279, 280*f*
External hordeolum (stye), 163–164
External (transcutaneous) levator advancement surgery, for ptosis, 219, 219*f*
Extraconal fat/surgical space (peripheral surgical space), 11, 115, 115*f*
Extraocular muscles, 11–12, 12*f*
damage to
during blepharoplasty, 234
during enucleation/evisceration, 130
in orbital floor/blowout fracture, 108, 109–110
in orbital roof fractures, 106
innervation of, 12, 14*f*, 15*f*
metastatic disease of, 99
nonspecific orbital inflammation involving, 63–64
orbital implants and, 131, 132
in ptosis, 212
in thyroid eye disease, 25, 52, 54, 54*f*, 56
Extraocular myopathy, in thyroid eye disease, 25, 52, 54, 54*f*, 56
Exuberant hyperkeratosis (cutaneous horn), 168
Eye, removal of. *See also* Anophthalmic socket; Enucleation; Evisceration; Exenteration
prevention of removing wrong eye and, 130
Eye movements. *See* Ocular motility
Eye socket. *See* Socket
Eyebrows
direct elevation of, 235
drooping of (brow ptosis), 234–235, 235*f*
dermatochalasis and, 229, 234, 235
follicles of, tumors arising in, 172, 172*f*, 173*f*
in trichotillomania, 165
Eyelashes (cilia), 153
entropion/ptosis of. *See also* Trichiasis
in anophthalmic socket, 136
in epiblepharon, 157*f*, 159, 159*f*
follicles of, 154*f*
tumors arising in, 172, 172*f*, 173*f*
misdirection of. *See* Trichiasis
in trichotillomania, 165
Eyelid crutches, for benign essential blepharospasm, 227
Eyelid hygiene
for canaliculitis, 284–285
for chalazia, 162
Eyelid imbrication syndrome, 164
Eyelid-sharing techniques, in eyelid repair, 161, 195
Eyelid splitting
for distichiasis, 160
for orbitotomy, 116*f*, 117–118
Eyelid springs, for paralytic lagophthalmos/upper eyelid paralysis, 226
Eyelid weights
for paralytic ectropion, 225–226
for paralytic lagophthalmos/upper eyelid paralysis, 226
Eyelids
aging affecting
orbital septum changes and, 149
suborbicularis oculi fat (SOOF) and, 152
anatomy of, 145–154, 146*f*, 147*f*, 148*f*, 150*f*, 152*f*, 154*f*
basal cell carcinoma of, 177–182, 178*f*, 179*f*
biopsy of, 179–180, 179*f*
for basal cell carcinoma, 179–180, 179*f*
for melanoma, 185–186
for sebaceous carcinoma, 184
canthal tendons and, 152*f*, 153
coloboma of, 160–161, 160*f*
congenital anomalies/disorders of, 155–162, 157*f*
conjunctiva of, 146*f*, 152
connective tissue structures of, 152–153
creases of, 146*f*, 147
for orbitotomy incision, 116–117, 116*f*, 117*f*, 119, 121
in ptosis, 210, 210*f*, 214*t*
cysts of
epidermal, 168–169, 168*f*, 169*f*
inclusion/sebaceous, 168, 168*f*
disorders of, 155–196. *See also specific type*
acquired, 162–165
congenital, 155–162, 157*f*
neoplastic, 165–187. *See also* Eyelids, tumors of
in thyroid eye disease, 25, 52, 52*f*, 54, 56, 59. *See also* Thyroid eye disease
traumatic, 187–190, 188*f*. *See also* Eyelids, trauma to
ectropion of, 197–201, 198*f*, 200*f*. *See also* Ectropion
congenital, 156, 157*f*
edema of, 164
in blepharochalasis, 230
in orbital floor/blowout fracture, 108
in thyroid eye disease, 54

emphysema of, in orbital floor/blowout fracture, 109
entropion of, 202–207, 203*f*, 204*f*, 205*f*, 206*f*, 207*f*. *See also* Entropion
congenital, 159–160, 160*f*
epithelium of
benign lesions of, 168–169, 168*f*, 169*f*
hyperplasias of, 166–168, 166*f*, 167*f*
in situ carcinoma of, 176–177, 177*f*
eversion of. *See* Ectropion
floppy, 164, 164*f*
folds of, 147
fusion of (ankyloblepharon), 157*f*, 158
horizontal laxity of
in involutional ectropion, 199
in involutional entropion, 202, 203
horizontal shortening/tightening of
for cicatricial ectropion, 201
for involutional ectropion, 199, 200*f*
for involutional entropion, 204
inversion of. *See* Entropion
keratosis of
actinic, 175–176, 176*f*
squamous cell carcinoma and, 176, 182
seborrheic, 167, 167*f*
lacerations of
canthal tissue involved in, 189
lid margin involved in, 188–189, 188*f*, 192–195, 193*f*, 194*f*
lid margin not involved in, 187–188, 191–192
ptosis caused by, 218
repair of, 188, 188–189, 188*f*, 189. *See also* Eyelids, surgery/reconstruction of
secondary, 189–190
lower
blepharoplasty on, 230–231, 231, 232–233, 232*f*
laser resurfacing as adjunct to, 237
vision loss after, 233
crease of, 147
for orbitotomy incision, 118
involutional entropion in, 202–204, 203*f*, 204*f*, 205*f*
reconstruction of, 192–195, 194*f*
retractors of, 146*f*, 151
in involutional ectropion, repair of, 200–201
in involutional entropion, 202–203
repair of, 204, 205*f*
reverse ptosis of, 212, 215
tarsal plate of, 152
vertical elevation of, for paralytic ectropion, 226
malpositions of, 197–224. *See also specific type*
margin of, 153
distance from corneal reflex and, in ptosis, 209–210, 210*f*, 214*t*
eversion of, 197–201, 198*f*, 200*f*. *See also* Ectropion
inversion of, 202–207, 203*f*, 204*f*, 205*f*, 206*f*, 207*f*. *See also* Entropion
lacerations of, 188–189, 188*f*
nevus involving, 173, 174*f*
repair of, 188–189, 188*f*, 192–195, 193*f*, 194*f*
sebaceous carcinoma arising in, 184
in nonspecific orbital inflammation, 64
orbital fat and, 146*f*, 149
orbital septum and, 146*f*, 149
orbital tumors/inflammation originating in, 94–95
plexiform neurofibroma involving, 77*f*, 78, 78*f*
protractors of, 147–149, 148*f*
spasms of (benign essential blepharospasm), 226–227, 227*f*
racial variations in, 147, 147*f*
reconstruction of. *See* Eyelids, surgery/reconstruction of
retraction of, 222–224, 222*f*
after blepharoplasty, 223, 234
in Parinaud syndrome, 223
in thyroid eye disease, 52, 52*f*, 54, 56, 59, 222–223, 223, 224
treatment of, 223–224
retractors of, 149–151, 150*f*
in involutional ectropion, repair of, 200–201
in involutional entropion, 202–203
repair of, 204, 205*f*
rhabdomyosarcoma involving, 82
skin of, 146–147, 146*f*
excessive removal of, in blepharoplasty, 234
redundancy of. *See* Dermatochalasis
splitting of. *See* Eyelid splitting
squamous cell carcinoma of, 182, 182*f*
actinic keratosis and, 176, 182
in situ (Bowen disease), 176
keratoacanthoma, 176–177, 177*f*
subcutaneous tissue of, 146–147, 146*f*
suborbicularis fat pads/suborbicularis oculi fat (SOOF) and, 146*f*, 152–153
midface rejuvenation surgery (SOOF lift) and, 242, 243*f*
surgery/reconstruction of, 191–196, 193*f*, 194*f*
for basal cell carcinoma, 180, 180–181
in blepharophimosis–ptosis–epicanthus inversus syndrome, 159
blepharoplasty, 230–234, 232*f*
for coloboma, 161
for defects involving eyelid margin, 188–189, 188*f*, 192–195, 193*f*, 194*f*
for defects not involving eyelid margin, 187–188, 191–192
for epicanthus, 159
for euryblepharon, 157–158
for eyelid retraction, 224
history and examination in patient considering, 197
laceration/trauma repair and, 188, 188–189, 188*f*, 189
secondary, 189–190
for lateral canthal defects, 195
for medial canthal defects, 195–196
after Mohs micrographic surgery, 181
principles of, 191
priorities in, 191
for ptosis repair, 218–222, 219*f*, 220*f*, 221*f*
in blepharophimosis–ptosis–epicanthus inversus syndrome, 159
for thyroid eye disease, 58, 59
symblepharon and, 208
tarsus of, 146*f*, 151–152, 152*f*
trauma to, 187–190, 188*f*
bite wounds (dog and human), 190
blunt, 187
burns, 190
penetrating, 187–189, 188*f*
ptosis caused by, 190, 218

repair of, 188, 188–189, 188*f*, 189. *See also* Eyelids, surgery/reconstruction of
secondary, 189–190
tumors of, 165–187
benign, 166–169, 166*f*, 167*f*, 168*f*
adnexal lesions, 169–172, 171*f*, 172*f*, 173*f*
epithelial hyperplasias, 166–168, 166*f*, 167*f*
epithelial lesions, 168–169, 168*f*, 169*f*
melanocytic, 172–175, 174*f*, 175*f*
biopsy in evaluation of, 179–180, 179*f*
clinical evaluation of, 165–166
malignant, 177–187
basal cell carcinoma, 177–182, 178*f*, 179*f*
in situ epithelial, 176–177, 177*f*
Kaposi sarcoma, 186, 186*f*
melanoma, 184–186, 185*f*
Merkel cell carcinoma, 187
predisposing factors and, 165
sebaceous adenocarcinoma (sebaceous gland carcinoma), 183–184, 183*f*
signs suggesting, 165
squamous cell carcinoma, 182, 182*f*
actinic keratosis and, 176, 182
in situ (Bowen disease), 176
keratoacanthoma, 176–177, 177*f*
mechanical ptosis caused by, 217–218
orbital involvement and, 94–95
premalignant
epidermal, 175–176, 176*f*
melanocytic, 177
upper
blepharoplasty on, 230, 231, 232, 232*f*
crease of, 150
for orbitotomy incision, 116–117, 116*f*, 117*f*, 119, 121
in ptosis, 210, 210*f*, 214*t*
drooping of. *See* Ptosis
excursion of, in ptosis, 210, 211*f*
fold of, 147, 150
paralysis of, 226
reconstruction of, 192, 193*f*
retractors of, 149–151, 150*f*
tarsal plates of, 151–152, 152*f*
vascular supply of, 154

Face. *See also under Facial*
aging affecting
pathogenesis of, 236
physical examination and, 197, 236–237
rejuvenation and, 235–247. *See also* Facial rejuvenation
anatomy of, 141–144, 142*f*, 143*f*, 144*f*, 145*f*
Face-lift. *See also* Facial rejuvenation
elevation of superficial musculoaponeurotic system (SMAS) and, 141, 142*f*, 245
Facial artery, 16*f*
Facial clefts, 36–38, 37*f*, 38*f*. *See also* Craniofacial malformations
nasolacrimal duct obstruction and, 259
Facial dystonia, 226–229, 227*f*
Facial fasciae
deep, 141
superficial, 141
Facial muscles, 16, 141, 141–143, 143*f*
Facial nerve. *See* Cranial nerve VII
Facial neurectomy, for benign essential blepharospasm, 228
Facial paralysis/weakness, 224–226
ectropion and, 198*f*, 224–226, 225*f*
after facial nerve ablation for benign essential blepharospasm, 228
hemifacial paralysis and, 229
upper eyelid paralysis and, 226
Facial rejuvenation, 235–247
botulinum toxin (cosmetic) for, 238–239
laser skin resurfacing for, 237–238
nonsurgical, 237–240, 239*f*, 240*f*
pathogenesis of aging face and, 236
physical examination of aging face and, 236–237
soft tissue dermal fillers for, 239–240, 239*f*, 240*f*
surgical, 241–247, 242*f*, 243*f*, 244*f*, 245*f*, 246*f*. *See also* Facial surgery
Facial surgery. *See also specific procedure and* Eyelids, surgery/reconstruction of
anatomy and, 141–144, 142*f*, 143*f*, 144*f*, 145*f*
history and examination in patient considering, 197, 236–237
preoperative considerations and, 236, 241, 245
rejuvenation procedures, 241–247, 242*f*, 243*f*, 244*f*, 245*f*, 246*f*
brow- and forehead-lift, endoscopic/pretrichial, 241, 242*f*, 243*f*
forehead rejuvenation, 241, 242*f*, 243*f*
lower face and neck rejuvenation, 245–247, 245*f*, 246*f*
midface rejuvenation, 241–245, 243*f*, 244*f*
neck liposuction, 246
platysmaplasty, 246–247, 246*f*
rhytidectomy, 245–246, 245*f*
Facial vein, eyelids drained by, 154
Family history/familial factors, in ptosis evaluation, 209
Fasanella-Servat ptosis repair procedure, 220
Fascia lata, autogenous and banked, for frontalis suspension, 221
Fascia lata sling, for paralytic ectropion, 226
Fascial cutaneous ligaments, 141
Fasciitis, necrotizing, of orbit, 48–49
Fat
orbital, 11, 146*f*, 149
dermatochalasis and, 229
eyelid lacerations and, 149, 187, 188
retro-orbicularis oculi (ROOF), 146*f*, 152, 153
suborbicularis oculi (SOOF/suborbicularis fat pads), 146*f*, 152–153
midface rejuvenation surgery (SOOF lift) and, 242, 243*f*
Fat-suppression techniques, in MRI, 28*f*, 29
Fibroblasts, orbital, in thyroid eye disease, 55
Fibroepithelial polyp (acrochordon/skin tag), 166, 166*f*
Fibrosarcoma, of orbit, 84
Fibrous dysplasia, of orbit, 84, 85*f*
secondary, 97
Fibrous histiocytoma, of orbit, 84
Fibrous tumor, solitary, of orbit, 84

Fine-needle aspiration biopsy (FNAB), of orbit, 124
in lymphoma, 88
in tumor evaluation, 33, 99
Fissures
orbital, 6*f*, 7, 7*f*, 8*f*, 9, 10*f*
inferior, 6*f*, 7*f*, 8*f*, 9
superior, 6*f*, 7, 7*f*, 9, 10*f*
palpebral, 153
in euryblepharon, 157
vertical height of, in ptosis, 210, 210*f*
Fistulas
arteriovenous, of orbit, 72–74, 72*f*, 73*f*
carotid-cavernous sinus, 72–73, 72*f*, 73*f*
direct, 72, 72–73
dural (indirect), 72, 73
lacrimal–cutaneous, congenital, 257, 258*f*
lacrimal gland, 257
Fitzpatrick skin type, 236–237
FLAIR (fluid-attenuated inversion recovery) technique, 29
Flaps
for canthal repair, 195, 196
after exenteration, 137
for eyelid repair, 190, 191, 192, 193*f*, 194, 194*f*, 195
in burn injury, 190
for symblepharon, 208
Floppy eyelid syndrome, 164, 164*f*
Flow cytometry, 124
in orbital lymphoma, 88
Fluid-attenuated inversion recovery (FLAIR) technique, 29
Fluorescein
for dye disappearance test, 269
for Jones I and Jones II tests, 269
for tear breakup time testing, 267
FNAB. *See* Fine-needle aspiration biopsy
Follicles, hair
of eyelash, 154*f*
tumors originating in, 172, 172*f*, 173*f*
Follicular center lymphoma, of orbit, 86
Foramen (foramina)
ethmoidal, anterior/posterior, 6*f*, 7*f*, 9
infraorbital, 6*f*
oculomotor, 12
optic, 10
rotundum, 6*f*, 8*f*
supraorbital, 6, 6*f*
zygomaticofacial, 6*f*, 8*f*
zygomaticotemporal, 6*f*
Forced duction test (traction test), in orbital floor/blowout fracture, 109
surgery and, 110
Forehead
drooping of (brow ptosis), 234–235, 235*f*
dermatochalasis and, 229, 234, 235
surgical rejuvenation procedures of, 241, 242*f*, 243*f*
Forehead flap
for canthal repair, 196
for eyelid repair, 193*f*
Forehead rejuvenation, 241, 242*f*, 243*f*
Foreheadplasty, 241, 242*f*
Foreign bodies, intraorbital, 112
MRI and, 30–31, 112
Fornices
contracture of, anophthalmic socket and, 133
socket contracture and, 135
depth of, in "giant fornix syndrome," 133
Fossae
anterior cranial, 7*f*
lacrimal/lacrimal gland, 6, 6*f*, 254, 254*f*
nasal, 18
pterygopalatine, 7*f*
for trochlea of superior oblique tendon, 6
*FOXL2* gene, in blepharophimosis–ptosis–epicanthus inversus syndrome, 155
Frames (spectacle), anophthalmic socket camouflage and, 136
Freckle
of eyelid, 174
Hutchinson melanotic (lentigo maligna/precancerous melanosis), 177
Frontal bone, 6, 6*f*, 7*f*
Frontal craniotomy, for orbital surgery, 124
Frontal (temporal) nerve, 10*f*, 13*f*, 14*f*, 15*f*, 16, 17*f*, 142*f*, 143, 144, 144*f*
Frontal sinuses, 7*f*, 18, 18–19, 19*f*
Frontalis muscle, 16, 141, 142*f*, 143*f*, 146*f*, 148*f*
Frontalis suspension, for ptosis repair, 220–221, 221*f*
anophthalmic socket and, 135
in blepharophimosis–ptosis–epicanthus inversus syndrome, 155
Frontoethmoidal (Lynch) incision, for orbitotomy, 116*f*, 119
Frontoethmoidal suture, 8, 9
Frontotemporal-orbitozygomatic approach, for orbital surgery, 124
Frontozygomatic suture, 6*f*, 7
Frozen section, in orbital tumor evaluation, 33
Full-thickness eyelid biopsy, 179*f*
Full-thickness pentagonal resection, for trichiasis, 208
Fungal infection, of orbit
aspergillosis, 50–51
exenteration in management of, 50, 136
zygomycosis/mucormycosis/phycomycosis, 50
exenteration in management of, 50, 136

Gadolinium, 29
GAGs. *See* Glycosaminoglycans
Galea aponeurotica, 141, 143*f*
Gasserian ganglion, 14*f*, 15*f*
GCA. *See* Giant cell arteritis
General anesthesia
for dacryocystorhinostomy, 279
for lacrimal probing, 260
Giant cell arteritis (GCA/temporal arteritis), 61
"Giant fornix syndrome," 133
Glabellar flap, for canthal repair, 196
Glands of Krause, 146*f*, 152, 252
Glands of Moll, 154*f*, 170
hidrocystoma arising in, 171, 171*f*
Glands of Wolfring, 146*f*, 152, 252
Glands of Zeis, 170
hordeolum caused by infection of, 163
sebaceous adenocarcinoma arising in, 183
Glioblastomas, optic nerve (malignant optic gliomas), 76

Gliomas, optic nerve/pathway/chiasm, 74–77, 75*f*
  malignant (glioblastomas), 76
  in neurofibromatosis, 74, 76, 78
Globe
  displacement of, in orbital disorders, 11–12, 23–24, 95, 95*f*
  orbital tumors/inflammation originating in, 94–95
  ptosis of, in orbital floor/blowout fracture, 109
  suspensory ligament of. *See* Lockwood ligament
Glycosaminoglycans (GAGs), in thyroid eye disease, 55
Goblet cells, 152
  mucin tear secretion by, 252
Gold eyelid weights
  for paralytic ectropion, 225–226
  for paralytic lagophthalmos/upper eyelid paralysis, 226
Goldenhar syndrome (oculoauricular dysplasia), 37
Gorlin syndrome (basal cell nevus syndrome), 178
GPA. *See* Granulomatosis, with polyangiitis
Gradient echo MR sequences, 29
Grafts
  for canthal repair, 195
  for cicatricial ectropion, 201, 202*f*
  for cicatricial entropion, 207
  dermis-fat, 132
    in children, 129
    in congenital anophthalmia/microphthalmia management, 36
    for exposure and extrusion of orbital implant, 134
    for superior sulcus deformity, 132–133
  after exenteration, 137
  for eyelid repair, 190, 191, 193, 193*f*, 194, 194*f*
    in burn injury, 190
  for eyelid retraction, 223, 224
  mucous membrane
    for cicatricial entropion, 207
    for contracted socket, 134
    for eyelid retraction, 224
    for symblepharon, 208
  for paralytic ectropion, 226
  scleral patch, for exposure and extrusion of orbital implant, 133
  for symblepharon, 208
  tarsoconjunctival
    for cicatricial entropion, 207
    for eyelid repair, 190
Granulocytic sarcoma (chloroma), 98–99
Granulomas, eosinophilic, orbital, 90
Granulomatosis, with polyangiitis (GPA/Wegener granulomatosis), 61–62, 62*f*
  screening/diagnostic tests for, 33–34
Graves hyperthyroidism/ophthalmopathy/eye disease, 51, 52, 53, 55, 56. *See also* Thyroid eye disease
Gray line, 149, 153, 154*f*
Group A β-hemolytic streptococcus, orbital necrotizing fasciitis caused by, 48
Guérin (Le Fort I) fracture, 103, 104*f*

*Haemophilus influenzae*
  orbital cellulitis caused by, 47
  preseptal cellulitis caused by, 44
*Haemophilus influenzae* type b (Hib) vaccine, cellulitis prevention and, 44
Hair follicles, of eyelid, 154*f*
  tumors arising in, 172, 172*f*, 173*f*
Hamartomas, of orbit, 39
Hand-Schüller-Christian disease, orbital involvement and, 90
Hard palate composite grafts
  for cicatricial entropion, 207
  for eyelid repair, 190
  for eyelid retraction, 224
  for paralytic ectropion, 226
Hashimoto thyroiditis, thyroid eye disease and, 52, 53, 56
Hasner, valve of, 253*f*, 254*f*
  nasolacrimal duct obstruction and, 255, 260
Hedgehog pathway inhibitors, for squamous cell carcinoma, 182
Helical (spiral) computed tomography, in orbital evaluation, 27
Hemangiomas
  of eyelid, infantile (capillary), 161–162
  of orbit
    cavernous, 68–69, 69*f*
    infantile (capillary), 67–68, 67*f*
Hemangiopericytoma, of orbit, 69
Hematic cyst, orbital, 112
Hemifacial microsomia, 37
Hemifacial paralysis, after facial nerve ablation for benign essential blepharospasm, 228
Hemifacial spasm (HFS), 228–229
Hemorrhages
  orbital, 74, 112
    after blepharoplasty, vision loss and, 233–234
    in orbital floor/blowout fracture, 108, 109
    from orbital lymphatic malformation, 70, 70*f*, 71
    postoperative, 121, 125
  retrobulbar, after blepharoplasty, vision loss and, 233
Hering's law, eyelid retraction and, 222, 223
Herpes simplex virus, skin infection after laser resurfacing caused by, 238
Hertel exophthalmometer, 24, 24*f*
HFS. *See* Hemifacial spasm
Hidrocystoma
  apocrine, 171, 171*f*
  eccrine, 170
High-grade lymphoma, of orbit, 86
Histiocytoma, fibrous, orbital, 84
Histiocytosis (Langerhans cell histiocytosis/histiocytosis X), orbital involvement and, 90
History
  orbital evaluation and, 21–22, 22*f*, 23*t*
  in periocular malpositions/involutional changes, 197
  in ptosis evaluation, 209
HIV infection/AIDS
  Kaposi sarcoma in, 186, 186*f*
  molluscum contagiosum in, 169
Hodgkin disease, orbital, 86
Hordeolum (hordeola), 163–164
  external (stye), 163–164
  internal, 162, 163
Horizontal eyelid shortening/tightening
  for cicatricial ectropion, 201
  for involutional ectropion, 199, 200*f*
  for involutional entropion, 204
Hormone therapy, for breast metastasis to orbit, 100
Horner muscle, 148

Horner syndrome, 18
congenital, 215
in neuroblastoma, 98
pharmacologic testing for, 212
ptosis and, 212
HPV. *See* Human papillomaviruses
Hughes/modified Hughes procedure, in eyelid repair, 194–195, 194*f*, 195
Human bites, eyelid injuries caused by, 190
Human papillomaviruses (HPV), eyelid infection/wart caused by, 167
Hutchinson melanotic freckle (lentigo maligna/precancerous melanosis), 177
Hyaluronan/hyaluronic acid
as dermal filler for facial rejuvenation, 239, 240*f*, 241*f*
in thyroid eye disease, 55
Hybridization, in orbital lymphoma, 88
Hydatid cyst, orbital infection caused by, 51
Hydroxyapatite orbital implant, 131, 131*f*. *See also* Orbital implant
Hypercholesterolemia, xanthelasma associated with, 169
Hyperglobus, 23
Hyperkeratosis, exuberant (cutaneous horn), 168
Hyperpigmentation, after laser skin resurfacing, 238
Hyperplasia
epithelial, of eyelid, 166–168, 166*f*, 167*f*
lymphoid, of orbit, 86–88, 88. *See also* Lymphoproliferative disorders
pseudoepitheliomatous, 167
sebaceous, 170
Hypertelorism (telorbitism), 23
in craniosynostosis, 37
with midline clefts, 37
Hyperthyroidism
Graves, 51, 52. *See also* Thyroid eye disease
treatment of, 58
Hypoesthesiam in infraorbital nerve distribution
in orbital floor/blowout fracture, 19, 109
after orbital surgery, 125
Hypoglobus, 23
Hypothyroidism, thyroid eye disease and, 52, 56

Ice-pack test, for myasthenia gravis, 217
Ichthyosis, congenital ectropion and, 156
Idiopathic orbital inflammation/inflammatory syndrome. *See* Nonspecific orbital inflammation
IgG4 disease, 60
IL. *See under Interleukin*
Immunoglobulin G (IgG)
IgG4 disease and, 60
in thyroid eye disease, 55
Implant, orbital, 131–132, 131*f*
in children, 129
after evisceration, 130
exposure and extrusion of, 130, 131, 133–134, 134*f*
contracted socket and, 134
migration of, 130, 131
for orbital floor/blowout fracture, 111
for superior sulcus deformity, 132
Incisional biopsy, 179*f*, 180
Incisions, for orbital surgery, 116–121, 116*f*
Inclusion cysts, epidermal, of eyelid, 168, 168*f*
IncobotulinumtoxinA, 238. *See also* Botulinum toxin
Indirect (dural) carotid-cavernous fistula, 72, 73
Indirect (blowout) fractures
of medial orbital wall, 8, 108
orbital cellulitis following, 47
of orbital floor, 108–112, 110*f*
diplopia after, 108
infraorbital nerve and, 19
surgery for, 111–112
indications for, 110–111
of orbital roof, in children, 106
Inert orbital implant, 131
Infantile (capillary) hemangioma
of eyelid, 161–162
of orbit, 67–68, 67*f*
and thrombocytopenia (Kasabach-Merritt syndrome), 67–68
Infection (ocular)
canalicular obstruction caused by, 274
lacrimal system, 284–286, 285*f*, 286*f*
Inferior infraorbital vein, 13*f*
Inferior meatus, 10, 18, 255. *See also* Inferior turbinate
Inferior oblique muscle, 11, 14*f*, 146*f*
innervation of, 12, 14*f*, 15*f*
Inferior ophthalmic vein, 14*f*
Inferior orbital fissure, 6*f*, 7*f*, 8*f*, 9
Inferior rectus muscle, 11, 13*f*, 14*f*, 15*f*, 146*f*
injury of, in orbital floor/blowout fracture, 108, 109–110
innervation of, 12, 14*f*, 15*f*
surgery of, for orbital floor/blowout fracture, 109–110
Inferior tarsal muscle, 151
Inferior turbinate/concha, 18, 253*f*, 254*f*
infracture of, for congenital nasolacrimal duct obstruction, 265
Inferolateral displacement of globe, in orbital disorders, 24
Inferomedial displacement of globe, in orbital disorders, 24
Inflammation (ocular)
canalicular obstruction caused by, 274
lacrimal gland tumors causing, 94, 274
nasolacrimal duct obstruction caused by, 278
orbital, 43–66, 43*t*. *See also* Nonspecific orbital inflammation
autoimmune, 43*t*
granulomatous, 43*t*
in histiocytic disorders, 90
infectious, 43*t*, 44–51
noninfectious, 51–66
vasculitic, 43*t*, 60–63, 62*f*
Informed consent, for facial rejuvenation surgery, 241
Infraciliary blepharoplasty incision, for orbitotomy, 118
Infracture of turbinates, for congenital nasolacrimal duct obstruction, 265
Infraorbital canal, 9
Infraorbital foramen, 6*f*
Infraorbital groove, 9
Infraorbital nerve, 12*f*, 17*f*, 145*f*
hypoesthesia in distribution of
in orbital floor/blowout fracture, 19, 109
after orbital surgery, 125
Infraorbital vein, inferior, 13*f*
Infratrochlear nerve, 14*f*, 15*f*, 145*f*
Inspection, in orbital disorders, 23–25, 24*f*, 25*f*

Insulin-like growth factor I, in thyroid eye disease, 55
Interferon-α, for infantile (capillary) hemangioma, 162
Intergroup Rhabdomyosarcoma Study Group, 83
Interleukin-6, thyroid eye disease and, 55
Interleukin-8, thyroid eye disease and, 55
Intermuscular septum, 11
Internal (transconjunctival) approach, in ptosis repair, 220, 220*f*
Internal carotid artery, 13, 14*f*, 15*f*, 154
Internal (endonasal) dacryocystorhinostomy (DCR), 279, 280*f*, 281*f*
  endoscopic, 280
Internal hordeolum, 162, 163
Intraconal fat/surgical space (central surgical space), 11, 115*f*, 116
Intranasal examination, for lacrimal drainage evaluation, 272
Intraocular pressure, elevated, in traumatic optic neuropathy, 113
Intraocular tumors
  canalicular obstruction and, 274
  enucleation for, 128
  exenteration for, 136
  nasolacrimal duct obstruction and, 278
Intraorbital foreign bodies, 112
  MRI and, 30–31, 112
Intraorbital region of optic nerve, 5, 11
  length of, 5*t*, 11
Intraorbital tissue expanders, in congenital anophthalmia/microphthalmia management, 36
Intubation, lacrimal
  for acquired nasolacrimal obstruction, 278
  for canalicular obstruction, 275
  for canalicular trauma, 283
  for congenital lacrimal drainage obstruction, 262–263, 264*f*
  for punctal/canalicular agenesis/dysgenesis, 259, 260
Involutional ectropion, 198*f*, 199–201, 200*f*
Involutional entropion, 202–204, 203*f*, 204*f*, 205*f*
Involutional stenosis, nasolacrimal obstruction caused by, 277
Iodine, radioactive (RAI)
  for block and replace therapy in thyroid eye disease, 58
  nasolacrimal duct obstruction and, 278
Iodine 131, for block and replace therapy in thyroid eye disease, 58
Irrigation, of lacrimal drainage system
  for acquired obstruction, 270*f*, 271
  for canalicular obstruction evaluation, 270*f*, 271, 271*f*
  for canalicular trauma, 283
  for congenital obstruction, 261–262, 261*f*, 262*f*, 263*f*
Isotretinoin, laser skin resurfacing contraindicated in patients taking, 238

Jaw-winking syndrome/ptosis, Marcus Gunn, 211, 215, 216*f*
Jones I (primary dye) test, 269
Jones II test, 269
Jones tubes, 195, 260, 275, 275–276, 276*f*
Junctional nevus, 173
Juvenile xanthogranuloma, 91

Kaposi sarcoma, 186, 186*f*
Kasabach-Merritt syndrome, 67–68
Keratoacanthoma, eyelid, 176–177, 177*f*
Keratosis
  actinic, 175–176, 176*f*
    squamous cell carcinoma and, 176, 182
  seborrheic, 167, 167*f*
Krause, glands of, 146*f*, 152, 252

Lacerations
  canalicular, 282–283
  eyelid
    lid margin involved in, 188–189, 188*f*, 192–195, 193*f*, 194*f*
    lid margin not involved in, 187–188, 191–192
    ptosis caused by, 218
    repair of, 188, 188–189, 188*f*, 189. *See also* Eyelids, surgery/reconstruction of
      secondary, 189–190
  lacrimal sac/nasolacrimal duct, 284
Lacrimal artery, 12*f*, 14*f*, 15*f*
  eyelids supplied by, 154
Lacrimal bone, 6*f*, 7*f*, 8, 8*f*, 254
Lacrimal canaliculi. *See* Canaliculi
Lacrimal–cutaneous fistula, congenital, 257, 258*f*
Lacrimal drainage system, 252–255, 253*f*, 254*f*. *See also* Nasolacrimal duct
  anatomy of, 252–255, 253*f*, 254*f*
  development of, 255
    abnormalities of, 257–259, 258*f*
  diagnostic tests for evaluation of, 269–272, 269*f*, 270*f*, 271*f*
  disorders of. *See also* Tearing
    acquired, 267–281
    congenital, 255, 259–267
    infectious, 284–286, 285*f*, 286*f*
    neoplastic, 287
      canalicular obstruction and, 274
      nasolacrimal duct obstruction and, 278
    traumatic, 282–284
  duplications in, 257–258, 258*f*
  irrigation of
    for canalicular obstruction evaluation, 270*f*, 271, 271*f*
    for canalicular trauma, 283
    for congenital lacrimal drainage management, 261–262, 261*f*, 262*f*, 263*f*
    for lacrimal drainage evaluation, 269–271, 270*f*, 271*f*
  obstruction of
    acquired, 267–281
      evaluation of, 267–272, 269*f*, 270*f*, 271*f*
      neoplastic causes of, 274
    in canalicular disorders
      acquired, 273–276, 276*f*
      congenital, 259–260
    congenital, 255, 259–267
      evaluation of, 259
    dacryocystocele and, 265–267, 266*f*
    diagnostic tests for evaluation of, 269–272, 269*f*, 270*f*, 271*f*
    examination in patient with, 259, 267–268
    history in patient with, 267
    lacrimal outflow evaluation in patient with, 268–269
    nasolacrimal duct obstruction
      acquired, 276–281, 277*f*, 280*f*, 281*f*
      congenital, 255, 259, 260–265, 261*f*, 262*f*, 263*f*, 264*f*

pseudoepiphora evaluation and, 267–268
in punctal disorders
acquired, 272–273
congenital, 259–260
reconstruction of, 275, 283
after medial canthal basal cell carcinoma removal, 180
therapeutic closure of, 281–282
Lacrimal ducts, 251
Lacrimal fossa/lacrimal gland fossa, 6, 6*f*, 254, 254*f*
lymphoproliferative lesions/lymphomas arising in, 88, 91
Lacrimal gland, 14*f*, 15*f*, 18, 251–252, 252*f*. *See also* Lacrimal system
accessory glands and, 146*f*, 152, 252
agenesis of, 257
anatomy of, 14*f*, 15*f*, 18, 251–252, 252*f*
congenital abnormalities of, 257
development of, 251, 255
abnormalities of, 257
ectopic, 257
hypoplasia of, 257
infection of. *See* Dacryoadenitis
nonspecific orbital inflammation involving, 64, 94
parasympathetic innervation of, 16, 251
prolapse of, 257
sarcoidosis involving, 63
tumors of, 91–94, 92*f*
epithelial, 91–94, 92*f*
exenteration for, 93, 136
nonepithelial, 94
Lacrimal gland fistula, 257
Lacrimal intubation
for acquired nasolacrimal obstruction, 278
for canalicular obstruction, 275
for canalicular trauma, 283
for congenital lacrimal drainage obstruction, 262–263, 264*f*
for punctal/canalicular agenesis/dysgenesis, 259, 260
Lacrimal nerve, 10*f*, 13*f*, 14*f*, 15*f*, 16, 17*f*, 145*f*
in reflex tear arc, 251–252
Lacrimal outflow evaluation, 268–269
dye disappearance test and, 269, 269*f*
Jones I and Jones II tests in, 269
Lacrimal plugs, for dry eye, 281–282
canalicular obstruction and, 274, 282
extrusion/migration of, 282
nasolacrimal duct obstruction and, 278, 282
Lacrimal probing
for acquired nasolacrimal duct/canalicular obstruction, 271–272, 273
for canalicular trauma, 283
for congenital dacryocystocele, 265
for congenital nasolacrimal duct obstruction, 260, 261–262, 261*f*, 262*f*, 263*f*
Lacrimal pump, 147, 255, 256*f*
large puncta affecting, 273
Lacrimal sac (tear sac), 253, 253*f*, 254, 254*f*
cast formation in (dacryoliths), 277, 277*f*
development of, 255
distension of
in dacryocystitis, 285
in dacryocystocele, 265–267, 266*f*
dacryolith causing, 277
in nasolacrimal duct obstruction, 249, 271
neoplasm causing, 278
evaluation of, 268
inflammation of, 285–286, 286*f*. *See also* Dacryocystitis
trauma to, 284
tumors of, 287
Lacrimal scintigraphy, for lacrimal drainage evaluation, 272
Lacrimal system. *See also specific structure*
anatomy of, 251–255, 252*f*, 253*f*, 254*f*
biopsy of, in dacryocystorhinostomy, 279
development of, 255
abnormalities of, 257–259, 258*f*
disorders of, 257–287. *See also* Tearing
acquired, 267–281
congenital, 259–267
developmental abnormalities, 257–259, 258*f*
infection, 284–286, 285*f*, 286*f*
neoplastic, 91–94, 92*f*, 286–287
therapeutic closure of drainage system for, 281–282
traumatic, 282–284
excretory apparatus of, 252–255, 253*f*, 254*f*, 255. *See also* Excretory lacrimal system; Lacrimal drainage system
intubation of
for acquired nasolacrimal obstruction, 278
for canalicular obstruction, 275
for canalicular trauma, 283
for congenital lacrimal drainage obstruction, 262–263, 264*f*
for punctal/canalicular agenesis/dysgenesis, 259, 260
physiology of, 255, 256*f*
secretory apparatus/function of, 251–252, 252*f*, 255. *See also* Lacrimal gland; Secretory lacrimal apparatus
tumors of, 91–94, 92*f*, 286–287
canalicular obstruction and, 274
nasolacrimal duct obstruction and, 278
Lacrimal vein, 12*f*
Lacrimation, 267. *See also* Tearing
in thyroid eye disease, 56
Lagophthalmos
after blepharoplasty, 234
paralytic, 226
in paralytic ectropion, 224, 226
in ptosis, 210, 210*f*
after repair, 222
Lamellar deficiency, surgery for eyelid retraction and, 224
Lamina papyracea, 8, 254
Langerhans cell histiocytosis (histiocytosis X), orbital involvement and, 90
Laser therapy (laser surgery)
canaliculoplasty, for canalicular reconstruction, 275
for infantile (capillary) hemangioma, 68, 162
for punctal occlusion, 282
for skin resurfacing, 237–238
for trichiasis, 208
Lash follicles, 154*f*
tumors arising in, 172, 172*f*, 173*f*
Lash margin entropion
in anophthalmic socket, 136
tarsal fracture operation for, 207, 207*f*
trichiasis in, 208
Lateral canthal defects, repair of, 195

Lateral canthal tendon, 7, 14*f*, 152*f*, 153
laxity in, in involutional ectropion, 199
trauma involving, 189
Lateral canthotomy. *See* Canthotomy
Lateral flare, in thyroid-related eyelid retraction, 223
Lateral orbital tubercle of Whitnall, 6*f*, 7, 7*f*
Lateral orbital wall, 7–8
Lateral orbitotomy, 120–121. *See also* Orbitotomy
incisions for, 116*f*, 120–121
Lateral rectus muscle, 11, 12*f*, 13*f*, 14*f*, 15*f*
innervation of, 12
Lateral tarsal strip procedure
for cicatricial ectropion, 201
for involutional ectropion, 199, 200*f*
for involutional entropion, 204
Le Fort (midfacial) fractures, 103, 104*f*
Lenses, anophthalmic socket camouflage and, 136
Lentigo (lentigines)
senile, 174
simplex (simple lentigines), 174
solar, 174
Lentigo maligna (Hutchinson melanotic freckle/precancerous melanosis), 177
Lentigo maligna melanoma, 177, 185
Letterer-Siwe disease, orbital involvement and, 90
Leukemia, orbital involvement and, 98–99
Levator anguli oris muscle, 141, 143*f*
Levator aponeurosis, 7, 14*f*, 15*f*, 146*f*, 149, 150, 150*f*
horns of, 150, 150*f*
laceration of, 188
ptosis and, 214, 214*f*, 214*t*, 218
repair of, for ptosis correction, 219, 219*f*
Levator labii superioris alaeque nasi muscle, 143, 143*f*
Levator labii superioris muscle, 143, 143*f*
Levator muscle (levator palpebrae superioris), 11, 13*f*, 14*f*, 15*f*, 146*f*, 149, 149–151, 150*f*
damage to, in enucleation/evisceration, 130
evaluation of function of, in ptosis, 210, 210*f*, 211*f*, 214*t*
external (transcutaneous) advancement of, for ptosis correction, 219, 219*f*
innervation of, 12, 151
laceration of, 188
in myasthenia gravis/myogenic ptosis, 213, 213*f*
in traumatic ptosis, 218
"Lid lag," in thyroid eye disease, 25, 52, 56
Lid margin. *See* Eyelids, margin of
Lidocaine, for dacryocystorhinostomy, 280
Ligaments. *See specific ligament*
Light, corneal reflex to, eyelid margin distance to (margin–reflex distance), in ptosis, 209–210, 210*f*, 214*t*
Lipid disorders, xanthelasma associated with, 169
Liposarcomas, of orbit, 84
Liposuction, neck, 246
LMs. *See* Lymphatic malformations
Local anesthesia
for dacryocystorhinostomy, 279
for lacrimal probing, 260
Lockwood ligament (suspensory ligament of Lockwood), 7, 150, 151
Long ciliary nerve, 14*f*, 15*f*, 16
Longitudinal relaxation time (T1), 28
Lorazepam, for benign essential blepharospasm, 228
Lower eyelid. *See* Eyelids, lower
Lower eyelid reverse ptosis, 212, 215
Lower face and neck rejuvenation, 245–247, 245*f*, 246*f*
Lubricants
for involutional entropion, 203
for paralytic ectropion, 224–225
Lung cancer, eye involvement and, 100
Lymph node biopsy
in eyelid melanoma, 185
in sebaceous adenocarcinoma, 184
Lymphangiomas. *See* Lymphatic malformations
Lymphatic malformations (LMs/lymphangiomas), 69–71, 70*f*
Lymphatics, eyelid, 154
Lymphedema, eyelid, 164
Lymphoid hyperplasia, reactive, of orbit, 86–88, 88
Lymphoid tissues, mucosa-associated (MALT), lymphoma of, 86
Lymphomas, orbital, 85–89, 87*f*
lacrimal gland origin and, 87*f*, 88, 91
mucosa-associated (MALT), 86
Lymphoproliferative disorders. *See also specific type*
of lacrimal gland, 94
of orbit, 85–91
histiocytic disorders, 90
lymphoid hyperplasia/lymphomas, 85–89, 87*f*
plasma cell tumors, 89–90
xanthogranuloma, 90–91
Lynch (frontoethmoidal) incision, for orbitotomy, 116*f*, 119
Lysozyme, serum levels of, in sarcoidosis, 34, 63

Madarosis, basal cell carcinoma associated with, 179
Magnetic resonance angiography (MRA)
in carotid-cavernous fistulas, 73
in orbital evaluation, 32
Magnetic resonance imaging (MRI)
in lacrimal drainage evaluation, 272
in orbital evaluation, 28–29, 28*f*, 30*f*
CT compared with, 29–31, 29*t*, 30*f*
dermoid cysts and, 40
T1- and T2-weighted images in, 28–29, 28*f*
Malignant melanoma. *See* Melanoma
Malignant mixed tumor, of lacrimal gland, 91, 93
MALT lymphoma. *See* Mucosa-associated lymphoid tissue (MALT) lymphoma
Mandibular ligament, 141
Mandibular nerve. *See* Cranial nerve V (trigeminal nerve), $V_3$
Mandibulofacial dysostosis (Treacher Collins–Franceschetti syndrome), 37, 37*f*
Map biopsy, conjunctival, pagetoid spread of sebaceous adenocarcinoma and, 184
Marcus Gunn jaw-winking syndrome/ptosis, 211, 215, 216*f*
Margin
ciliary, 153
lid. *See* Eyelids, margin of
Margin–reflex distance ($MRD_1$ and $MRD_2$), in ptosis, 209–210, 210*f*, 214*t*
Marginal arterial arcades, eyelids supplied by, 16*f*, 146*f*, 154

Marginal entropion
in anophthalmic socket, 136
tarsal fracture operation for, 207, 207*f*
trichiasis in, 208
Marginal mandibular nerve, 142*f*, 143, 144*f*
Masseter muscle, 142*f*, 143
Masseteric ligament, 141
Maxilla/maxillary bone, 6*f*, 7*f*, 8, 8*f*
fracture of, 103, 104*f*
Maxillary nerve. *See* Cranial nerve V (trigeminal nerve), $V_2$
Maxillary sinuses, 7*f*, 9, 18, 19, 19*f*
Mechanical ectropion, 198*f*, 201
Mechanical ptosis/blepharoptosis, 217–218
Media, clear, traumatic vision loss with, 112–114
Medial canthal defects, repair of, 195–196
Medial canthal tendon, 152*f*, 153, 254
laxity in, in involutional ectropion, 199
trauma involving, 189
Medial canthal tumors
basal cell carcinoma, 180
canalicular obstruction and, 274
reconstructive surgery after removal of, 195–196
Medial orbital fractures, 8, 106–108, 107*f*
Medial orbital wall, 5, 5*t*, 8
fracture of, 8, 106–108, 107*f*
Medial rectus muscle, 11, 12*f*, 13*f*, 14*f*, 15*f*
innervation of, 12, 14*f*, 15*f*
Medial spindle procedure, for involutional ectropion, 199, 200*f*
Median forehead flap, for eyelid repair, 193*f*
Medications. *See* Drugs
Meibomian glands, 146*f*, 154, 154*f*, 162, 170
chalazion/hordeolum caused by infection of, 162, 163
sebaceous adenocarcinoma arising in, 183
in tear-film lipids/tear production, 252
Meige syndrome, 228
Melanocytes, 172, 173
tumors arising from
benign, 172–175, 174*f*, 175*f*
malignant (melanoma), 184–186, 185*f*
Melanocytic tumors, of eyelid
benign, 172–175, 174*f*, 175*f*
malignant (melanoma), 184–186, 185*f*
nevi, 173–174, 174*f*
premalignant, 177
Melanocytosis, dermal/oculodermal (nevus of Ota), 175, 175*f*
Melanoma, 184–186, 185*f*
acrolentiginous, 185
enucleation for, 128
exenteration for, 136
of eyelid, 184–186, 185*f*
lentigo maligna, 177, 185
nodular, 185, 185*f*
oculodermal melanocytosis and, 175
superficial spreading, 185
Melanosis, precancerous (lentigo maligna/Hutchinson melanotic freckle), 177
Melasma, 173
Meningiomas, 78–82, 79*f*, 80*f*
malignant, 81
optic nerve sheath, 79, 80*f*, 81
orbital, 78–82, 79*f*, 80*f*
sphenoid wing, 79, 79*f*, 81
Meningoceles, 37
Meningoencephaloceles, 37
Mental nerve, 145*f*
Mentalis muscle, 141, 143*f*
Merkel cells/Merkel cell carcinoma, 187
Mesenchymal tumors, orbital, 82–85, 82*f*, 85*f*
malignant, 84
Metastatic eye disease, of orbit, 98–101, 98*f*, 99*f*, 100*f*
in adults, 99–101, 99*f*, 100*f*
in children, 98–99, 98*f*
management of, 101
Methicillin-resistant *Staphylococcus aureus* (MRSA)
dacryoadenitis caused by, 284
preseptal cellulitis caused by, 45
Methimazole, for block and replace therapy in thyroid eye disease, 58
Methylprednisolone, for thyroid eye disease, 59
MG. *See* Myasthenia gravis
Micrographic surgery, Mohs
for canthal tumors, 195–196
for eyelid tumors
basal cell carcinoma, 180, 180–181
sebaceous adenocarcinoma, 184
squamous cell carcinoma, 182
Microphthalmia, 35–36, 127
with cyst, 36
treatment of, 36
Middle lamellar deficiency, surgery for eyelid retraction and, 224
Middle meatus, 18, 254
Middle turbinate/concha, 18, 253*f*
Midface rejuvenation/elevation, 241–245, 243*f*, 244*f*, 245*f*
Midfacial (Le Fort) fractures, 103, 104*f*
Mikulicz syndrome, 94
Milia, 168
Mimetic muscles, 141, 141–143, 143*f*
facial nerve supplying, 16, 143–144, 144*f*
Miniplates
for canthal repair, 195
for orbital fracture, 108
Minus (concave) lenses, anophthalmic socket camouflage and, 136
Mitomycin C, in dacryocystorhinostomy, 281
Mixed tumor
benign (pleomorphic adenoma)
of eyelid, 170
of lacrimal gland, 91, 92–93, 92*f*
malignant, of lacrimal gland, 91, 93
MMCRs. *See* Müller muscle–conjunctival resections
Mohs micrographic surgery
for canthal tumors, 195–196
for eyelid tumors
basal cell carcinoma, 180, 180–181
sebaceous adenocarcinoma, 184
squamous cell carcinoma, 182
Moll, glands of, 154*f*, 170
hidrocystoma arising in, 171, 171*f*
Molluscum contagiosum, of eyelid, 169, 169*f*
Monocanalicular stents
for lacrimal trauma, 283
for nasolacrimal intubation, 263, 264*f*

Monocular elevation deficiency (double-elevator palsy), 213
*Moraxella,* orbital cellulitis caused by, 47
Morning glory disc anomaly, 37
Morpheaform basal cell carcinoma, 178–179, 178*f*, 180. *See also* Basal cell carcinoma
Motility disorders. *See* Ocular motility, disorders of
MPO-ANCA. *See* Myeloperoxidase autoantibodies
MRA. *See* Magnetic resonance angiography
$MRD_1/MRD_2$. *See* Margin–reflex distance
MRI. *See* Magnetic resonance imaging
MRSA. *See* Methicillin-resistant *Staphylococcus aureus*
Mucins, tear film, 252
Mucoceles
  dacryocystitis and, 286
  lacrimal sac (dacryocystocele), 265–267, 266*f*
  orbital invasion by, 95, 95*f*
Mucocutaneous junction, eyelid, 153, 154*f*
Mucopyoceles, orbital invasion by, 95
*Mucor* infection (mucormycosis/zygomycosis/phycomycosis), orbit involved in, 50
  exenteration in management of, 50, 136
Mucosa-associated lymphoid tissue (MALT) lymphoma, of orbit, 86
Mucous membrane graft
  for cicatricial entropion, 207
  for contracted socket, 134
  for eyelid retraction, 224
  for symblepharon, 208
Muir-Torre syndrome, 170
Müller muscle (superior tarsal muscle), 146*f*, 149, 151
  in Horner syndrome, 215
  internal (transconjunctival) resection of, for ptosis correction, 220, 220*f*
    anophthalmic socket and, 135
Müller muscle–conjunctival resections (MMCRs), for ptosis repair, 220, 220*f*
Multicentric basal cell carcinoma, 179. *See also* Basal cell carcinoma
Multifocal eosinophilic granuloma of bone, 90
Muscle relaxants, for benign essential blepharospasm, 228
Muscle of Riolan, 149, 153, 154*f*
Mustardé flap/procedure, for eyelid repair, 194*f*, 195
Myasthenia gravis (MG), 216–217
  diagnosis of, edrophonium chloride in, 217
  ptosis in, 209, 212, 216–217
  thyroid eye disease and, 56
Myectomy, for benign essential blepharospasm, 228
Myelogenous leukemia, orbital involvement and, 99
Myelohyoid muscle, 143
Myeloperoxidase autoantibodies (MPO-ANCA), in granulomatosis with polyangiitis (Wegener granulomatosis), 62
Myogenic ptosis, 213–214, 213*f*, 214*t*
Myopathies, extraocular, in thyroid eye disease, 25, 52, 54, 54*f*, 56
Myositis, orbital, nonspecific orbital inflammation and, 63–64
Myxedema, pretibial, thyroid eye disease and, 56

Nasal artery, 16*f*
Nasal bone, 6*f*
Nasal cavity, 18
Nasal conchae (turbinates), 18, 253*f*, 254*f*
  infracture of, for congenital nasolacrimal duct obstruction, 265
Nasal endoscopy
  for lacrimal drainage evaluation/obstruction, 272
  for orbital decompression, 122
Nasal fossae, 18
Nasal nerve
  dorsal, 17*f*
  external, 145*f*
Nasal orbital fat pad, 149
Nasal septum, 18
Nasalis muscles, compressor and dilator, 143*f*
Nasociliary nerve, 10*f*, 12*f*, 13*f*, 14*f*, 15*f*, 16, 17*f*
Nasolacrimal canal, 8*f*, 10, 19
  balloon catheter dilation of
    for acquired nasolacrimal duct obstruction, 278
    for congenital nasolacrimal duct obstruction, 263–265
Nasolacrimal duct (NLD), 10, 18, 253*f*, 254–255, 254*f*. *See also* Lacrimal drainage system
  development of, 255
  irrigation of
    for acquired obstruction evaluation, 270*f*, 271
    for congenital obstruction management, 261–262, 261*f*, 262*f*, 263*f*
  obstruction of (NLDO). *See also* Tearing
    acquired, 276–281, 277*f*, 280*f*, 281*f*
      balloon catheter dilation for, 278
      dacryocystorhinostomy for, 278–281, 280*f*, 281
      etiology of, 277–278, 277*f*
      intubation and stenting for, 278
      irrigation in evaluation of, 270*f*, 271
      probing in evaluation of, 271–272
    congenital, 255, 259, 260–265, 261*f*, 262*f*, 263*f*, 264*f*
      balloon dacryoplasty (balloon catheter dilation) for, 263–265
      dacryocystorhinostomy for, 265
      intubation for, 262–263, 264*f*
      irrigation for, 261–262, 261*f*, 262*f*, 263*f*
      lacrimal–cutaneous fistula and, 258
      probing for, 260, 261–262, 261*f*, 262*f*, 263*f*
      turbinate infracture for, 265
    dacryocystitis and, 260, 285, 286
    functional, 271
    management of, 259, 278–281, 280*f*, 281*f*
  stenosis of, 271
    involutional, 277
  trauma to, 278, 284
Naso-orbital/naso-orbital-ethmoidal (NOE) fractures, 106–107, 107*f*
  nasolacrimal duct obstruction and, 278
NBX. *See* Necrobiotic xanthogranuloma
Neck
  anatomy of, 143
  rejuvenation surgery on, 245–247, 245*f*, 246*f*
    liposuction, 246
    platysmaplasty, 246–247, 246*f*
Necrobiotic xanthogranuloma (NBX), 90, 91
Necrotizing fasciitis, of orbit, 48–49
Neural tumors. *See also specific type*
  orbital, 74–82

Neurectomy, facial, for benign essential blepharospasm, 228
Neurilemoma (schwannoma), 82
Neuroblastoma, of orbit, 98, 98*f*
Neurofibromas, 77–78, 77*f*, 78*f*
discrete, 77–78
of orbit, 77–78, 77*f*, 78*f*
plexiform, 77, 77*f*, 78, 78*f*
eyelid involvement/ptosis and, 77*f*, 78, 78*f*
of orbit, 77, 77*f*, 78, 78*f*
Neurofibromatosis 1 (von Recklinghausen), 77*f*, 78, 78*f*
eyelid involvement/ptosis and, 77*f*, 78, 78*f*
optic pathway/optic nerve gliomas and, 74, 76, 78
orbital involvement and, 77*f*, 78, 78*f*
Neurogenic ptosis, 215–217, 216*f*
Neuropathy, optic. *See* Optic neuropathy
Nevi. *See* Nevus
Nevus, 173–174, 174*f*
blue, 175
of Ota (dermal/oculodermal melanocytosis), 175, 175*f*
Nevus cells, 172, 173
tumors arising from, 173–174, 174*f*. *See also* Nevus
Newborns
ectropion in, 156, 157*f*
milia in, 168
NLD. *See* Nasolacrimal duct
NLDO. *See* Nasolacrimal duct, obstruction of
NO SPECS scoring system, for thyroid eye disease, 57
Nodular basal cell carcinoma, 178, 178*f*. *See also* Basal cell carcinoma
Nodular melanoma, 185, 185*f*
NOE fractures. *See* Naso-orbital/naso-orbital-ethmoidal (NOE) fractures
Nonaxial displacement of globe, in orbital disorders, 24
Nonepithelial tumors, 94
orbital invasion by, 97, 97*f*
Non-Hodgkin lymphomas. *See also* Lymphomas
orbital, 85–89, 87*f*
Nonspecific orbital inflammation (NSOI/orbital pseudotumor/idiopathic orbital inflammation/ orbital inflammatory syndrome), 43, 43*t*, 63–66, 64*f*
lacrimal gland masses and, 64, 94
plasma cell–rich, 89
Nose, 18. *See also under Nasal*
inferior meatus of, 10, 18, 19, 255
middle meatus of, 18, 254
orbital tumors originating in, 95–98, 95*f*, 96*f*, 97*f*
superior meatus of, 19
NSOI. *See* Nonspecific orbital inflammation

Oblique muscles, 11, 12*f*, 13*f*, 14*f*, 15*f*, 146*f*. *See also specific muscle*
innervation of, 12, 14*f*, 15*f*
Observation
in management of epicanthus, 159
in management of optic nerve glioma, 76
in management of orbital lymphoma, 89
in management of traumatic vision loss, 114
Occipital nerves, 145*f*
Ocular adnexa, 169–170
benign lesions of, 169–172, 171*f*, 172*f*, 173*f*
lymphoproliferative lesions of, 85–91
Ocular motility
control of, extraocular muscles in, 11–12, 12*f*
disorders of, 25
in carotid-cavernous fistulas, 73
in orbital floor/blowout fracture, 108–109
surgery and, 110
orbital mass causing, 25
after orbital surgery, 125
in thyroid eye disease, 25, 52, 54, 56
evisceration and, 129, 130
ocular prostheses and, 132
orbital implants and, 131, 132
in ptosis, 212
Ocular myasthenia gravis, 217. *See also* Myasthenia gravis
Ocular prostheses, 36, 132
anophthalmic ectropion and, 135, 137
Oculoauricular dysplasia (Goldenhar syndrome), 37
Oculodermal/dermal melanocytosis (nevus of Ota), 175, 175*f*
Oculomotor foramen, 12
Oculomotor nerve. *See* Cranial nerve III
Oculomotor nerve palsy. *See* Third nerve (oculomotor) palsy
Oil glands, of eyelid, 170
lesions originating in, 170. *See also under Sebaceous*
OnabotulinumtoxinA, 238. *See also* Botulinum toxin
Operating microscope, for intraorbital surgery, 121
Ophthalmia, sympathetic
enucleation in prevention of, 128
evisceration and, 130
incidence of, 128
Ophthalmic artery, 10*f*, 12*f*, 13, 13*f*, 14*f*, 15*f*
eyelids supplied by, 154
orbit supplied by, 12*f*, 13
Ophthalmic lenses, anophthalmic socket camouflage and, 136
Ophthalmic nerve. *See* Cranial nerve V (trigeminal nerve), $V_1$
Ophthalmic pathology, of orbit, 32–33
Ophthalmic vein, 10*f*, 12*f*, 13–14, 13*f*, 14*f*, 15*f*
Ophthalmopathy, Graves/dysthyroid. *See* Thyroid eye disease
Optic canal, 6*f*, 7*f*, 8, 10, 19
decompression of, for traumatic vision loss, 114
Optic foramen, 10
Optic nerve (cranial nerve II), 12*f*, 13*f*, 14*f*, 15*f*
glioma of. *See* Optic nerve (optic pathway/chiasm) glioma
intraorbital region of, 5, 11
length of, 5*t*, 11
orbital varices affecting, 71
in thyroid eye disease, 52, 54, 56, 59
trauma to, 10, 113
Optic nerve glioblastoma (malignant optic glioma), 76
Optic nerve (optic pathway/chiasm) glioma (pilocytic astrocytoma), 74–77, 75*f*
malignant (glioblastoma), 76
in neurofibromatosis, 74, 76, 78
Optic nerve sheath meningioma, 79, 80*f*, 81
Optic neuropathy
orbital varices and, 71
thyroid eye disease and, 52, 54, 56, 59
traumatic, 113

Optic strut, *6f*, 10, *13f*
Optical (ocular) media, clear, traumatic vision loss with, 112–114
Optics, cosmetic, for anophthalmic socket, 136
Optociliary shunt vessels (retinociliary venous collaterals), 22, *22f*
Orbicularis oculi muscle, 16, 141, *143f*, *146f*, 147–149, *148f*, *154f*
  in involutional entropion, 203, 204
  in lacrimal pump, 147, 255, *256f*
  myectomy for benign essential blepharospasm and, 228
  spasm of, entropion caused by, 205–206
Orbicularis oris muscle, *143f*
Orbit. *See also under Orbital*
  abscesses of, 47, *47f*
  anatomy of, 5–19
  angiography/arteriography in evaluation of, 32
  anophthalmic socket and, 35
  apertures in walls of, *6f*, *7f*, *8f*, 9–10
  basal cell cancer involving, 180, 181
  biopsy of, 32–33
    fine-needle aspiration, 33, 88
    in nonspecific orbital inflammation, 65–66
    in rhabdomyosarcoma, 82, 83
  bones of, 5–6, *6f*, *7f*, *8f*
  cellulitis affecting. *See* Orbital cellulitis
  congenital/developmental disorders of, 35–41, *37f*, *38f*, *39f*, *41f*
  CT in evaluation of, 26–27, *26f*, *27f*, *30f*
    MRI compared with, 29–31, *29t*, *30f*
  cysts of
    dermoid, 39–40, *39f*
    epidermoid, 39
    with microphthalmia, 36
  dimensions of, 5, *5t*
  disorders of. *See also specific type*
    congenital/developmental anomalies, 35–41, *37f*, *38f*, *39f*, *41f*
    evaluation of, 21–41
      auscultation in, 26
      biopsy in, 32–33
      history in, 21–22, *22f*, *23t*
      inspection in, 23–25, *24f*, *25f*
      laboratory studies in, 33–34
      palpation in, 25–26
      physical examination in, 23–26, *24f*, *25f*
      primary imaging studies in, 26–31, *26f*, *27f*, *28f*, *29t*, *30f*
      secondary imaging studies in, 32
    globe displacement and, 11–12, 23–24, 95, *95f*
    granulomatous, *43t*
    infections, *43t*, 44–51
    inflammations, 43–66, *43t*. *See also* Nonspecific orbital inflammation
    neoplastic, 67–101. *See also* Orbit, tumors of
    pain and, 21. *See also* Pain, orbital
    periorbital changes and, 22, *22f*, *23t*
    pulsation and, 26
    rate of progression of, 21–22
    vasculitic, *43t*, 60–63, *62f*
  emphysema of, in orbital floor/blowout fracture, 109
  fissures in. *See* Orbital fissures
  floor of, 8–9, *8f*
    fractures of, 108–112, *110f*
  foreign bodies in, 112
    MRI and, 30–31, 112
  fractures of, 103–112
    midfacial (Le Fort) fractures, 103, *104f*
    zygomatic/zygomaticomaxillary complex (quadripod), 103–105, *105f*
  hemorrhages in, 74, 112
    after blepharoplasty, vision loss and, 233–234
    in orbital floor/blowout fracture, 108, 109
    from orbital lymphatic malformation, 70, *70f*, 71
    after surgery, 121, 125
  hypoplasia of, in microphthalmia, 36
  inflammation of, 43–66, *43t*. *See also* Nonspecific orbital inflammation
    autoimmune, *43t*
    granulomatous, *43t*
    in histiocytic disorders, 90
    infectious, *43t*, 44–51
    vasculitic, *43t*, 60–63, *62f*
  lacrimal gland neoplasia and, 287
  lateral wall of, 7–8
  leukemic infiltration of, 98–99
  lymphoproliferative lesions of, 85–91
  malformations of, 67–101
  medial wall of, 5, *5t*, 8
    fracture of, 8, 106–108, *107f*
  MRI in evaluation of, 28–29, *28f*, *30f*
    CT compared with, 29–31, *29t*, *30f*
  myositis affecting, nonspecific orbital inflammation and, 63–64
  nerves of, 16–18, *17f*
  neuroblastoma involving, 98, *98f*
  optic nerve in, 5
    length of, *5t*
  paranasal sinuses and, 5, *7f*, 18–19, *19f*
  periorbital structures and, 11, 18–19, *19f*. *See also* Periorbita
    disorders causing changes in, 22, *22f*, *23t*
  roof of, 6
    fractures of, 106
  sebaceous carcinoma involving, 184
  septum of, 5, *146f*, 149
    lacerations of, 188
  soft tissues of, 11–18
  surgery of, 115–125. *See also specific procedure*
    decompression, 121–123, *122f*, *123f*. *See also* Orbital decompression
    incisions for, 116–121, *116f*
    for orbital floor/blowout fracture, 111–112
      indications for, 110–111
    orbitotomy, 116–121. *See also* Orbitotomy
    postoperative care and, 124
    special techniques in, 124
    surgical spaces and, 115–116, *115f*, *116f*
  teratoma of, 41
  in thyroid eye disease, 51–60, *52f*, *53f*, *54f*, *57t*
  tight, 113
  topography of, 5–9, *6f*, *7f*, *8f*
  trauma to, 103–114
    foreign bodies, 112
    fractures, 103–112

hemorrhages, 74, 112
midfacial (Le Fort) fractures, 103, 104*f*
orbital fractures, 103–112
vision loss with clear media and, 112–114
tuberculosis affecting, 49, 49*f*
tumors of, 67–101
computed tomography in evaluation of, 27
congenital, 39–41, 39*f*, 41*f*
enucleation for, 128
exenteration for, 136
inspection in evaluation of, 23, 24, 25
lacrimal gland involvement and, 91–94, 92*f*
lymphoproliferative, 85–91
mesenchymal, 82–85, 82*f*, 85*f*
metastatic, 98–101, 98*f*, 99*f*, 100*f*
in adults, 99–101, 99*f*, 100*f*
in children, 98–99, 98*f*
management of, 101
neural, 74–82
palpation in evaluation of, 25
pathologic examination of, 32–33
secondary, 94–98
eyelid carcinoma and, 96–97, 96*f*
vascular (vascular tumors/malformations/ fistulas), 67–74
ultrasonography of, 31
vascular system of, 13–16, 14*f*, 15*f*, 16*f*
venography in evaluation of, 32
volume of, 5*t*
augmentation of, for anophthalmia/ microphthalmia, 36
loss of, in anophthalmic socket, 129
Orbital apex, 5, 6*f*, 10*f*, 13*f*
fracture of, 106
Orbital apex syndrome
in nonspecific orbital inflammation, 64
in zygomycosis, 50
Orbital cellulitis, 46–48, 46*f*, 46*t*, 47*f*
Orbital decompression, 121–123, 122*f*, 123*f*
complications of, 125
for orbital hemorrhage, 112
for thyroid eye disease, 52, 58, 59, 121
for traumatic vision loss, 113
for vision loss after blepharoplasty, 233
Orbital fat, 11, 146*f*, 149
dermatochalasis and, 229
eyelid lacerations and, 149, 187, 188
Orbital fibroblasts, in thyroid eye disease, 55
Orbital fissures, 6*f*, 7, 7*f*, 8*f*, 9, 10*f*
inferior, 6*f*, 7*f*, 8*f*, 9
superior, 6*f*, 7, 7*f*, 9, 10*f*
Orbital implant, 131–132, 131*f*
in children, 129
after evisceration, 130, 131–132
exposure and extrusion of, 130, 131, 133–134, 134*f*
contracted socket and, 134
migration of, 130, 131
for orbital floor/blowout fracture, 111
for superior sulcus deformity, 132
Orbital inflammatory syndrome. *See* Nonspecific orbital inflammation
Orbital orbicularis muscle, 146*f*, 147, 148–149, 148*f*
myectomy for benign essential blepharospasm and, 228
Orbital pseudotumor. *See* Nonspecific orbital inflammation
Orbital varices, 71
Orbital veins, eyelids drained by, 154
Orbitectomy, for lacrimal gland tumors, 93
Orbitomalar ligament, 141
Orbitopathy
in IgG4 disease, 60
thyroid/thyroid-associated/Graves. *See* Thyroid eye disease
Orbitotomy, 116–121
incisions for, 116–121, 116*f*
inferior approach for, 118
lateral approach for, 120–121
medial approach for, 116*f*, 118–120, 120*f*
for specimen collection, 32
in rhabdomyosarcoma, 82
superior approach for, 116–118, 117*f*
Orphenadrine, for benign essential blepharospasm, 228
Osteocutaneous ligaments, 141
Osteoma, orbital, 84
secondary, 97, 97*f*
Osteosarcoma, of orbit, 84
Osteotomy, for dacryocystorhinostomy, 279
Ota, nevus of. *See* Nevus, of Ota

Pagetoid spread, of sebaceous carcinoma, 183, 184
Pain, orbital, 21
in cellulitis, 45, 46
enucleation/evisceration for, 128
in necrotizing fasciitis, 48
in nonspecific orbital inflammation, 64
in orbital floor/blowout fracture, 108
after surgery, 125
in thyroid eye disease, 56
Palatine bone, 7*f*, 8, 8*f*
Palpation, orbital, 25–26
Palpebral artery, 16*f*
Palpebral fissures, 153
in euryblepharon, 157
vertical height of, in ptosis, 210, 210*f*
Palpebral orbicularis muscle, 147
myectomy for benign essential blepharospasm and, 228
Papillomas
eyelid, 166, 166*f*
lacrimal sac, 287
Paralytic ectropion, 198*f*, 224–226, 225*f*
Paralytic lagophthalmos, 226
Paranasal sinuses, 5, 7*f*, 18–19, 19*f*
*Aspergillus* causing infection of, 50–51
nasolacrimal duct obstruction caused by disorders of, 277
orbital cellulitis caused by infection of, 19, 44, 46, 47
orbital tumors originating in, 95–98, 95*f*, 96*f*, 97*f*
osteoma involving, 84
preseptal cellulitis caused by infection of, 44
silent sinus syndrome caused by infection of, 95–96, 96*f*
tuberculous infection of, orbital involvement and, 49
Parasites, orbital infection caused by, 51
Parasympathetic ganglia/nerves/pathway
orbit supplied by, 14*f*, 15*f*, 16, 17*f*
in reflex tear arc, 251

Parinaud syndrome, eyelid retraction in, 223
Parotid gland, 142*f*, 144*f*
Parotideomasseteric fascia, 142*f*, 143
Parotidocutaneous ligament, 141
Pedicle flap, 191
  for canthal repair, 195
Pegged porous orbital implant, 131, 131*f*. *See also* Orbital implant
Penetrating injuries. *See also* Trauma
  canthal soft tissue, 189
  eyelid, 187–189, 188*f*. *See also* Lacerations, eyelid
  preseptal cellulitis caused by, 44
Pentagonal resection, for trichiasis, 208
Pericytes, in hemangiopericytoma, 69
Periocular tissues, malpositions/involutional changes and, 197–247. *See also specific type*
  blepharochalasis, 230
  blepharoplasty and, 230–234, 232*f*
  blepharoptosis (ptosis), 209–222, 210*f*, 211*f*, 213*f*, 214*f*, 216*f*, 218*f*, 219*f*, 220*f*, 221*f*
  brow ptosis, 234–235, 235*f*
  dermatochalasis, 229–230, 229*f*
  ectropion, 197–201, 198*f*, 200*f*
  entropion, 202–207, 203*f*, 204*f*, 205*f*, 206*f*, 207*f*
  eyelid retraction, 222–224, 222*f*
  facial dystonia, 226–229, 227*f*
  facial paralysis, 224–226, 225*f*
  facial rejuvenation and, 235–247
    nonsurgical, 237–240, 239*f*, 240*f*
    surgical, 241–247, 242*f*, 243*f*, 244*f*, 245*f*, 246*f*
  history/examination in evaluation of, 197
    aging face and, 236–237
  pathogenesis of aging face and, 236
  symblepharon, 208
  trichiasis, 208–209
Periorbita (periorbital structures), 11, 18–19, 19*f*. *See also specific structure*
  cellulitis affecting, 44–48, 46*f*, 46*t*, 47*f*. *See also* Orbital cellulitis; Preseptal cellulitis
  ecchymosis of, 22, 22*f*
    in neuroblastoma, 98, 98*f*
    in orbital floor/blowout fracture, 108
    in orbital roof fracture, 106
  innervation of, 16, 16*f*
  involutional changes in, 229–230, 229*f*
  orbital diseases causing changes in, 22, 22*f*, 23*t*
Peripheral arterial arcade, eyelids supplied by, 16*f*, 146*f*, 154
Peripheral surgical space (extraconal fat/surgical space), 11, 115, 115*f*
Phleboliths, orbital varices and, 71
Photophobia, in thyroid eye disease, 56, 58
Phycomycetes infection (phycomycosis/mucormycosis/zygomycosis), orbit involved in, 50
  exenteration in management of, 50, 136
Pigmentations/pigment deposits, after laser skin resurfacing, 238
Pilar (trichilemmal) cyst, 168
Pilocytic astrocytoma. *See* Optic nerve (optic pathway/chiasm) glioma
Pilomatricoma (pilomatrixoma), 172, 173*f*
Plasma cell–rich pseudotumors, 89
Plasma cell tumors, of orbit, 89–90
Plasmacytoma, of orbit, 89
Platysma muscle, 141, 142*f*
Platysmaplasty, 246–247, 246*f*
Pleomorphic adenoma (benign mixed tumor)
  of eyelid, 170
  of lacrimal gland, 91, 92–93, 92*f*
Pleomorphic rhabdomyosarcoma, 83
Plexiform neurofibromas, 77, 77*f*, 78, 78*f*
  eyelid involvement/ptosis and, 77*f*, 78, 78*f*
  of orbit, 77, 77*f*, 78, 78*f*
Plus (convex) lenses, anophthalmic socket camouflage and, 136
Polyangiitis, with granulomatosis (GPA/Wegener granulomatosis), 61–62, 62*f*
  screening/diagnostic tests for, 33–34
Polyarteritis nodosa, 62–63
Polyethylene orbital implant, 131, 131*f*. *See also* Orbital implant
  exposure of, 134*f*
Polymerase chain reaction, 124
  in orbital lymphoma, 88
Pork tapeworm *(Taenia solium)*, orbital infection caused by, 51
Porous polyethylene orbital implant, 131, 131*f*. *See also* Orbital implant
Posterior ciliary arteries, 14*f*, 15*f*
Posterior lamellar deficiency, surgery for eyelid retraction and, 224
Posterior superior alveolar nerve, 17*f*
Postoperative care of ophthalmic surgery patient, orbital surgery and, 124
Postseptal venous drainage system, 154
Posttraumatic cellulitis
  orbital, 47
  preseptal, 44, 45
Precancerous eyelid lesions
  epidermal, 175–176, 176*f*
  melanocytic, 177
Precancerous melanosis (lentigo maligna/Hutchinson melanotic freckle), 177
Precorneal tear film, 252. *See also* Tear film (tears)
Prednisone
  for nonspecific orbital inflammation, 65
  for thyroid eye disease, 58
Pregnancy, cavernous hemangioma growth during, 68
Premalignant eyelid lesions
  epidermal, 175–176, 176*f*
  melanocytic, 177
Preoperative assessment/preparation for surgery
  blepharoplasty, 231
  facial rejuvenation surgery, 236, 241, 245
  lower face and neck rejuvenation, 245
Preorbital orbicularis muscle, 146*f*, 147, 148–149, 148*f*
Preperiosteal approach, for midface lift, 242–243, 243*f*
Preseptal cellulitis, 44, 44–46
Preseptal orbicularis muscle, 146*f*, 147, 148, 148*f*
  in involutional entropion, 203, 204
Preseptal tissues, 147
Preseptal venous drainage system, 154
Pretarsal orbicularis muscle, 14*f*, 146*f*, 147, 147–148, 148*f*
  gray line and, 149, 153, 154*f*

Pretarsal tissues, 147
Pretibial myxedema, thyroid eye disease and, 56
Pretrichial incision, for brow- and forehead-lift, 241, 243*f*
Primary anophthalmia, 35
Primary dye test (Jones I test), 269
Prisms, anophthalmic socket camouflage and, 136
Probing of lacrimal system
  for acquired nasolacrimal duct/canalicular obstruction, 271–272, 273
  for canalicular trauma, 283
  for congenital dacryocystocele, 265
  for congenital nasolacrimal duct obstruction, 260, 261–262, 261*f*, 262*f*, 263*f*
Procerus muscle, 16, 141, 143*f*, 148*f*
Propranolol, for infantile (capillary) hemangioma, 68, 161
Proptosis (exophthalmos/exorbitism), 23, 24, 25*f*
  in carotid-cavernous fistulas, 73
  in cavernous hemangioma, 68, 69*f*
  in craniosynostosis, 37
  dermoid cyst causing, 40
  in lymphatic malformation–associated hemorrhage, 70, 70*f*, 71
  in meningioma, 79, 79*f*, 81
  in neurofibromatosis, 78
  in nonspecific orbital inflammation, 64
  in optic nerve glioma, 74, 75*f*
  orbital mass causing, 24, 95
  orbital varices and, 71
  in orbital zygomycosis, 50
  in rhabdomyosarcoma, 82
  in teratoma, 41
  in thyroid eye disease, 24, 52, 52*f*, 54
Prostaglandin $E_2$, thyroid eye disease and, 55
Prostate cancer, eye/orbital metastases and, 101
Prostheses, ocular, 36, 132
  anophthalmic ectropion and, 135, 137
Proton density, 28
Protractors, eyelid, 147–149, 148*f*
  spasms of (benign essential blepharospasm), 226–227, 227*f*
Pseudoepiphora, evaluation of, 267–268
Pseudoepitheliomatous hyperplasia, 167
Pseudoproptosis, 24–25
Pseudoptosis, 218, 218*f*
Pseudostrabismus, in epicanthus, 158
Pseudotumor
  orbital. *See* Nonspecific orbital inflammation
  plasma cell–rich, 89
Pterygoid venous plexus, eyelids drained by, 154
Pterygopalatine fossa, 7*f*
Ptosis (blepharoptosis), 209–222
  acquired, 209, 214*t*
    aponeurotic, 214, 214*f*, 214*t*
    eyelid position in downgaze and, 211, 214*t*
    mechanical, 218
    myogenic, 213
    neurogenic, 215–216
  ancillary tests in evaluation of, 212
  anophthalmic, 135
  aponeurotic, 214, 214*f*, 214*t*
  apparent (pseudoptosis), 218, 218*f*
  in blepharochalasis, 230
  in blepharophimosis–ptosis–epicanthus inversus syndrome, 155, 212
  botulinum toxin causing, 216
  classification of, 213–218
  congenital, 209, 214*t*
    amblyopia in, 211–212
    eyelid position in downgaze and, 211, 214*t*
    mechanical, 217–218
    myogenic, 213, 213*f*, 214*t*
    neurogenic, 215, 216*f*
  as cosmetic vs functional issue, 212, 218–219
  in dermatochalasis, 229, 229*f*
  downgaze exacerbating, 209
  enucleation/evisceration and, 130
  evaluation of, 209
  eyelid position in downgaze and, 211, 214*t*
  in Horner syndrome, 212
    pharmacologic testing for, 212
  Marcus Gunn jaw-winking, 211, 215, 216*f*
  mechanical, 217–218
  in monocular elevation deficiency (double-elevator palsy), 213
  in myasthenia gravis, 209, 216–217
    edrophonium chloride test and, 217
  myogenic, 213–214, 213*f*, 214*t*
  neurogenic, 215–217, 216*f*
  in orbital floor/blowout fracture, 109
  pharmacologic testing in, 212
  physical examination of patient with, 209–212, 210*f*, 211*f*
  reverse, lower eyelid, 212, 215
  in rhabdomyosarcoma, 82
  synkinesis in, 211
  traumatic, 190, 218
    amblyopia and, 190
  treatment of, 218–222, 219*f*, 220*f*, 221*f*
    anophthalmic socket and, 135
    complications of, 222
  visual field testing in, 212
Ptosis, brow, 234–235, 235*f*
  dermatochalasis and, 229, 234, 235
Ptosis repair, 218–222, 219*f*, 220*f*, 221*f*. *See also specific procedure*
  in blepharophimosis–ptosis–epicanthus inversus syndrome, 155
  complications of, 222
  cosmetic vs functional, 212, 218–219
Pulsation, orbital, 26
Punch (incisional) biopsy, 179*f*, 180
Puncta. *See* Punctum
Punctal occlusion/plugs, for dry eye, 281–282
  canalicular obstruction and, 274, 282
  extrusion/migration of, 282
  nasolacrimal duct obstruction and, 278, 282
Punctoplasty, 272, 273
Punctum (puncta), 252–253, 253*f*, 254*f*
  agenesis/dysgenesis of, 259–260
  aplasia/hypoplasia of, 258
  disorders of, 272–273
  duplication of, 257
  large, 273
  malposition of, 273

stenosis and occlusion of, 258, 272, 273
surgical closure of, 282
Pupillary defects
afferent
in meningioma, 81
in optic nerve glioma, 74
in traumatic optic neuropathy, 113
in ptosis, 212
Pupils, examination of, in ptosis, 212
Pyoceles
in dacryocystitis, 286
orbital invasion by, 95

Quadripod (zygomaticomaxillary complex) fractures, 103–105, 105*f*
Quickert sutures, for involutional/spastic entropion, 203, 203*f*, 206

Race
dermal melanocytosis (nevus of Ota) and, 175
eyelid crease/fold and, 147, 147*f*
sarcoidosis and, 63
Radiation therapy
for basal cell carcinoma of eyelid, 181
contracted socket and, 134
for infantile (capillary) hemangioma, 68
for lacrimal gland tumors, 93
for lacrimal sac tumors, 287
for optic nerve glioma, 77
for optic nerve sheath meningioma, 81
for orbital lymphoma, 89
for rhabdomyosarcoma, 83, 84
for thyroid eye disease, 59
Radioactive iodine (RAI)
for block and replace therapy in thyroid eye disease, 58
nasolacrimal duct obstruction and, 278
Radiofrequency ablation, for trichiasis, 208
RAI. *See* Radioactive iodine
Reactive lymphoid hyperplasia, of orbit, 86–88, 88
REAL (Revised European American Lymphoma) classification, 85, 86
Reconstructive surgery
for canalicular obstruction, 275
eyelid, 191–196, 193*f*, 194*f*. *See also* Eyelids, surgery/reconstruction of
after basal cell carcinoma surgery, 180, 181
for blepharophimosis–ptosis–epicanthus inversus syndrome, 155
for coloboma, 161
for epicanthus, 159
for euryblepharon, 157–158
for eyelid defects involving eyelid margin, 188–189, 188*f*, 192–195, 193*f*, 194*f*
for eyelid defects not involving eyelid margin, 187–188, 191–192
lateral canthal defects and, 195
for lower eyelid defects, 192–195, 194*f*
medial canthal defects and, 195–196
after Mohs micrographic surgery, 181
principles of, 191
priorities in, 191
secondary repair after trauma and, 189–190
for upper eyelid defects, 192, 193*f*
socket, 134, 136. *See also* Anophthalmic socket
Rectus muscles, 11, 12*f*, 13*f*, 14*f*, 15*f*, 146*f*. *See also specific muscle*
entrapment of, in orbital floor/blowout fracture, 108, 109–110
innervation of, 12, 14*f*, 15*f*
surgery of
eyelid position changes after, 222, 223
for orbital floor/blowout fracture, 110, 111
in thyroid eye disease, 25, 54
Reflex blepharospasm, 227
Reflex tear arc, 251, 252*f*
Refractive errors, in ptosis, 211–212
Rejuvenation surgery, facial, 241–247, 242*f*, 243*f*, 244*f*, 245*f*, 246*f*. *See also specific procedure*
Relaxation times, in MRI, 28
Retinal artery occlusion, central (CRAO), hyaluronic filler injection causing, 239, 240*f*
Retinoblastoma
enucleation for, 128
exenteration for, 136
malignant mesenchymal tumors in children with, 84
Retinociliary venous collaterals (optociliary shunt vessels), 22, 22*f*
Retraction, eyelid, 222–224, 222*f*
after blepharoplasty, 223, 234
in Parinaud syndrome, 223
in thyroid eye disease, 52, 52*f*, 54, 56, 59, 222–223, 223, 224
treatment of, 223–224
Retractors, eyelid, 149–151, 150*f*
lower eyelid, 146*f*, 151
in involutional ectropion, repair of, 200–201
in involutional entropion, 202–203
repair of, 204, 205*f*
upper eyelid, 149–151, 150*f*
Retrobulbar hemorrhage, after blepharoplasty, vision loss and, 233
Retro-orbicularis oculi fat (ROOF), 146*f*, 152, 153
Revised European American Lymphoma (REAL) classification, 85, 86
Rhabdomyosarcoma, of orbit, 82–84, 82*f*
*Rhizopus*/*Rhizopus* infection, orbital, 50
Rhytidectomy, 245–246, 245*f*
Ring sign, in nonspecific orbital inflammation, 64
Riolan, muscle of, 149, 153, 154*f*
Risorius muscle, 141, 143*f*
Rituximab, for thyroid eye disease, 58
ROOF (retro-orbicularis oculi fat), 146*f*, 152, 153
Rosenmüller, valve of, 253, 254*f*
Rosenthal fibers, in optic nerve gliomas, 76
Rotation/rotational flap, for eyelid repair, 191, 192

Salmon patches, in orbital lymphoma, 86, 87*f*
Sarcoidosis, 63
screening/diagnostic tests for, 34, 63
Sarcoma
granulocytic (chloroma), 98–99
orbital, 84
exenteration for, 136
secondary, 97
Schirmer tests, in pseudoepiphora, 268
Schwann cells, in neurofibroma, 77
Schwannoma (neurilemoma), 82

Sclera, nonspecific orbital inflammation involving, 64
Scleral graft
for cicatricial entropion, 207
for exposure and extrusion of orbital implant, 133
Scleral shells, for cosmesis/pain, 128
Scleritis
in granulomatosis with polyangiitis (Wegener granulomatosis), 61
nonspecific orbital inflammation and, 64
Sclerosing agents, for lymphatic malformation, 71
Sclerosing nonspecific orbital inflammation, 65, 66
Screening/diagnostic tests
of lacrimal drainage function, 269–272, 269*f*, 270*f*, 271*f*
in orbital disorders, 33–34
for thyroid eye disease, 33, 57*t*
Sebaceous adenomas, 170
Sebaceous carcinoma/adenocarcinoma, 183–184, 183*f*
Sebaceous cysts (epidermal inclusion cysts), of eyelid, 168, 168*f*
Sebaceous glands of eyelid, 170
tumors/lesions of
benign, 170
malignant, 183–184, 183*f*
Sebaceous hyperplasia, 170
Seborrheic keratosis, 167, 167*f*
Sebum, in chalazion formation, 162
Secondary anophthalmia, 35
Secretory lacrimal apparatus, 251–252, 252*f*. *See also* Lacrimal gland
anatomy of, 251–252, 252*f*
development of, 255
abnormalities of, 257
disorders of, 257–287
Sedatives, for benign essential blepharospasm, 228
Semicircular flap
for canthal repair, 195
for eyelid repair, 161, 192, 193*f*, 194*f*, 195
Senile lentigo, 174
Sentinel lymph node (SLN) biopsy
in eyelid melanoma, 185
in sebaceous adenocarcinoma, 184
Seventh nerve (facial) palsy/paralysis. *See* Facial paralysis/weakness
Shave biopsy, 179*f*
Short ciliary nerves, 12*f*, 14*f*, 15*f*, 16, 17*f*
Silent sinus syndrome, 95–96, 96*f*
Silicone plugs, for dry eye, 281–282. *See also* Lacrimal plugs
Silicone rods, for frontalis suspension, 221
Silicone stent, for nasolacrimal intubation, 262, 263. *See also* Lacrimal intubation
Silicone suspension sling, for paralytic ectropion, 226
Simple lentigines (lentigo simplex), 174
Single-fiber electromyography, in myasthenia gravis, 217
Sinus surgery, in orbital cellulitis, 48
Sinus thrombosis, cavernous, orbital infection/cellulitis and, 48
Sinuses
ethmoid, 8, 8*f*, 18, 19, 19*f*
frontal, 7*f*, 18, 18–19, 19*f*
maxillary, 7*f*, 9, 18, 19, 19*f*
osteoma involving, 84
paranasal, 5, 7*f*, 18–19, 19*f*
*Aspergillus* causing infection of, 50–51
nasolacrimal duct obstruction caused by disorders of, 277
orbital cellulitis caused by infection of, 19, 44, 46, 47
orbital tumors originating in, 95–98, 95*f*, 96*f*, 97*f*
preseptal cellulitis caused by infection of, 44
silent sinus syndrome caused by infection of, 95–96, 96*f*
tuberculous infection of, orbital involvement and, 49
sphenoid, 7*f*, 8, 8*f*, 18, 19, 19*f*
Sinusitis
allergic aspergillosis, 51
orbital cellulitis caused by, 19, 44, 46, 47
orbital tumors/inflammation and, 95, 95*f*
preseptal cellulitis caused by, 44
silent sinus syndrome and, 95–96, 96*f*
tuberculous, orbital infection and, 49
Sjögren syndrome, lacrimal lymphoepithelial lesions in, 94
Skin
disorders of, in xanthogranuloma, 91
eyelid, 146–147, 146*f*
excessive removal of, in blepharoplasty, 234
redundancy of. *See* Dermatochalasis
tumors of. *See also* Eyelids, tumors of
medial canthal/lacrimal drainage involvement and, 180
facial, aging affecting, 236–237
laser resurfacing of, 237–238
Skin cancer, eyelid involvement and, 165
melanoma, 184–186, 185*f*
Skin grafts. *See* Flaps; Grafts
Skin-muscle flap, for eyelid repair, 192
Skin tag (acrochordon), 166, 166*f*
SLN biopsy. *See* Sentinel lymph node biopsy
SMAS. *See* Superficial musculoaponeurotic system
Smoking
basal cell carcinoma and, 177
thyroid disease and, 52, 56, 58
Snapback test, 199, 203
Socket contraction, 134–135, 135*f*. *See also* Anophthalmic socket
Socket expansion, for anophthalmia/microphthalmia, 36
Sodium morrhuate, for lymphatic malformation, 71
Soft tissue dermal fillers, in facial rejuvenation, 239–240, 239*f*, 240*f*
Soft-tissue histiocytosis, diffuse, 90
Solar lentigo, 174
Solitary fibrous tumor, of orbit, 84
SOOF (suborbicularis oculi fat), 146*f*, 152–153
SOOF (suborbicularis oculi fat) lift, 242, 243*f*
Spasm
essential blepharospasm/benign essential blepharospasm (BEB), 226–228, 227*f*
hemifacial (HFS), 228–229
Spastic/acute spastic entropion, 203, 204*f*
Spectacle lenses/frames, anophthalmic socket camouflage and, 136
Sphenoethmoidal recess, 18

Sphenoid bone, 6, 6*f*, 7, 7*f*, 8, 8*f*
in metastatic disease, 99, 99*f*
Sphenoid sinuses, 7*f*, 8, 8*f*, 18, 19, 19*f*
Sphenoid wings, 6, 6*f*, 7, 7*f*, 8, 8*f*
meningiomas of, 79, 79*f*, 81
Sphenopalatine ganglion, 14*f*, 15*f*
Spindle procedure, medial, for involutional ectropion, 199, 200*f*
Spiral (helical) computed tomography, in orbital evaluation, 27
Squamous cell carcinoma
of eyelid, 182, 182*f*
actinic keratosis and, 176, 182
in situ (Bowen disease), 176
keratoacanthoma, 176–177, 177*f*
of lacrimal sac, 287
of orbit, secondary, 96–97, 96*f*
Squamous cell papilloma
of eyelid (acrochordon/skin tag), 166, 166*f*
of lacrimal sac, 287
Stab incisions (adits), for neck liposuction, 246
Stallard-Wright incision, for orbitotomy, 116*f*, 120–121
*Staphylococcus aureus*
chalazion caused by, 162
methicillin-resistant (MRSA)
dacryoadenitis caused by, 284
preseptal cellulitis caused by, 45
Stent placement. *See also* Lacrimal intubation
for canalicular obstruction, 274, 275
for canalicular trauma, 283
for nasolacrimal duct obstruction, 262–263, 264*f*, 278
for punctal occlusion/stenosis, 272
Steroids. *See* Corticosteroids
Strabismus
in infantile (capillary) hemangioma, 68, 161
in orbital floor/blowout fracture, 109, 111
in rhabdomyosarcoma, 82
in thyroid eye disease, 54
Strabismus surgery, thyroid eye disease and, 52, 58
*Streptococcus*, group A β-hemolytic, orbital necrotizing fasciitis caused by, 48
Stye (external hordeolum), 163–164
Subarachnoid surgical space, 115*f*, 116
Subciliary incision, for orbitotomy, 116*f*
Subcutaneous fat/tissue, eyelid, 146–147, 146*f*
Subcutaneous (vintage) rhytidectomy, 245
Suborbicularis fat pads (suborbicularis oculi fat/SOOF), 146*f*, 152–153
midface rejuvenation surgery (SOOF lift) and, 242, 243*f*
Subperiorbital (subperiosteal) surgical space, 115, 115*f*
Subperiosteal abscess, 47, 47*f*
Subperiosteal approach, for midface lift, 243, 244*f*
Sub-Tenon (episcleral) surgical space, 115, 115*f*
Sunlight. *See* Ultraviolet light
Superficial basal cell carcinoma, 179. *See also* Basal cell carcinoma
Superficial cervical fascia, 143
Superficial facial fascia, 141
Superficial mimetic muscles, 141
Superficial musculoaponeurotic system (SMAS), 141, 142*f*
cosmetic surgery and, 141, 142*f*, 245
elevation/refixation of, in rhytidectomy, 245, 245*f*
Superficial spreading melanoma, 185
Superficial temporal fascia (temporoparietal fascia), 141, 142*f*, 144
Superior displacement of globe, in orbital disorders, 24
Superior meatus, 19
Superior oblique muscle, 11, 12*f*, 13*f*, 14*f*, 15*f*, 146*f*
innervation of, 12
Superior oblique tendon, 14*f*, 15*f*
fossa for trochlea of, 6
Superior ophthalmic vein, 10*f*, 12*f*, 13–14, 14*f*, 15*f*
Superior orbital fissure, 6*f*, 7, 7*f*, 9, 10*f*
Superior rectus muscle, 11, 13*f*, 14*f*, 15*f*, 146*f*
innervation of, 12
Superior sulcus deformity, anophthalmic socket and, 132–133, 133*f*
Superior tarsal muscle of Müller, 146*f*, 149, 151
in Horner syndrome, 215
internal (transconjunctival) resection of, for ptosis correction, 220, 220*f*
anophthalmic socket and, 135
Superior transverse (Whitnall) ligament, 7, 14*f*, 15*f*, 146*f*, 150, 150*f*, 251
Superior turbinate/concha, 18
Supraorbital artery, 14*f*, 15*f*, 16*f*
eyelids supplied by, 154
Supraorbital ethmoids, 19
Supraorbital foramen/notch, 6, 6*f*
Supraorbital nerve, 14*f*, 15*f*, 142*f*, 145*f*
Supratrochlear artery, 16*f*
Supratrochlear nerve, 14*f*, 15*f*, 142*f*, 145*f*
Surgical spaces, orbital, 115–116, 115*f*, 116*f*
Suspensory ligament of Lockwood (Lockwood ligament), 7, 150, 151
Sutures (surgical), Quickert, for involutional/spastic entropion, 203, 203*f*, 206
Sweat glands, of eyelid, 170
tumors originating in, 170, 171, 171*f*
Switch flap, for eyelid repair, 193*f*
Symblepharon, 208
Sympathetic nerves/pathway, orbit supplied by, 16–18, 17*f*
Sympathetic ophthalmia
enucleation in prevention of, 128
evisceration and, 130
incidence of, 128
Syndactyly, in Apert syndrome, 38*f*
Syndromic congenital craniofacial anomalies, 35–38, 37*f*, 38*f*. *See also specific type and* Craniofacial malformations
Syndromic craniosynostosis, 37–38, 38*f*
Synkinesis
aberrant nerve regeneration and, 211, 229
in Marcus Gunn jaw-winking syndrome/ptosis, 211, 215, 216*f*
Syringoma, 170, 171*f*

T1 (longitudinal relaxation time), 28
T1-weighted images, 28–29, 28*f*
T2 (transverse relaxation time), 28
T2-weighted images, 28–29
$T_4$. *See* Thyroxine
T-cell lymphomas, orbital, 86
*Taenia solium* (pork tapeworm), orbital infection caused by, 51
Tapeworms, orbital infection caused by, 51

Tarsal ectropion, 200
Tarsal fracture operation, for cicatricial entropion, 207, 207*f*
Tarsal kink, 159
Tarsal muscles
inferior, 151
superior (Müller), 146*f*, 149, 151
in Horner syndrome, 215
internal (transconjunctival) resection of, for ptosis correction, 220, 220*f*
anophthalmic socket and, 135
Tarsal plates/tarsus, 146*f*, 151–152, 152*f*
sebaceous adenocarcinoma arising in, 183, 184
Tarsal-sharing procedures, for eyelid repair, 192
Tarsal strip procedure
for cicatricial ectropion, 201
for involutional ectropion, 199, 200*f*
for involutional entropion, 204
Tarsoconjunctival flap, for eyelid repair, 193, 193*f*, 194, 194*f*
Tarsoconjunctival grafts
for cicatricial entropion, 207
for eyelid repair, 190, 192, 192–193, 193*f*, 194*f*, 195
Tarsorrhaphy
for eyelid burns, 190
for eyelid retraction, 223
for paralytic ectropion, 225–226, 225*f*
Tarsus. *See* Tarsal plates/tarsus
Tear breakup time, in pseudoepiphora evaluation, 267–268
Tear film (tears), 255, 256*f*
composition of, 252
evaluation of, in ptosis, 211
hypersecretion of (lacrimation), 267. *See also* Tearing
precorneal, 252
Tear function tests, 269–272, 269*f*, 270*f*, 271*f*. *See also specific test*
Tear meniscus, in pseudoepiphora evaluation, 267
Tear sac. *See* Lacrimal sac
Tear secretion, basal, testing, 268
Tearing/epiphora, 267. *See also specific cause and* Lacrimal drainage system, obstruction of
acquired, 267–281
evaluation of, 267–272, 269*f*, 270*f*, 271*f*
congenital, 259–267
evaluation of, 259
diagnostic tests for evaluation of, 269–272, 269*f*, 270*f*, 271*f*
examination in patient with, 267–268
history in patient with, 259, 267
lacrimal outflow evaluation in patient with, 268–269
in nasolacrimal duct obstruction
acquired, 276–281, 277*f*, 280*f*, 281*f*
congenital, 260–265, 261*f*, 262*f*, 263*f*, 264*f*
pseudoepiphora evaluation and, 267–268
punctal disorders causing, 272–273
weakened blink and, 255
Tears (artificial), for paralytic ectropion, 224–225
TED. *See* Thyroid eye disease
Telecanthus, 23
in blepharophimosis–ptosis–epicanthus inversus syndrome, 155
Telorbitism (hypertelorism), 23
in craniosynostosis, 37
with midline clefts, 37
Temporal arteritis (giant cell/GCA arteritis), 61
Temporal artery, 16*f*
eyelids supplied by, 154
Temporal artery biopsy, in giant cell arteritis, 61
Temporal fascia
deep, 141, 142*f*, 144
superficial (temporoparietal fascia), 141, 142*f*, 144
Temporal fat pad, 142*f*
Temporal flare, in thyroid-related eyelid retraction, 223
Temporal (frontal) nerve, 10*f*, 13*f*, 14*f*, 15*f*, 16, 17*f*, 142*f*, 143, 144, 144*f*
Temporal orbital fat pad, 149
Temporal veins, eyelids drained by, 154
Temporalis muscle, 142*f*, 143, 143*f*
Temporoparietal fascia (superficial temporal fascia), 141, 142*f*, 144
Tensor fascia lata, autogenous and banked, for frontalis suspension, 221
Tenzel semicircular rotation flap/modified Tenzel flap, for eyelid repair, 192, 195
Teratomas, orbital, 41
Thermal cautery, for punctal occlusion, 282
Third nerve (oculomotor) palsy, ptosis in, 215, 215–216
Three-dimensional computed tomography, in orbital evaluation, 27, 27*f*
Thrombocytopenia, hemangiomas and (Kasabach-Merritt syndrome), 67–68
Thymoma, in myasthenia gravis, 216–217
Thyroid-associated ophthalmopathy/orbitopathy. *See* Thyroid eye disease
Thyroid-binding inhibitory immunoglobulins, in thyroid eye disease, 53
Thyroid disease
screening/testing for, 33, 57*t*
smoking and, 52, 56, 58
thyroiditis, 52, 53, 56
Thyroid eye disease (TED), 51–60, 52*f*, 53*f*, 54*f*, 57*t*
antithyroid antibodies and, 53
clinical presentation and diagnosis of, 52, 52*f*, 53–54, 53*f*, 54*f*, 56, 57*t*
epidemiology of, 55–56
eye movements/extraocular myopathy and, 25, 52, 54, 54*f*, 56
eyelid abnormalities and, 25, 52, 52*f*, 54, 56
management and, 59
retraction, 52, 52*f*, 54, 56, 59, 222–223, 223, 224
myasthenia gravis and, 56
optic neuropathy in, 52, 54, 56, 59
pathogenesis of, 55
prognosis of, 56–60
proptosis and, 24, 52, 52*f*, 54
radioactive iodine treatment affecting, 58
smoking and, 52, 56, 58
thyroid function tests in, 33, 57*t*
treatment of, 56–60, 57*t*
von Graefe sign in, 25, 52
Thyroid function tests, 33, 57*t*
Thyroid orbitopathy/ophthalmopathy. *See* Thyroid eye disease
Thyroid-stimulating hormone (TSH). *See* Thyrotropin

Thyroid-stimulating immunoglobulins (TSIs), in thyroid eye disease, 33, 53
Thyroiditis, Hashimoto, thyroid eye disease and, 52, 53, 56
Thyrotoxic exophthalmos. *See* Thyroid eye disease
Thyrotropin (thyroid-stimulating hormone/TSH)
  receptor for
    antibodies to, in thyroid eye disease, 33, 53
    in thyroid eye disease, 33, 53
      radioactive iodine treatment and, 58
  serum levels of, 33
Thyroxine ($T_4$)
  for block and replace therapy in thyroid eye disease, 58
  serum levels of, 33
Tight orbit, 113
Timolol, for infantile (capillary) hemangioma, 68, 161
Tissue expanders, intraorbital, in congenital anophthalmia/microphthalmia management, 36
Tomography, computed. *See* Computed tomography
Topography, orbital, 5–9, 6*f*, 7*f*, 8*f*
Traction test (forced duction test), in orbital floor/blowout fracture, 109
  surgery and, 110
Tram-tracking/tram-track sign, in optic nerve sheath meningioma, 80*f*, 81
Transcaruncular incision
  for orbital decompression, 122
  for orbitotomy, 116*f*, 120
Transconjunctival incision
  for lower blepharoplasty, 232
  for orbital decompression, 122, 122*f*
  for orbitotomy
    inferior approach, 116*f*, 118, 119*f*
    medial approach, 116*f*, 119–120, 120*f*
    superior approach, 117
  for ptosis repair, 220, 220*f*
Transcranial orbitotomy, coronal incision for, 117
Transcutaneous incision
  for levator advancement, in ptosis correction, 219, 219*f*
  for orbital decompression, 121
  for orbitotomy
    inferior approach, 118
    medial approach, 116*f*, 119
    superior approach, 116–117, 117*f*
Transnasal endoscopy
  for lacrimal drainage evaluation/obstruction, 272
  for orbital decompression, 122
Transposition flaps
  for canthal repair, 195
  for eyelid repair, 191
Transverse ligament, superior (Whitnall), 7, 14*f*, 15*f*, 146*f*, 150*f*, 251
Transverse relaxation time (T2), 28
Trapdoor fracture, 109–110, 110*f*
Trauma
  canalicular, 282–283
    obstruction caused by, 274
  canthal soft tissue, 189
  cellulitis caused by
    orbital, 47
    preseptal, 44, 45
  eyelid, 187–190, 188*f*. *See also* Eyelids, trauma to
  lacrimal system, 282–284
  nasolacrimal duct obstruction caused by, 278
  optic canal fracture caused by, 10
  optic neuropathy caused by, 113
  orbital, 103–114. *See also* Orbit, trauma to
  ptosis caused by, 190, 218
    amblyopia and, 190
  sympathetic ophthalmia and, enucleation in prevention of, 128
Traumatic optic neuropathy, 113
Traumatic vision loss with clear media, 112–114
Treacher Collins–Franceschetti syndrome (mandibulofacial dysostosis), 37, 37*f*
Trichiasis, 208–209
  in cicatricial entropion, 208
  in involutional entropion, 203
Trichilemmal (pilar) cyst, 168
Trichilemmomas, 172
*Trichinella spiralis* (trichinosis), orbital infection caused by, 51
Trichoepithelioma, 172, 172*f*
Trichofolliculoma, 172
Trichotillomania, 165
Trigeminal ganglion, 16, 17*f*
Trigeminal nerve. *See* Cranial nerve V
Trochlea, 14*f*, 15*f*
Trochlear nerve. *See* Cranial nerve IV
TSH (thyroid-stimulating hormone). *See* Thyrotropin
TSH-R. *See* Thyrotropin (thyroid-stimulating hormone/TSH), receptor for
TSIs. *See* Thyroid-stimulating immunoglobulins
Tuberculosis, ocular involvement in
  dacryoadenitis, 284
  orbital, 49, 49*f*
Tumors. *See also specific type and structure or organ affected and* Intraocular tumors
  canalicular obstruction and, 274
  nasolacrimal duct obstruction and, 278
Turban tumors, 171
Turbinates (conchae), nasal, 18, 253*f*, 254*f*
  infracture of, for congenital nasolacrimal duct obstruction, 265
Turkey gobbler defect, 236

Ulcerative basal cell carcinoma, 178*f*. *See also* Basal cell carcinoma
ULE. *See* Upper eyelid excursion
Ultrasonography/ultrasound (echography), in orbital evaluation, 31
Ultraviolet light (ultraviolet radiation), eye disorders/injury associated with
  actinic keratosis, 176
  basal cell carcinoma, 177
  eyelid tumors, 177, 182
  lentigines, 174
  melanoma, 184
Unifocal eosinophilic granuloma of bone, 90
Upgaze, disorders/limitation of
  monocular deficiency (double-elevator palsy) and, 213
  in orbital floor/blowout fracture, 108
    surgery and, 110
Upper eyelid. *See* Eyelids, upper
Upper eyelid excursion (ULE), in ptosis, 210, 211*f*

Valve of Hasner, 253*f*, 254*f*
nasolacrimal duct obstruction and, 255, 260
Valve of Rosenmüller, 253, 254*f*
Varices, orbital, 71
Vascular malformations, orbital, 67–74
Vascular system
of eyelids, 154
of orbit, 13–16, 14*f*, 15*f*, 16*f*
Vascular tumors, of orbit, 67–74
Vasculitis. *See also specific type and* Arteritis
orbital manifestations of, 43*t*, 60–63, 62*f*
Venography, in orbital evaluation, 32
Venous malformations (varices), orbital, 71
Verruca vulgaris (wart), of eyelid, 167, 167*f*
Vertical deviations, orbital floor/blowout fracture and, 108–109
surgery and, 110
Vertical diplopia, in orbital floor/blowout fracture, 108
surgery and, 110
Vertical eyelid splitting, for orbitotomy, 116*f*, 117–118
Vertical palpebral fissure height, in ptosis, 210, 210*f*
Vertical rectus muscles, surgery of, eyelid position changes after, 222, 223
Vidian nerve, 14*f*, 15*f*
VISA classification, for thyroid eye disease, 57
Vision loss/impairment
after blepharoplasty, 233–234
in meningioma, 81
in optic nerve glioma, 74
in orbital floor/blowout fracture, 109
after orbital surgery, 125
in ptosis, 209, 210, 211–212, 212, 214, 218–219
in thyroid eye disease, 56, 59–60
traumatic, with clear media, 112–114
in xanthogranuloma, 91
Vismodegib, for orbital infiltrative basal cell carcinoma, 181
Visual acuity
postoperative, 124
in ptosis, 209, 211–212
Visual field defects, in ptosis, 209, 212, 214
Visual field testing, in ptosis, 212
von Graefe sign, 25, 52
von Recklinghausen disease. *See* Neurofibromatosis 1
Vortex veins, 14*f*, 15*f*

Wart (verruca vulgaris), of eyelid, 167, 167*f*
Watchful waiting. *See* Observation
Wegener granulomatosis (granulomatosis with polyangiitis/GPA), 61–62, 62*f*
screening/diagnostic tests for, 33–34
White-eyed blowout fracture, 108
Whitnall ligament (superior transverse ligament), 7, 14*f*, 15*f*, 146*f*, 150, 150*f*, 251
Whitnall tubercle, 6*f*, 7, 7*f*
Wolfring, glands of, 146*f*, 152, 252
Worm's-eye view position, 24, 25*f*

Xanthelasma, of eyelid, 169, 169*f*
Xanthogranuloma, of orbit, 90–91
Xeroderma pigmentosum, 178

Y-V-plasties
for blepharophimosis–ptosis–epicanthus inversus syndrome, 155
for epicanthus, 159

Z-plasties
for blepharophimosis–ptosis–epicanthus inversus syndrome, 155
for epicanthus, 159
for eyelid repair, 190
for symblepharon, 208
Zeis, glands of, 170
hordeolum caused by infection of, 163
sebaceous adenocarcinoma arising in, 183
Zinn, annulus of, 11, 12–13, 13*f*, 14*f*, 15*f*, 16
ZMC fractures. *See* Zygomaticomaxillary complex (ZMC) fractures
Zygoma. *See* Zygomatic bone
Zygomatic bone, 6*f*, 7, 7*f*, 8, 8*f*
fractures of, 103–105, 105*f*
Zygomatic ligament, 141
Zygomatic nerve, 9, 14*f*, 15*f*, 17*f*, 142*f*, 144*f*
Zygomaticofacial canal, 9
Zygomaticofacial foramen, 6*f*, 8*f*
Zygomaticofacial nerve, 14*f*, 15*f*, 17*f*, 143, 145*f*
Zygomaticomaxillary complex (ZMC) fractures (quadripod fractures), 103–105, 105*f*
Zygomaticotemporal canal, 9
Zygomaticotemporal foramen, 6*f*
Zygomaticotemporal nerve, 14*f*, 15*f*, 17*f*, 145*f*
in reflex tear arc, 251
Zygomaticus muscles, major and minor, 141, 143*f*
Zygomycetes infection (zygomycosis/mucormycosis/phycomycosis)
orbit involved in, 50
exenteration in management of, 50, 136